Dr. Edythe Ashmore.
S. C. O. March 4, 1901.

THE

PRACTICE and APPLIED THERAPEUTICS

—OF—

..OSTEOPATHY..

—BY—

CHARLES HAZZARD, PH. B. D.O.,

Professor of the Practice and of the Principles
of Osteopathy.

AMERICAN SCHOOL OF OSTEOPATHY.

KIRKSVILLE, MISSOURI.

PART I.

GENERAL METHODS.

PREFACE.

The matter contained in this volume was delivered as a course of lectures. In order that the classes might have lectures in printed form as the work progressed, they were printed and distributed in weekly lots, but in such form that at the end of the course they could be bound and preserved. The work being printed piecemeal in this way explains why there occur various blank pages through the book. They will, however, be found useful for annotations.

As the lectures were delivered in conjunction with daily quizzes in the symptomatology of the diseases considered, the standard texts upon Practice of Medicine being used, it was manifestly desirable to omit from this work all the matter so easily accessible in those writings. This plan left the author free to devote these pages entirely to osteopathic considerations, intending that this work should be used in conjunction with any standard text of medical practice.

No special attempt has been made to follow the usual classification of diseases closely, for various reasons. Likewise, no effort has been made to cover every disease known. It is hoped, however, that the effort to represent the osteopathic view of disease and the osteopathic mode of treatment, even upon this limited scale, may not have been in vain.

CHARLES HAZZARD.

Kirksville, Mo., Jan. 15, 1901.

ERRATA.

p.	10,	div.	XIV,	read	"supine"	for	"prone."
"	19,	"	I,	"	"	"	"
"	20,	"	VIII,	"	"	"	"
"	20,	"	IX (1)	"	"	"	"
"	22,	"	II,	"	"	"	"
"	23,	"	II,	"	"	"	"
"	24,		line 7,	"	"	"	"
"	27,		" 5,	"	"	"	"
"	30,	div	VI,	"	"	"	"
"	30,	"	VII,	read	"prone"	"	"supine."
"	30,	"	VIII,	"	"	"	"
"	30,	"	IX,	"	"supine"	"	"prone."
"	32,	"	(4)	"	"	"	"
"	32,		last line	"	"points"	"	"portion."
"	35,		line 8,	"	"supine"	"	"prone."
"	36,	div.	VI	"	"	"	"
"	227,	"	3,	"	"superior"	"	"inferior."

CHAPTER I.

EXAMINATION OF THE SPINE.

Inspection, percussion and palpation are the methods employed by the practitioner. Of these, the latter is used almost entirely. Attention must be given to the position of the patient, changing it as required for the best detection of the various lesions for which examination is being made. For example, lateral deviations of vertebræ and departures from normal curvature of the spine are best detected while the patient is sitting. Points of separation between spinous processes, thickening of posterior spinal ligaments, rigidity of the spine, etc., are most readily made out while the patient is lying upon the side.

The back must be bared in examination. For ladies, a loose gown buttoned down the front and back may be conveniently used.

By the methods mentioned above the examiner searches for certain definite lesions, as follows:

INSPECTION reveals the color of the skin; rashes, which may indicate disease; the presence of curvature; unequal muscular development; scars, strains, and excoriations leading to inquiry regarding accident, injury, operation or the use of poultice.

Inspection may be made with the patient sitting.

PALPATION is our most important method of examination, the trained touch revealing to the Osteopath most of the lesions which he regards as the causes of disease.

With the patient sitting slightly bent forward, the arms folded loosely or the hands resting lightly on the knees, the examiner stands behind the patient and passes his two index fingers, or the index and second fingers of the examining hand, carefully down the opposite sides of the vertebral spines, he notes:

I. Single vertebræ or groups of vertebræ which may be *deviated laterally* from normal position. In such case there is usually, though not always, tenderness in the tissues upon the side of deviation, owing to the irritation by the process.

II. *Lateral swerving* or sagging of any portion of the spine.

III. Any *exaggeration, deviation from or lessening of the normal curves* of the spine. The most common of these are a flattening of the spine anteriorly at the dorsal curve between the shoulders, a flattening of the spine posteriorly at the lumbar curve, these two lesions together causing the so called "straight spine."

IV. Sharp friction, made by passing the hand quickly down the spine, reddens the tips of the spinous processes so that one may then count them or note their alignment.

V. The flat of the hand is passed down over the posterior aspect of the *sacrum* and detects any flattening or bulging thereof. It is also passed over the posterior superior *iliac spines*, noting their degree of prominence and comparing them with each other relatively to the sacrum.

VI. The cushions of the examining fingers are pressed deeply into the *sacro-iliac spaces* to detect any abnormal tension in the superficial or deep tissues.

VII. The index finger follows the course of the *coccyx* to its tip, noting any lateral, anterior, or posterior deviation.

VIII. The index finger is carefully passed down the spine upon the *spinous processes*, pressure being made firmly upon each, to detect either *anterior or posterior projection* of vertebræ.

IX. The *temperature* of the back is found by passing the palm of the hand evenly over it. Vaso-motor disturbances, resulting in lowered or increased temperatures of certain areas, may be thus discovered. Frequently a cold area may be traced diagonally backward and upward along the course of the spinal nerves toward the seat of some lesion

The patient is now placed upon his side in an easy position, the examiner stands at the front of the patient, and passing his hands over to the spine, continues the examination.

X. The cushion of the examining finger, which is held at right angles to the spinal column, is carefully pressed deeply into the space between each successive pair of spinous processes. It discovers any *separation* or *approximation* of processes, thus of vertebrae.

Points of anatomical weakness are frequently found at the junction of the *twelfth dorsal* with the first lumbar vertebra, also at the junction of the *fifth lumbar* with the sacrum.

The *fifth lumbar* is often prominent posteriorly, but is also very apt to be luxated anteriorly.

XI. The examining hand is passed slowly along the spinal column to note any general or local thickening and increased tension in the posterior spinal ligaments which results is partially obliterating the space between the spinous processes, and in producing the so-called *"smooth spinal column."*

XII. The examining fingers are pressed firmly into the spinal muscles and moved transerversely to the course of their fibres for the purpose of detecting any abnormal *hardening or contracturing* of them. Contractures generally affect certain sets of fibres rather than the muscle as a whole. They may be situated in the *superficial* or in the *deep* muscles, and may be *primary* or *secondary* according as they are produced by direct or indirect lesion of the fibres.

XIII. The body of the patient is braced against that of the practitioner, who places the fingers of both hands upon the under side of the row of spinous processes, (the patient lying on his side) and draws the spine forcibly toward him, noticing whether the *spine* be *rigid*, or too greatly *relaxed*.

It must be borne in mind that bony lesions are not alone important. *Ligamentous lesions* are quite as much so, and though they are not so generally discernible as are the former, the student must not forget that following upon and consequent to bony lesion they may bring pressure upon important structures, may thus interfere with the functions of blood-vessels, nerves, etc., and become a fruitful source of ill..

PERCUSSION, PRESSURE AND MOTION may be employed in the examination of the spine, and may sometimes reveal deep tenderness or pain in the tissues which has escaped notice by the other methods.

Upon motion, certain *sounds* are heard in various parts of the column, due to the motion of parts upon each other. These seem to occur most frequently in the neck, between the articular processes, and in the lumbar region, between the bodies of the vertebræ. They may occur anywhere along the spine and are of diagnostic value in indicating relaxation of ligaments, interference with blood-supply, resulting in insufficient secretion of synovial fluid, or malposition of bony parts.

CHAPTER II

Treatment of the Spine.

In this chapter it is proposed to outline the general method of procedure in spinal treatment. As no specific case or disease is now under consideration, the student must bear in mind that the treatments described are general methods of work and that, in any given case, he would find it necessary to select and combine these different modes in a manner best calculated to enable him individually to reach the case.

As far as practicable the specific lesions mentioned in chapter I will be considered, and treatments appropriate to their reduction will be given.

These treatments are all manipulative. They have as their object the righting of what is mechanically wrong. They are therefore mechanical of necessity, and are founded upon the necessities of the human mechanism when deranged.

In treatment, the practitioner may have in view either or both of *two objects*. He works to right the spine itself, and to affect it alone, or he works upon the spine to affect some other part of the body pathologically connected with the part of the spine in question.

I. The patient lies upon the *ventral aspect* of the body in as comfortable a position as possible. The head turns easily to one side, and the arms hang down loosely at the sides of the table. The practitioner must see that the patient thoroughly *relaxes* the muscles of the whole body. He now, standing at the side of the patient, uses the palms of the hands or the cushions of the fingers to thoroughly manipulate and relax all the spinal muscles. In treating the muscles upon the side toward him, he works from one end of the spinal column to the other, in a direction at right angles to the general direction of the muscular fibres. He treats the muscles of the opposite side by spreading them away from the spinous processes.

In this way all *contractures* of the muscles are released, *flabby muscles* are toned, *blood and nerve* mechanisms are freed and upbuilt. Thus removing of contractures is sometimes a necessary preliminary step to the diagnosis of deeper lesions which may have been masked by them.

II. The patient lies upon his *side*, the practitioner stands at the side of the table, in front of the patient, with one hand he grasps the uppermost arm of the patient just above the elbow; with the other hand he holds under the spinous processes of any portion of the spine under treatment. Now, using the *arm as a lever*, he pushes it downward and forward, at the same time springing the spine toward him.

This treatment releases tension in all deep structures, restores free-play between bony parts, and removes pressure from blood-vessels and nerves. It may be applied in all cases of *curvature, sagging* or swerving of a portion of the spine, *lateral deviations* of vertebrae, in *separating* or *approximating* vertebrae, etc.

III. Practically the same effect may be obtained upon the lower portion of the spine as follows: with the patient still upon the side, his thighs and legs are flexed, and fixed by pressure of the abdomen of the practitioner against them. Both hands are now free and spring the spine strongly upward toward him, or manipulate the muscles: or

IV. With the patient still lying upon his side, the practitioner leans over him, placing his forearms, one against the iliac crest and the other against the shoulder. He now with his forearms pushes these two points further apart, while with both hands he springs the middle portions of the spine toward him, or manipulates the muscles.

It will be observed that the treatments described under II, III and IV above all may be used to thoroughly stretch any portion of the spine by laterally directed force. In this way deeper stretching of all spinal structures may be accomplished within the limits of safety than by stretching the spine as a whole by *longetudinal traction*.

V. The latter is applied with the patient lying upon his back; the practitioner, standing at the head of the table, passes one hand beneath the occiput, the other beneath the chin, and draws toward him. The required degree of resistance is offorded by the weight of the patient or by an assistant holding the ankles.

The neck must not be rotated during this forcible tension, and jerking must be avoided.

VI. The principle of *exaggeration of the lesion* is one that may be applied to the treatment of many bony luxations. It consists in so manipulating the parts as to tend to further increase their malposition, and in then applying pressure to them in such a direction as to force them back toward normal position at the same time as the part in question is released from its condition of exaggeration.

This motion releases tension, loosens adhesion, and gains the benefit of the natural recoil of the structures from their exaggerated position.

VII. With the patient prone and the practitioner *kneeling upon the table* at one side of the patient, or with a knee upon either side, direct pressure may be applied, from above downward, to all spinal parts. This position of relaxation is favorable for forcing vertebrae or the heads of ribs into place and for the stretching of the deep and anterior spinal *ligaments*.

VIII. The patient lies *across the table* with the abdomen and anterior chest resting upon it, the arms and head hanging loosely down upon one side and the legs upon the other. The practitioner may stand at either side of the table (or kneel upon it,) and work for results as in VII, with the additional advantage that the arms, neck, or limbs may be manipulated at will in the course of the treatment.

IX. The patient sits, the practitioner stands in front, slightly to one side. He passes the arm nearest the patient back of the neck, and slips his hand under the opposite axilla. This bends the neck and upper spine forward and swings the opposite side of the thorax backward, thus *rotating the spine*. By using the free hand as a fixed point at various points along the spine, its successive portions may be thoroughly rotated and all of its structures loosened.

X. The patient sits; the practitioner stands behind, pushing the head forward and to one side with one hand, while with the other he makes fixed points along the upper spine, upon the side from which the head has been forced. The head is now swung forward and to the side opposite its first position while the hand brings pressure upon the fixed points, one after the other. This motion makes use of *the neck as a lever* of the first class, the fulcrum being formed by the hand at the fixed point, with the lesion (weight) below, and the power (hand applied to the head) above. It is a method of "exaggeration the lesion," and is especially useful for the reduction of lateral luxations in the upper part of the spine.

XI. The patient sits and *clasps his hands around his neck*; the practitioner stands behind, passes his arms beneath the axillæ and his palms behind the patient's wrists, which he grasps in his hands. He now places one foot upon the stool and presses the flat of the knee against the back at one side of the spinous processes. As the practitioner straightens his body and draws the patient back against his knee the neck and upper dorsal spine are bent forward, the middle and lower portions of the spine are pressed forward by the knee, the scapulæ travel back and up, and all of the ribs, except the first three or four pairs which are sprung forward and downward, are drawn strongly backward and upward.

This treatment thoroughly stretches most of the spinal ligaments, costo-spinal ligaments, muscles of the back of the neck, scapulæ, and of the spine. It also brings tension upon most of the intervertebral, the costo-vertebral, the costo-sternal, acromio claricular and claviculo sternal articulations.

XII. With the patient sitting, the practitioner, standing behind, may place one *knee beneath the patient's axilla*, thus raising and fixing the shoulder and the ribs of one side of the thorax. This relieves the spine of the weight of these structures and affords the practitioner two free hands with which he may manipulate the spine or opposite side of the thorax, using the neck and other arm of the patient as levers, if desired.

XIII. The ligaments of the *posterior lumbar* and of the *sacro-iliac regions* may be thoroughly relaxed by bending the body of the patient, who is sitting far forward between his well separated knees.

XIV. The same object is accomplished with the patient prone, while the legs and thighs are both forcibly flexed to their limit.

XV. To *stretch the posterior scapular, rhomboid, and levator anguli scapulae* muscles, the patient lies upon his back, while the practitioner slips one hand beneath the shoulder and grasps the spinal edge of the scapula, which has been approximated as closely as possible to the spinal column. The other hand holds the arm of the patient just above the elbow, and the arm is raised and pushes across the chest, the patient's hand being in this way forced across well into to the opposite axilla.

XVI. With the same position of the patient, the *anterior scapular muscles* may be reached by thrusting the fingers of one hand deeply beneath the spinal edge of the scapula, while the other hand grasps the point of the shoulder. Now the whole lateral half of the shoulder-girdle may be rotated, the first hand continually working deeper beneath the scapula.

XXII. A thorough *"breaking up"* of the lower dorsal and lumbar regions of the spine is accomplished as follows: The patient lies prone; the practitioner stands at the side and passes one arm beneath the thighs of the patient, just above the knees which he raises just free of the table, moving them horizontally from side to side. At the same time his free hand is applied to the part of the spine in question, the thumb upon one side of the spinous processes, the fingers upon the other. The thumb and fingers make lateral pressure upon the spine, alternating with, and in a contrary direction to, the movement of the limbs.

This treatment loosens and separates the vertebræ, releases tension of muscles and ligaments, and upbuilds nerve and blood action.

Very many more treatments might be described, but enough general treatments have been given to reach all parts of the spine and to correct the lesions that are likely to be met with in practice. These treatments may be combined, or may be taken for the basis of new ones which the practitioner may often find necessary to work out in order to reach some special lesion or to treat some special case.

In this portion of the text, the treatments can of necessity be described, and their application be given, only in a general way. They are outlines of methods of procedure, and the application of the principles embodied in them must be made to the specific lesion met with in a given case by the practitioner.

The lesions described in Chapter I, such as lateral deviation of a vertebra or lateral swerving of a portion of the column; vertebræ separated or approximated; anterior or posterior luxations of vertebræ; the "smooth spine"; the loss of normal curvature; the rigid or relaxed spine, etc., may all be reduced by various applications of these treatments.

Generally speaking, the results attained by the use of these treatments are, the relaxation of contractured muscles; the release of tension in nerve, muscle, ligament or other fibrous structure; the reduction of bony lesion; the removal of obstruction from, and the renewal of, blood and nerve currents.

XVIII. The *fifth lumbar* vertebra, after luxation, may be restored in various ways. The *posterior displacement* is the most frequent. In this case one may place the patient upon his side, flex the knees against the abdomen, fix the fifth lumbar by holding beneath it with one hand, while with the other beneath the thighs the weight of the body is rotated about the fixed point. Recent dislocations may be adjusted in this way without difficulty. In long standing cases continued treatment is necessary, the work of relaxation of parts etc., in preparation for its reduction, being performed in part by the application of principles already described.

With the patient upon his back and the body below the fifth lumbar protruding over the foot of the table, the practitioner standing between the limbs and holding one under each arm, places both hands beneath the pelvis, makes a fixed joint at the fifth lumbar, and by the movement of his own body, rotates the lower part of the patient's body about the fixed point.

With the patient upon his back, the practitioner standing at one side, the clenched hand is placed beneath the body at one side of the fifth lumbar spine. The leg and thigh are now strongly flexed by the free hand, external circumduction of the thigh is made, and the weight of the body is thrown onto the fixed joint. In some cases this treatment is sufficient for replacing the bone.

In case the vertebra be *anterior* the above treatments may be applied to the case for the purpose loosening all the ligaments.

Also the principle of exaggerating the lesion may be applied by making a fixed point of the practitioner's knee at the fifth lumbar, the patient sitting. The patient's body is bent backward against the fixed point and then rotated forward. Also, with the patient sitting and the fifth lumbar fixed with one hand, the free arm grasps the body of the patient and rotates it about the fixed point. The bodies of the vertebra may be thus warped or slightly moved upon each other, drawing the bone back to place.

In many long standing cases of bony lesion, the strengthening of the surrounding muscles and ligaments must take place and be depended upon to hold the ground gained as the part is gradually, during a course of treatment, brought back towards its normal position.

XIX. In case the *sacrum* be found to be *anterior or posterior* from its normal position, this is a matter partly relative to the position of the innominate bones, luxations of which will be discussed later.

In cases of posterior protrusion, after relaxation of the sacro-iliac ligaments, pressure may be made with the knee directly upon the sacrum from behind, with the patient either sitting or lying upon his side. At the same time the pelvis and the upper parts of the body are drawn strongly backwards.

XX. In restoring the *coccyx* to normal position both external and rectal treatment may be necessary. In some cases external treatment alone will be sufficient. The sacro-coccygeal articulation is generally quite pliable. In *external* treatment attention must be first given to the relaxation of the muscles and fibrous tissues concerned. The bone may then be grasped and moved or sprung from either side toward the median line, may be forced anteriorly, or the finger may be gently inserted beneath its tip and may draw it back toward its natural position.

Rectal treatment should not be given oftener than once a week or ten days. The patient lies upon his side or bends over a table. The index finger, anointed with vaseline or other oil is inserted, palm down, into the rectum. It is then turned palm up, laid along the hollow of the coccyx, and swept from side to side, to free the action of blood-vessels and nerves. With the finger in the rectum and the thumb outside, the bone may be grasped and moved toward any position necessary. As a rule its restoration to a normal position is only gradually accomplished.

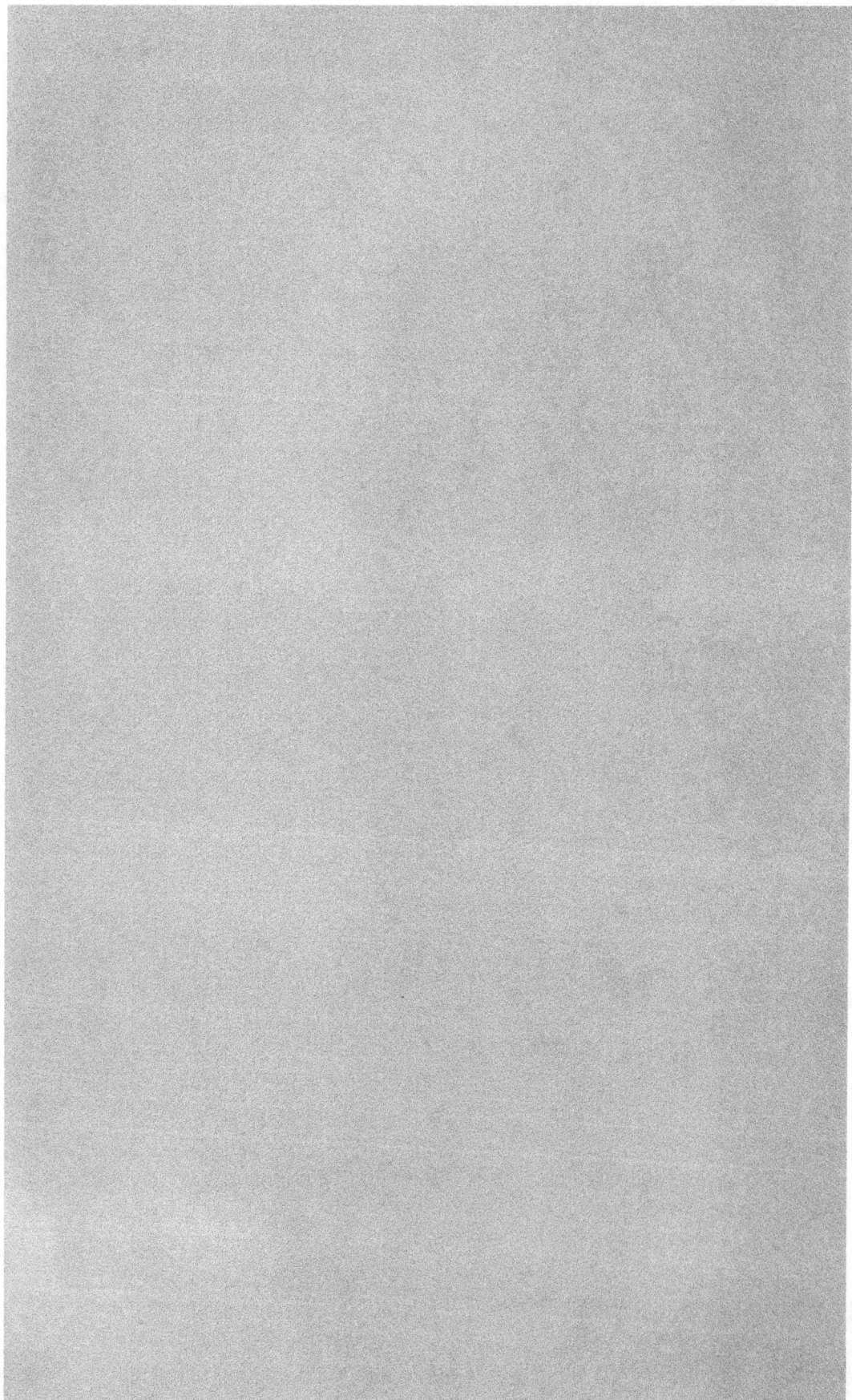

CHAPTER III.

Examination of the Neck.

Inspection and palpation are the two physical methods used in examination of the neck.

Inspection reveals scars due to wounds, and suggests a history of accident or operation. The general conformation of the neck should be noted.

Upon the *anterior aspect* may be seen enlargement due to increase in the size of the tonsils or of the lymphatic glands; abnormal pulsations or engorgement of the blood-vessels; an enlarged thyroid gland.

Upon the *posterior aspect* may be found enlargement of the muscles or thickening of the tissues. Frequently an inequality of the tissues in and below the sub-occipital fossæ, due to thickening or to bony lesion, occurs.

Any unnatural position in which the head may be held should be noted.

Palpation is here, as elsewhere, the important method of examination. For convenience the *anterior structures* may be examined first. The patient lies prone, relaxing the neck as much as possible. This object may be aided by the practitioner, placing one hand upon the forehead and gently rolling the head from side to side, while with the other he lightly manipulates the muscles of the neck.

A. Anterior Structures.

I. The *tonsils* are located by pressure of the fingers just below the angles of the inferior maxillary bone. Any enlargement or tenderness of the organ is to be noted.

II. *Tender points*, frequent in catarrhal conditions, are found by deep pressure behind the angles of inferior maxillary.

III. The *hyoid bone* is located by pressing all the soft tissues just below the jaw toward the median plane of the body. This causes a prominence of the greater cornu upon the opposite side of the throat, which may be easily detected by the index finger.

The finger remains upon the cornu and pushes it back toward the opposite side, thus making prominent the greater cornu of that side. With the index finger and thumb upon the cornua, it may be moved about and a diagnosis of its position be made.

IV. The *hyoid muscles*, superior and inferior, are now carefully palpated to discover contracture, hypertrophy, congestion or tenderness in them. In public speakers, singers, and others liable to throat disease the superior hyoid muscles are often in pathological condition.

V. From the hyoid region palpation is carried down over the *thyroid* and *cricoid cartilages*, noting whether their condition be normal, and is extended along the shoulder to the root of the neck. In this examination the parts are grasped between the thumb and fingers of the examining hand and are moved from side to side. At the same time deep but gentle pressure is made at either side of the larynx and trachea in order to note any undue *tenderness in the laryngeal nerves* as generally revealed by an impulse upon the part of the patient to cough or swallow, *immobility* or *harshness* of *sound* upon motion of these parts as above abnormal tension in the related muscles and other tissues.

VI.   Enlargement or wasting of the *thyroid gland* or enlargement of the *cervical lymphatic glands* must be noted.

VII.   The *sterno-mastoid* muscle is made prominent by causing the patient to turn his head to the opposite side. Pressure deep behind the anterior border of this muscle impinges upon the *pneumogastric* nerve. *Tenderness* in it upon pressure may accompany liver or stomach disease.

VIII.   The *phrenic nerve* arises from the third, fourth, and fifth cervical nerves, and may, at its points of origin, be pressed backward against the bony column. It may be reached also by deep pressure with the thumb or finger in the angle formed by the posterior edge of the sterno-mastoid muscle with the upper margin of the clavicle. This pressure must be directed from above diagonally downward and forward toward the sternum.

IX.   *Pressure of the head directly downward* upon the spinal column with *rotation*, will sometimes discover deep pain at points of lesion.

X.   The posterior structures of the neck may be tested for abnormal tension by flexing the head upon the thorax, the patient prone.

XI.   The palms of the hands may be passed evenly over the surface of the neck to examine for variations of *temperature*. Hot or cold areas may be found. It is common to find an area of increased temperature at the base of the skull behind.

B. Posterior and Lateral Structures.

I.   With the patient sitting, the practitioner passes the examining hand down along the back of the neck. Just below the occiput is a depression in which he may feel the upper end of the *ligamentum nuchae* and the inner borders of the trapezius muscles. With the head bent slightly forward and the examining fingers pressed deeply into this space abnormal tension of these structures may be noted.

II.   The *second cervical spine* is the first bony prominence felt below the occiput. The spines of the *third, fourth* and *fifth* are made out with difficulty, as they recede from the surface anteriorly. The next prominent spine is that of the *sixth*, the next of the *seventh*. The latter is prominent, but not so much so as the first dorsal, from which it must be carefully distinguished.

Anterior, posterior, or lateral deviations of the cervical vertebræ may be diagnosed by this examination of the spinous processes.

III.   Anterior dislocations of the upper three cervical vertebrae may be sometimes noted by examining for the prominence caused by the body upon the posterior wall of the pharynx.   This is done by passing the finger over these bodies.

IV.   The position of the *atlas* is examined as follows: The patient lies upon his back and the practitioner stands at the head of the table.   The transverse processes are located by thrusting the palms of the examining fingers deeply into the space between the angle of the inferior maxillary bone and the tip of the mastoid process.   A finger is placed upon each transverse process which is usually prominent.   Normally these processes should be midway between the angle of the jaw and the tip of the mastoid process.   If they are too far forward, too far backward, to one side, or if one be forward and the other backward, the diagnosis is readily made by comparison of the position of the processes relatively to the points mentioned, and the corresponding displacement of the atlas is discovered.

V.   Lateral deviations of vertebrae in the neck are best found by examining the *articular processes.*

The head, with the patient lying upon his back, is turned to one side, making prominent the row of articular processes upon the opposite side. The second cervical spine is now readily located by its prominence behind, and the finger traces from it around to the *articular processes of the second,* lying at about the same level, but slightly above.   A finger is held upon this process and the head is turned to the opposite side.   The other articular process of the second is then located in the same way.   They are now compared while moving the head slightly from side to side, and lateral deviations or tenderness in the tissues are easily made out.   With these two points fixed, the head may be gently turned from side to side, and the examining fingers travel down over the successive articular processes, careful examination being made of the position of each.

VI.   Deep pressure may be made from the anterior surface of the neck back upon the anterior aspect of the *transverse processes* and diagnosis of anterior luxation be made.

VII.   *Crepitus* and abnormal mobility of bony parts indicates fracture.

VIII,   The patient lies, and the practitioner stands at one side of the head, turns the head slightly to one side and passes the examining hand transversely to the course of the muscle fibers, noting any *contractures* of the muscles, superficial or deep.

IX.   He then stands at the head of the table and examines both sides of the neck at the same time, a hand upon each stde, carefully *comparing* both sides with especial reference to any abnormality either of bone or of other tissue.

X.   Careful examination should be made for thickening of the *tissues* of the neck just *below the occuput.*

XI.   The *scaleni muscles* are made prominent upon one side by drawing the head to the opposite side. They are normally hard to the touch, and care should be taken in the diagnosis of contracture. Tenderness is often found upon pressure, as in cases of rheumatism.

Their contracture often results in drawing the *first two ribs upward* out of place.

XII. The *brachial plexus* of nerves emerges from between the scalenus anticus and the scalenus medius muscles, below the level of the fifth cervical vertebra. The head is inclined to the side to relax these muscles, and deep pressure is made at this point to impinge the plexus. Tenderness is thus revealed.

XIII. *Tender areas* are often found upon pressure in the *sub-occipital fossae*. They are due to irritation of the *great* and *small occipital* and *great auricular* nerves. It is through manipulation of these nerves largely that effects are gotten upon the *superior cervical* ganglia and upon the *medulla*. They are located at a *point* about two inches from the middle of the posterior margin of the mastoid process, in a line at right angles thereto extending toward the median plane of the neck posteriorly.

XIV. The *superior cervical ganglion* lies in front of the transverse processes of the second and third cervical vertebrae, and may be reached by direct pressure through the tissues. The method of locating the transverse process of the second cervical has been given under V of this chapter. Deep pressure from the anterior aspect of the neck may press this ganglion back against these processes.

The *middle cervical ganglion*, lying in front of the transverse processes of the sixth and seventh cervical vertebrae, may be likewise reached.

The transverse process of the seventh cervical vertebra is readily located by deep lateral pressure at the outer third of the supra-clavicular fossa.

Lesions of the atlas and axis are by far the most important occurring in this region of the body, and account for many serious diseases of the head and its parts, such as blindness, insanity, etc. The lesions of the neck hold an important relation also to diseases in other parts of the body.

Comparatively little treatment is given directly to the head and its parts. These are treated largely through the removal of lesion in the neck. Hence the importance of most thorough and careful attention to its examination.

The *value of gently moving a part* while under examination in order to relax tissues, to insinuate the examining fingers more deeply into them, and to develop the latent lesion through investigation of its relations to its neighboring parts during movement must not be overlooked.

CHAPTER IV.

TREATMENT OF THE NECK.

Treatment of the neck, as of other parts, is, in its specific application, always *removal of lesion*. The following general description of methods of work in treating the neck is for the purpose of laying before the student in a simple manner the general principles involved in our work. Later specific application of these general principles and methods will be made.

I. With the patient *supine* prone, the guiding hand is laid upon his forehead and the head is rolled gently from side to side a few times to aid in relaxing the muscles. The fingers of the operating hand are laid, palm down, upon the *muscles of the throat* on the side opposite to the practitioner. As the head is moved away from the practitioner these muscles are loosened through the shortening of that side of the neck. At the same time, the operating hand draws these muscles toward the median plane of the neck. The head may be now moved from side to side, while the fingers upon one side of the throat and the thumb upon the other manipulate the tissues. All the tissues of the anterior aspect of the throat may be included in this treatment, contracture and tension at any given point being thus removed. The treatments must be gentle in order that sensitive necks may not be irritated.

The operating hand must not be rubbed over the tissues, but they must be moved by the motion of the hand.

Holding or pressing gently but continuously against a contracture while the head is being slowly moved about will relieve the tension and remove the lesion.

II. The ligaments of the temporo-maxillary articulations, and the muscles and blood-vessels below the inferior maxillary bone may be relieve of tension, and be restored to free action by *springing the mouth open* againstd resistance.

The patient lies upon his back and the practitioner stands at the head of the table, placing the palms of his thumbs upon the malar prominences and the palms of the fingers beneath the jaw. The patient is now directed to open the mouth widely and then to gradually close it. Resistance is made by the operating hands to the first motion, and the fingers press the superior hyoid muscles downward and forward toward the median plane of the neck during the second motion.

The ligaments of temporo-maxillary articulations may be sprung by thrusting a finger deeply into each glenoid fossa after the patient has opened his mouth, nolding them there while the mouth is shut.

III. The *hyoid bone* may be held between the thumb and finger and be moved vertically and laterally, stretching the hyoid muscles.

IV. Pressure may be in some measure applied to the *pneumogastric*, *glosso-pharyngeal* and *spinal-accessory nerves* by deeply pressing the finger upward and inward behind the angle of the jaw, in the direction of the jugular foramen.

The *pneumogastric* nerve may be manipulated by deep pressure behind the anterior border of the sterno-mastoid muscle.

These three nerves are also influenced by manipulation upon their closely related nerves, the sub-occipital, great occipital, small occipital, and great auricular, reached in the sub-occipital fossæ as above described.

V. Pressure upon the *phrenic nerve* may be applied at the points described in Chapter III.

VI. The *sterno-mastoid* muscle may be manipulated following the method described for treatment of muscles of the throat under I of this chapter.

The muscle upon one side may be stretched by turning the head toward that side and slightly upward, thus increasing the distance between the mastoid process and the sterno-clavicular origin of the muscle.

VII. The *lateral and posterior muscles* of the neck may all be treated in a manner similar to that described under I of this chapter.

The practitioner may also stand at the head of the table, and with the palms of the hands upon each side and the back of the neck, gently grasp handfulls of the muscles, manipulate them thoroughly while slowly moving the head in all directions. Pressure and manipulation, together with motion, all gently and patiently applied, will relax the most obstinate contracture, loosen all deep fibrous structures, free blood-vessels and nerves, and prepare the way for what is usually the real object of the treatment, the reduction of *bony lesions*.

VIII. With the patient ~~prone~~ supine the head is pushed as far as may be easily done without resistance, first to one side and then to the other, and it is noticed whether it turns as *far to one side as to the opposite side*. Inequality between the two sides indicates lesion usually upon the side toward which the head turns least easily.

After relaxation of the tissues, turning the head to its limit toward each side will sometimes aid in the reduction of bony lesion, especially with the aid of pressure applied to force the part into its place.

IX. (1) In lesion of the *atlas* the patient lies prone and the practitioner, standing at the head of the table, holds the head between the hands, with a thumb or finger upon each transverse process. The head is now moved in a direction to exaggerate the lesion, and with traction, rotation, and pressure upon the processes, the atlas is forced toward its position.

(2) The operator may stand at the side of the head, one hand upon the forehead and the other pressed firmly just below the skull, in the region of the lateral arch of the atlas. Exaggeration of the lesion, rotation and strong pressure aid in replacing the part.

(3.) The patient sits and the practitioner, standing in front, places one knee beneath the chin, while the hands grasp the sides and back of the head. Exaggeration of the lesion, traction, pressure, and rotation are now applied as before.

(4.) The patient sits and an arm is passed about his head, the bend of the elbow coming beneath the occipital protuberance and the hand beneath the chin. The head is now forcibly raised with the idea of moving it upon the spine in the desired direction, while the free hand makes pressure upon the spine in the direction necessary to aid in reposition.

These various treatments may be applied to any of the usual lesions of the atlas. The same principles may be applied to the different malpositions of any of the cervical vertebrae, generally patience and time are necessary to the gradual restoration of the bones to place. Much attention must be given to the thorough and gradual loosening of all parts in preparation for replacement.

X. The axis is generally displaced laterally. The tissues upon its transverse and articular processes are quite tender and contractures are found in the muscles about it. Exaggeration of lesion, rotation and pressure usually restore it to place.

XI. The *scaleni muscles* may be stretched by pressing the head down toward the side in question, pressing the fingers behind the clavicle upon the first rib to force and hold it down, while the head is now drawn to the opposite side.

XIII. Thorough loosening of all cervical tissues may be accomplished by a somewhat *"spiral" treatment.* The patient lies, the guiding hand is placed upon the forehead, and the other hand is slipped beneath the neck and grasps it.

The head and neck are now raised slightly, the head being rotated in one direction, while, as far as possible, exactly the opposite motion is given the neck. The hand travels up and down the neck, treating its different portions alike.

CHAPTER V.

Osteopathic Points Concerning the Head and its Parts.

As stated, the chief lesions affecting the head and its parts occur in the neck, and have already been described. More detailed points in examnation and treatment of these important structures will be considered in lectures upon their specific diseases in the second part of this work. The present chapter will embrace only general Osteopathic points.

Inspection and Palpation are the methods of examination. By the former one notes the size and shape of the skull, the complexion, expression, eyes, etc. By palpation he notes the presence of tumors or other growths, open fontanelles, etc.

A. The Eye.

Those lesions most frequently affecting these organs occur at the atlas and axis.

I. The *conjunctiva lining the lids* may be examined. The lower lid is drawn out and down, pressure being made at the same time below it, causing it to become prominent.

The upper lid is turned back by grasping the edge slightly toward the outer canthus and raising the lid, while at the same time pressure is made upon it from above near the inner canthus. This inverts the tarsal cartilage and exposes the membrane.

If while this lid is turned back the lower one is also treated as above, both together stand out more prominently and may be observed together.

Granulations appear as minute white or pale red elevations.

II. With the patient prone, direct pressure is made, with the palms of the fingers, upon the eye-balls, pressing them directly back into the orbits. This impinges nerves, blood-vessels, muscles and all the orbital structures. It presses excess of blood from the vessels, and tones the muscles, nerves and the structures of the intra-ocular mechanism.

III. *Tapping* of the eyeball has much the same effect. It is performed by placing the palms of one or two fingers over the closed eye, and lightly tapping them with the index finger. Toning of the nerves, of the ball and its structures, and of the optic nerve is thus accomplished.

IV. *Granulations* are crushed by squeezing them between the fingers and thumb, the finger being inserted beneath the lid.

U. In *pterygia*, the small blood-vessels formed upon and in the conjunctiva as feeders, may be broken up by drawing the back portion of the edge of the finger-nail across them. Care must be taken not to wound the conjunctiva.

VI. In *strabismus* the weakened or tensed muscle may be treated by pressing the fingers into the orbit about the eye-ball.

B. THE FIFTH NERVE.

This nerve is reached at various points about the head, as it sends many branches out over the head and face. Its treatment is especially important in headaches, neuralgias, diseases of the eye, nose, etc., for the reason that it carries vaso-motor and trophic fibres to these parts.

I. Its *supra-orbital* branch may be traced from the supra-orbital foramen out over the forehead to the temple. It forms an angle of about fifty degrees with the superciliary ridge. It may be felt under the skin like a fine whip-cord, and it may be manipulated along its course by passing the fingers transversely across it.

II. The *infra-orbital* and *mental* branches may be manipulated at their respective foramina.

By clinching the fingers beneath the malar process several branches of the former may be impinged

The tissues over the foramina and along the courses of all of these different branches should be thoroughly relaxed to remove irritation.

III. A *supra trachlear* branch is located slightly to one side of the midline of the forehead, a *lachrymal* branch about the middle of the upper eyelid, a *temporal* branch external to the outer canthus of the eye, an *infra-trachlear* branch upon the nose opposite the inner canthus, and a *nasal* branch at the lower third of the side of the nose.

All are subcutaneous and are readily manipulated after knowing where to locate them.

With the EAR, as with the eye, lesion of the atlas, axis, or upper cervical region is the most usual cause of disease.

The NOSE, apart from neck treatment, is sometimes treated by local manipulation.

I. Manipulating and loosening all the tissues along the sides of the nose affects the blood-supply of its mucous membrane through branches of the fifth nerve. It will also operate to free the channel of the *nasal duct*.

II. With the patient ~~prone~~ supine, the palm of the hand is placed upon the forehead, the other hand is laid upon the first, and the practitioner, bending over the head of the table, brings his weight upon the patient's forehead. This pressure is continued several seconds and repeated a few times. It *frees the nostrils* and in acute colds frequently at once restores freedom of breathing through the nose.

The affect is probably gotten by the pressure affecting the branches of the fifth nerve upon the forehead.

III. In colds and catarrh pain in the *frontal sinus* may be relieved by *tapping* with the knuckles upon the frontal bone over the sinus.

The MOUTH and THROAT are sometimes treated internally by sweeping the palm of the index finger from the mid-line of the posterior portion of the hard palate outward and downward over the soft palate, pillars of the fauces, and tonsils. The uvula may also be touched. The nerves and blood-vessels of this region are thus toned.

THE TEMPRO-MAXILLARY ARTICULATIONS are examined. Inequality in their action is discovered by standing behind the head of the patient, who is lying ~~prone~~ *supine*. The mouth is opened and closed, and deviation of the mid-line of the chin from the median plane of the body noted. Deviation of this nature indicates luxation of one of the articulations, the jaw usually deviating away from the side of the lesion.

I. The ligaments of the articulation may first be loosened as described under II of Chapter IV. Pressure upon the opposite jaw while the patient is closing the mouth will bring the condyle back into place.

II. Sometimes it is necessary to place a small cork or piece of wood between the posterior molar teeth upon the affected side. Pressure is now made beneath the chin, tending to close the mouth, and the jaw is slipped into place. The corks may be inserted at the same time between the molars of both sides in case of bilateral luxation.

Treatment I, may be alternately applied in such case.

Opening the mouth against resistance (II, Chap. IV), manipulation of the throat to free the action of the carotid arteries, and treatment of the superior cervical region (XIII, Chap. III) are, together with *removal of specific lesions*, the chief methods of treatment in diseases of the eye, ear, nose and throat. They produce affects by building up the blood-supply.

CHAPTER VI.

Examination of the Thorax.

From an Osteopathic point of view, and not at present considering the contents of the thoracic cavity, the examination of the thorax consists mainly in discovering, by palpation and inspection, whether its bony structures are all in position.

Ligamentous and muscular lesions, also lesions of blood-vessels, nerves and centers are closely associated with bony lesions.

The relations of the thorax to the spine and to its contained viscera cause its lesions to be among the most important ones found in the body. Lesion of the spine, especially of its thoracic portion, often seriously affects the thorax proper.

INSPECTION reveals change in the *general conformation* of the thorax. It is made with relation to the spine, and effects of spinal irregularities are considered. *Flattening* or *prominence* of the ribs, either in portions of the thorax or affecting it as a whole; restriction or increase in the *movements* of the thorax, upon one or both sides; color of the skin, eruptions, scars, etc., are all noted.

The patient may sit, lie, or stand during inspection, as most convenient.

PALPATION, the more important method, proceeds in conjunction with further inspection, and is used in the detection of the various special lesions to be described.

I.   With the patient standing or sitting, the palms of the hands are passed evenly over the anterior and posterior aspects of the chest *comparing side with side*; region with region.   The *temperature* is also noted.

II.   The *precardial* region is examined for any protrusion or retraction of the thoracic wall, significant with relation to heart disease.

III.   Each lateral half of the chest is examined for change or lessening of its antero-posterior diameter, considering the direction of the component ribs as well.   Lessening of this diameter, and a tendency of the ribs to greater obliquity in direction, reveals a *flattened side* or sides of the chest. This shows spinal lesion generally, also disturbed ligaments, blood-vessels, nerves, etc., of all related parts.   In this case the whole side is *dropped down* and the *ilio-costal* space is lessened.

IV.   The same lesion may affect a portion of the thorax.   Often a *flattening of the ribs posteriorly beneath the scapula* is found.

Protrusions of retractions of one area of the chest generally correspond with the reverse condition in the corresponding anterior or posterior area. This is not true in case of slipping of the ribs downward.

V.   Marked depression in the *supra* or *infra-clavicular* regions are significant in the diagnosis of tuberculosis of the lungs.

VI. With the patient lying on his side, the *palm of the hand is swept along the lateral and postero-lateral aspects of the chest*, from the shoulder downwards. Changes in the position of the ribs individually, or in the conformation of the side of the thorax in question are thus readily made out, mainly by detection of changes in the angles of the ribs from normal.

The STERNUM must be examined.

I. It may be as a whole, *protruded or retracted*, following a change in the general shape of the thorax.

II. Luxation between the *first and second parts*, anteriorly or posteriorly, may occur.

III. The *ensiform* may be displaced laterally.

THE CLAVICLE AND CORACOID.

The latter is located as the first bony prominence at the outer end of the infra-clavicular fossa. Its relation to the clavicle is to be noted.

The clavicle may be luxated at either its sternal or acromial articulation. The sternal end may be upward, anteriorly or posteriorly from its normal position. The acromial end may be displaced downward toward the coracoid or upward upon the acromion process. Sometimes it is tilted so that one's fingers may be thrust far behind its upper edge.

LUXATION OF RIBS.

One of the main objects of examination of the thorax is to locate misplaced ribs. Departures from normal conformation of spine are at once indications of lesion of the several ribs. Hence, following the general examination as outlined above, each rib in particular must be scrutinized. Landmarks for the location of the various ribs should be employed.

I. Ribs are frequently *separated* or *approximated* beyond normal limits. These conditions are discovered by placing the patient upon his side and following the successive intercostal spaces with the tip or side of the examining finger. In the latter lesion the tissues are tender along the course of the intercostal space, due to irritation of the sensory branches of the intercostal nerves.

II. The same examination would reveal *rotation of a rib upon its horizontal* axis. In such case the intercostal space is *unequally widened or narrowed*. As a rule the twisting is about the head as a fixed point, and the lower margin of the rib is turned out prominently. Then the intercostal space next below is narrowed posteriorly and widened anteriorly. The anterior end is tended downward, luxating the costo-chondral and the chondro-sternal articulations, as it deranges the costal cartilage. The reverse rotation of the rib may take place, making prominent the upper edge, throwing the anterior end upward, etc.

III. By various lesions of the ribs, the *cartilages are twisted, distorted*, or *torn loose*.

In such case tender points are found upon pressure at the costo-chond-ral or chondro-sternal articulations. The cartilage may be _bulged forward_ by protrusion of the rib, causing a prominent tender point. It may be _retracted_, causing a slight depression.

With the patient lying prone, the examining fingers may be carefully passed over the successive pairs of cartilages and these lesions be noted.

The FIRST RIB is located by deep pressure _behind the middle or inner one third of the clavicle._ If the latter has been found _in situ_, comparison with it may be made to determine whether the rib be up or down. By deep pres-sure the rib may be traced well back toward its head, which is masked by the posterior cervical muscles. Pressure may be brought upon the head at the level of the seventh cervical spine, one and one-half inch laterally therefrom.

The _sternal end_ of the rib is located just below the claviculo-sternal ar-ticulation. Its cartilage and may be traced well outward an inch or more before disappearing beneath the clavicle.

In case it may be luxated upward, the cartilage is retracted, leaving a flat area or a depression at the cartilage. If downward, a protrusion of the cartilage at the edge of the sternum is usual. In either case the cartilage and the tissues about the rib are sensitive to pressure.

The first and second intercostal spaces are wider than the others.

The SECOND RIB is located opposite the junction of the first and second parts of the sternum. Prominence or depression of its cartilage, and tend-erness in the tissues about it are caused in the same way as in the case of the first. Its head is located and pressure brought upon its region at a point one and one-half inches external to the first dorsal spine.

The ELEVENTH AND TWELFTH RIBS are more frequently luxated down-wards because of their anterior ends being unsupported and because of traction upon the latter by the quadratus lumborum muscle. Their free ends are readily located except when irritation from them, or other cause, has irritated the overlying muscles, causing hypertrophy or contracture. In such case they must be located from the tenth rib.

The free end of the eleventh lies well forward, thus distinguishing it from the twelfth.

They may be so displaced downward as to be almost vertical; may overlap the iliac crest, or may be luxated upwards, the free end of the twelfth lying beneath the eleventh or that of the eleventh beneath the tenth.

Frequently a luxated rib guides one to a spinal lesion.

Displaced ribs cause disease by mechanical interference with internal viscera, by irritation of surrounding soft tissues, by dragging ligaments, im-pinging nerves, or occluding blood-vessels.

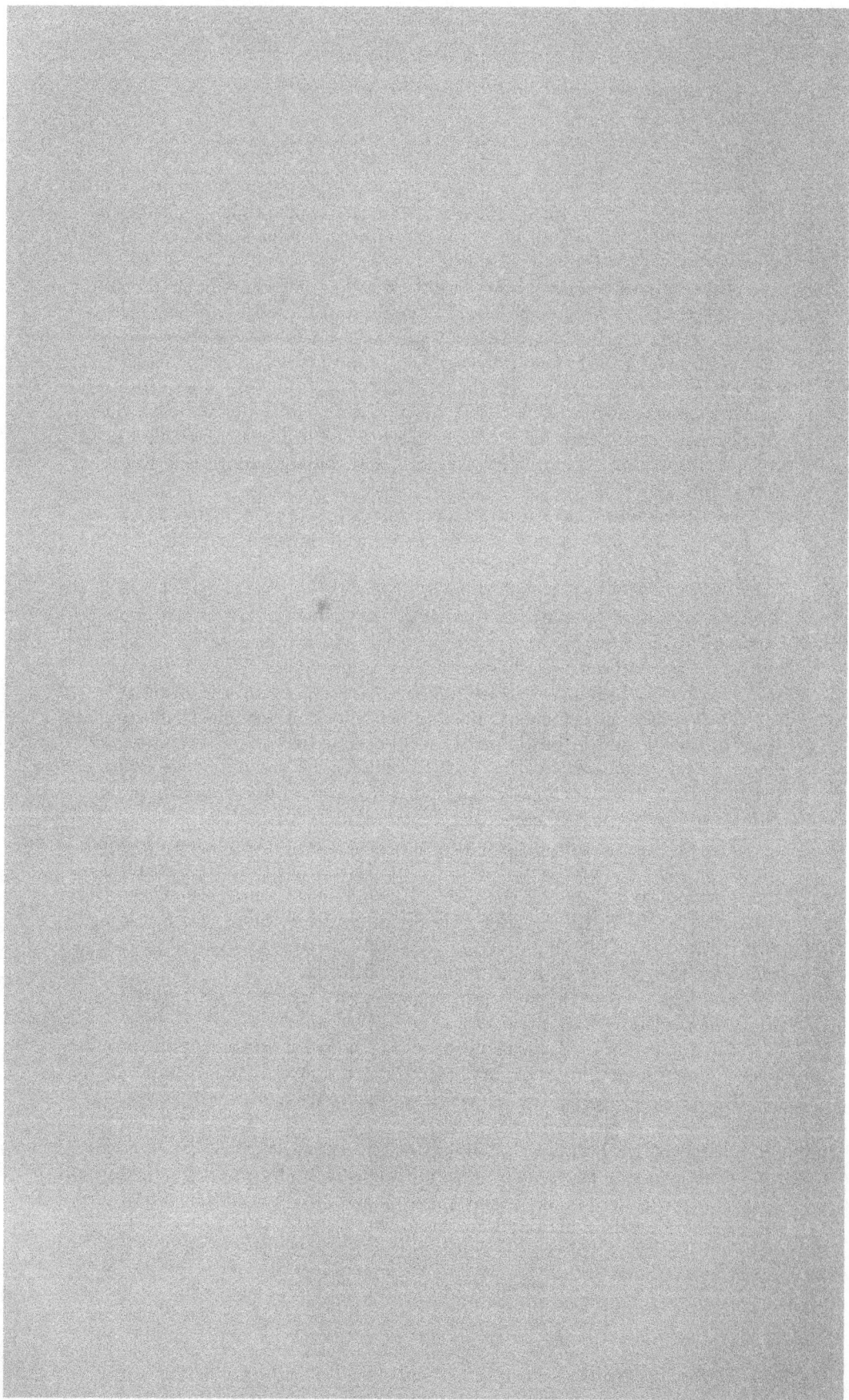

CHAPTER VII.

TREATMENT OF THORACIC LESIONS.

The thoracic portion of the spinal column is anatomically a part of the thorax, but has already been discussed under another head.

Osteopathic treatment of the thorax is directed generally to the restoration of the ribs and other bony portions to correct mechanical relations. It includes with this, work upon ligamentous, cartilaginous, and muscular lesions, which are usually secondary to bony lesion. Thus while osteopathic treatment of the thorax consists largely in the putting of ribs into proper position, this work is always done with an eye to those other lesions, and effects all surrounding tissues; muscles and ligaments; nerves and vessels; centers and viscera.

Thoracic is inseparable from spinal work, owing to the intimate anatomical relations of these parts.

There are various ways of setting ribs. Many of them rest upon the principle that the head of the rib, being but slightly movable, is the fixed point; that pressure upon the angles tends to move them about this fixed point; and that this pressure may be guided and aided by elevation of the arm or rotation of the shoulder, bringing traction upon the pectoral and latissimus dorsi muscles, etc., which are attached to the ribs.

In some treatments, the sternal end is made the fixed point and the parts are manipulated accordingly; in some, both ends of the rib are fixed, etc.

Exaggeration of lesion, fixing of a fulcrum, traction upon attached tissues, and rotation of related parts are principles applied to the work.

I. With the patient sitting upon the side of the table, the practitioner, standing in front, passes an arm about the body of the patient, extending his hand past the spine behind, and pressing with the fingers upon the angles of the ribs of the further side. With the other hand he raises the patient's arm, of the side in question, in front of the body and high over the head, rotating it downward and backward. This brings traction upon the pectoral muscles and soft tissues of the whole anterior aspect of the side of the chest, elevates the entire side, and effects particularly the ribs upon the angles of which pressure is made.

This motion may be repeated, the pressing hand traveling down the back to each successive rib in need of treatment.

This treatment elevates all the ribs and tones all the connected muscles, ligaments, vessels, nerves, etc.

II. The patient sits upon the stool; the practitioner stands behind, and, resting one foot upon the stool, makes a fixed point of his knee at the angle of the rib under treatment. One hand holds beneath the lower edge of the ribs, in front, while the other elevates and rotates the arm as in I.

Or the first hand may press down upon the upper edge of the rib, in front, while the arm is drawn from in front downwards to the side of the body, and backwards.

In these ways the ribs may be forced downward or upward.

III. With the patient sitting or lying upon his side, the rib is thrown into action by the patient's taking a full breath. The operating hands are applied, one at either end of the rib in question, and advantage is taken of the relaxation of tissues and the motion of the rib which take place as the patient expels the breath. The whole rib is manipulated at this time toward its normal position.

This treatment is aided in some cases by pushing the rib still further from its normal position before an attempt is made to restore it to place. In this way the principle of exaggeration of the lesion is called into play.

IV. Treatment II may be applied with the patient lying upon his side instead of sitting. Here the practitioner stands behinds, rests one foot upon the table, bending his limb so as to bring the flat of his knee against the angle of the rib. The treatment then proceeds as in II. The arm may be rotated either forward and up, or downward and back, pressure being made at either margin or at the sternal end of the rib as desired. This treatment allows the practitioner more latitude than does II.

Great caution must be exercised in any application of the knee to the chest, either anteriorly or posteriorly. Active work with it should be avoided, use being made of it only as a fixed point.

V. A fixed point may be made of the flat of the knee at the sternal end of the rib; the arm of the patient upon the same side is manipulated for traction as before, while the other operating hand is passed over the patient's opposite shoulder and applied to the spinal region of the rib. This treatment is applicable to luxations of the heads of ribs. The patient is sitting.

VI. With the patient prone, the practitioner stands at one side and reaches across the patient to manipulate the ribs of the opposite side. One hand is slipped beneath the back and applied as a fixed point to the angles of any ribs in question; with the other hand the patient's arm is rotated as before for traction.

VII. With the patient lying supine, the practitioner, standing at one side, reaches across the body and makes a fixed point of his elbow upon the angles of the rib. At the same time the hand of the same arm grasps the patient's forearm upon that side drawing it back and up. Thus, while the rib is in action the pressure of the elbow forces the head into place.

VIII. With the patient lying supine, pressure with the operating hands may be brought vertically downward upon heads or angles of ribs, springing them into place.

IX. With the patient lying prone, the practitioner stands at the side of the table and raises the patient's arm of the same side to a level with the shoulder. With the arm thus horizontal, traction is made upon it, away from the body, and in such a direciion as to bring longitudinal tension upon the costal cartilages. The other hand manipulates the cartilage to reduce any twist or anterior prominence of it.

X. With the patient sitting, the practitioner stands facing him, making pressure with one hand upon the sternal end of the rib in question. The other arm is passed about the patient's body, and locates and brings pressure upon the head of the same rib. With both ends of the rib thus fixed, the motion of the practitioner's body is used to rotate the patient's trunk about these fixed points, at the same time manipulation is directed to the restoration of the rib to position.

It may be said that as a rule the setting of a rib requires time and patience, though in many cases this may be accomplished at once. It is rarely the performance of a set motion that does this work. On the contrary, the practitioner, with his hands in position and the parts under his control as described in any particular treatment, must continue his efforts, with varying traction, pressure, rotation, etc. Movements of the patient's whole trunk, bending, turning, raising the parts, etc., may all contribute to the gradual relaxation and yielding of the parts to the persistent, well directed, and carefully judged efforts of the Osteopath.

In the case of the FIRST AND SECOND RIBS many of the general principles and treatments, as already described, may be applied. Special methods, however, are generally necessary to replace them. As already stated, these ribs are usually luxated upwards, but may as well be displaced downwards.

I. Upward Displacements.

(1) The scaleni muscles are first relaxed and stretched (Chap. IV, div. XI), the head is now bent toward the shoulder of the affected side, and and pressure is brought directly downward upon the upper margin, the sternal or spinal end of either or both ribs (Chap. VI). In this way, either rib may be lowered as a whole or at either end.

(2) With the patient lying upon his back, the practitioner stands at the head of the table; presses the palm of the thumb down upon the upper margin of the first rib; with the other hand he raises the arm of the patient upon the side in question, and pushes it across the chest at the level of the shoulder, thus relaxing the tissues at side of the neck, and elevating the clavicle so that the thumb may be thrust more deeply behind it. Pressure may be applied anywhere along the upper margin of the rib, lowering it to its normal position.

II. Downward Displacements.

(1) With the patient sitting, the practitioner stands behind and brings pressure with his fingers upon the inferior margin of the first or second rib (see p. 27). At the same time the head is bent to the opposite side, bringing traction upon the rib through the scaleni muscles, and rotated back-

wards. This rotation tends to bring more traction upon the anterior end through the scalenus anticus (in case of the first rib). This treatment may be used to elevate either rib.

(2) The treatment as described under II and IV of this chapter may be used.

(3) With the patient sitting and the practitioner standing in front, pressure may be made by the fingers below the region of the head of the first or second rib, (see p. 27), while the head is bent to the opposite side and rotated forward. This rotation tends to bring more traction upon the posterior ends of the first and second ribs through increased traction respectively of the scalenus medius and scalenus posticus muscles.

(4) In case of anterior protrusion of the cartilages (see p. 27), pressure may be brought upon them while treatment (I) above is being given.

Or the patient's arm is raised to the level of his shoulder and drawn backwards, bringing traction upon the cartilages, while pressure is applied to them.

The first two ribs may be *separated*, to some extent, as follows: The patient lies prone and a hand is slipped beneath his shoulder, bent to form a fulcrum beneath the two ribs; the patient's arm is grasped at the elbows raised, and bent strongly across the anterior chest at the level of the shoulder. This tends to drive the two ribs sternum-ward, and to separate them anteriorly owing to the intercostal space being wider at its anterior end than at the other.

THE ELEVEN AND TWELFTH RIBS.

A. DOWNWARD DISPLACMENTS.

A preliminary step must be taken in the relaxation of all muscles and tissues about the ribs, especially of the quadrati lumborum muscles. This is easily accomplished by manipulation of the tissues. A special method of *stretching the quadrati* is as follows: The patient lies upon his side and the practitioner stands in front. He grasps the arm of the patient and draws it diagnonally forward, at the level of the shoulder, in a direction away from the pelvis. At the same time his other hand makes pressure upon the anterior iliac crest in a direction diagonally backward, i. e., in a direction exactly the opposite from that in which the arm is drawn. This stretches the muscle diagonally and rotates the lumbar portion of the spine. The motion is now reversed by standing in front of the pelvis, grasping the crest of the ilium, and drawing it diagonally forward in a direction away from the shoulder. At the same time the other hand holds the bent arm rigid at the side and pushes it in a direction opposite from that of the traction applied to the pelvis. This motion gives the opposite diagonal stretch to the quadratus lumborum, and rotates the lumbar region of the spine.

The eleventh or twelfth rib itself is readily manipulated upwards or downward by taking advantage of three portion;(1)The head usually remains a fixed point, (2) Pressure made upon the outer aspect of the rib in the region of its angle (or turn in case of the twelfth, which lacks the angle) may be so directed as to move or rotate the rib upward or downward about the fixed point, (3) The free end may be readily moved upward or downward by the pressure of a finger, and this pressure, combined with pressure in the opposite direction applied at the angle, readily rotates the rib about its vertical axis.

One hand easily spans the rib, leaving the other hand free to manipulate the body and aid the operation. The thumb is pressed against the free end of the rib and forces it upward or downward while the fingers of the same hand bring pressure in the opposite direction at the angle of the rib. In this way the rib is rotated about the head as a fixed point and may be raised or lowered as desired.

I. With the patient lying upon his side, his knees flexed and supported against the abdomen of the practitioner, the operating hand manipulates the rib as above described, forcing it upward. At the same time the free arm has grasped the limbs, raised them slightly to rotate the pelvis and lower lumbar spine, and thrusts them downward in extension to stretch the soft tissues and aid in increasing the distance between ribs and pelvis.

II. This movement may be varied,grasping the limbs in the same way and drawing them and the pelvis over the side of the table, rotating them downward about the edge of the table,extending the limbs and rotating them upward and onto the table. The rib is manipulated as in I. This is a strong treatment, and applies great force to the rib.

III. With the patient sitting, a hand is applid to each end of the rib. The patient takes a full breath to throw the rib into activity; pressure is so applied as to exaggerate the lesion, and the rib is finally pressed upward to its normal position as the patient exhales.

IV. The patient lies upon his side; one operating hand grasps the iliocostal tissues and draws them diagonally downward and forward in the direction in which the rib points. The other hand is placed upon the angle of the rib and pushes it in the same direction. In this way the tissues are stretched and the lesion exaggerated. The motion is finished by an upward turn of the hands, the former pressing the end of the rib upward, the latter forcing the shaft of the rib upwards.

B. Upward Displacements.

In these cases the anterior ends of the ribs are upward under the rib above. All tissues are first relaxed as before, and the free end is located by deep pressure beneath the ribs and tissues. The rib may be manipulated as before described.

Treatments I, II and III may be applied equally as well to the reduction of upward displacements; the appropriate pressure being made to force the rib downward.

The STERNUM, if PROTRUDED or RETRACTED as a whole, is restored to normal through the general shaping of the thorax by methods already described. The *ensiform appendix*, being cartilaginous, is usually easily sprung by pressure and trained toward its normal position.

In case of luxation between the *first* and *second parts* of the sternum, traction is brought upon the first part through the deep cervical tissues and the sterno-mastoid muscle of either side by rotation of the head backward and to one side. At the same time pressure is made upon the prominent end of the first or second part, reducing it.

The CLAVICLE may be restored from any of its usual mal-positions as follows: The patient lies prone and the practitioner stands at the head of the table, slightly to one side. The fingers of the operating hand are pressed, palm up, behind the clavicle, the tissues being relaxed by slightly raising the shoulder. The free hand now grasps the arm of the patient just above the elbow and pushes the bent arm across the chest, up over the face, above the head, and rotates it down to the side again. This motion has raised the clavicle and allowed the fingers to be pressed deeply behind it. They may be applied particularly to the *sternal end*. The elevation of the shoulder has widened the anterior end of the costo-clavicular space and allowed the fingers to be brought well forward toward the sternal end. As the arm is now rotated outward, the increase of distance between the sternal and acromial attachments of the bone draws it down hard upon the fingers between it and the rib, forcing it upward from either an *anterior or posterior downward dislocation*.

In case the *sternal end* had been dislocated *upward* on the sternum, the motion would have been the same, except that during the outward rotation of the arm pressure would have been made above the sternal end to force it downward.

In case the *acromial end* had been *downward or upward* the same motion would be applied, with the operating hand directed to that end of the bone. During the outward rotation of the arm the bone would be grasped between the fingers behind and the thumb in front and moved upward or downward from its displacement.

Here, as in case of the ribs, it is less probable that the performance of a single set motion would accomplish the work than that insistent, though not violent, traction, pressure, rotation, etc., according to the manner of the described treatment, would secure the result.

CHAPTER VIII.

GENERAL OSTEOPATHIC POINTS IN REGARD TO THE ABDOMEN AND ITS PARTS.

Many of the specific lesions affecting the abdomen and its contained viscera occur in the spine and thorax and are of kinds already described. Much of the treatment for diseases of these parts is upon such lesions. The subject of examination and treatment of the various organs will be considered more in detail in relation to their specific diseases. The aim of this chapter is to give general methods of examination and general osteopathic points concerning these parts.

POSITION:—The patient lies prone; the thighs are flexed and the feet rest upon the table; the head and chest are slightly elevated by the inclined head of the table. In this position the abdominal muscles are relaxed. The sides of the body are disposed alike to avoid unequal tension upon the tissues.

Inspection, palpation, percussion are the physical methods employed.

INSPECTION reveals enlargement due to gas or fluid, tumor, muscular contraction, etc.; color, distended or retracted walls, restricted or increased motion, pulsation or engorgement of blood vessels, etc.

PALPATION reveals change in temperature; tumors, superficial or deep, fluid or solid; tenseness or flabbiness of the abdominal walls; enlargements and displacements of organs, etc.

PERCUSSION reveals the limits of organs, pressure of tumors, fluids or gases, etc.

AUSCULATION reveals the gurgling of gases, fetal sounds, lubrication of the bowel, etc.

I. A *general treatment* of the abdomen is sometimes necessary for general relaxation of the abdominal walls, often as a preliminary step toward further examination. With the patient in position as above, the practitioner stands at the side of the table and with the palm of the hand manipulates the tissues to relax them. Care should be taken to avoid pressure with the tips of the fingers or other rude work which causes the tissues to contract. The hand should be warm and the manipulation gentle but thorough.

II. Direct manipulation, including pressure and various movements, is often made upon the various abdominal organs. Specific directions for the treatment of any given organ are reserved until specific diseases of these organs are considered. But speaking in general of abdominal manipulation as one of the methods in the repertoire of the Osteopath, care must be taken to make clear the difference between such manipulation and massage. Here the mode of motion is relatively insignificant. The manipulation is not for the general effect following a thorough abdominal massage, but is corrective; directed to the specific end of restoring to proper mechanical relations an organ or organs definitely ascertained to be in need of mechanical adjustment. Here, as elsewhere in the body, this work removes pressure from, or interference with, blood-vessels and nerves. For example, osteopathic treatment of the colon is not made for general manipulative effect, but is directed to raising and straightening a sigmoid too much bent or folded. Thus it removes a mechanical obstruction to bowel action, but also lets free pelvic circulation and nerve action impeded by such a condition.

Or manipulation of the colon raises from its unnatural position the gut which has prolapsed and become wedged down among the pelvic viscera, where it has destroyed harmony of the functions. Osteopathic manipulation in this way is specific; corrective; based upon mechanical principles, and is applied by a practitioner who knows what causes such abdominal conditions and how to correct them.

III. With the patient in position as above, or standing or sitting bent well forward, the fingers are inserted deeply beneath the viscera in each iliac fossa. They are now drawn directly upward, raising all the pelvic and abdominal viscera, freeing the action of the femoral and pelvic vessels and nerves.

In case the patient has bent forward he straightens the body again at the same time the viscera are raised.

IV. With the patient lying upon the right side, the practitioner stands behind the pelvis and presses the fingers deeply into the iliac fossa upon the side of the sigmoid nearest the median plane of the body. He now raises the sigmoid flexure upward and slightly outward over the flaring ilium. This raises the gut from the pelvis, relieves kinking, and frees the circulation of the part.

The movement may be repeated for the caecum.

V. With the patient in the dorsal position, the practitioner stands at the side and places the palms of the hands over the false ribs and cartilages, one on either side, heel out and fingers directed toward the median plane of the body. Pressure is now made evenly upon the sides, springing the ribs and cartilages down upon the viscera beneath. As the pressure is directed inward the ribs and cartilages are forced toward the mid-line and pressed down upon the viscera. Repeating this motion at intervals of a few seconds thoroughly tones the nerve plexuses and blood-flow of the upper abdominal viscera.

VI. *Deep pressure is made upon the solar plexus* as follows: The patient lies prone, the practitioner stands at the side and lays the palmar surface of the distal phalanges of one hand over the pit of the stomach, at the level of the tips of the seventh and eighth ribs. Pressure with the second hand upon the first is gradually applied, the hand sinking deeper into the tissues until very deep pressure has been made. The plexus may now be manipulated by a slight circular movement of the hand. This treatment tones the action of the solar plexus, etc.   It should be gently and gradually applied, but the pressure must be considerable.

VII.   Deep pressure as above at any point will cause a purely nervous pain to lessen or disappear, while it increases a pain due to inflammation.

VIII.   Displaced ribs sometimes mechanicaliy depress viscera, and must then be replaced by methods already described,

IX. The fundus of the gall bladder is reached by deep pressure beneath the tip of the ninth rib on the right ride.   Thence the course of the bile duct to the duodenum is in the shape of a reversed "S," the upper limb lying above and to the right of the umbilicus, the lower limb encircling the umbilicus upon the right and opening into the duodenum from one to two inches below the umbilicus.   Manipulation aids in emptying the bladder and in passing gall stones along the duct.

Abdominal treatment is geneaally in conjunction with treatment upon specific lesion occurring in the spine, thorax, etc.   It must be given carefully, as there are many diseases, e. g., typhoid, in which rough abdominal treatment might cause serious injury.   It is directed to a specific end and restores mechanical relations of parts, frees nerve and blood mechanisms, removes muscular contracture, etc.

CHAPTER IX.

EXAMINATION AND TREATMENT OF LESIONS OF THE PELVIS.

Importance of pelvic lesion can scarcely be overestimated on account of its relations to the spine above, to its contained viscera, and to the lower portions of the body. This chapter does not deal with diseases of the pelvic organs, but with bony and ligamentous lesions of the pelvis which are so significant from the osteopathic standpoint, as causes of disease in the pelvic viscera in the limbs, or in the body above.

A. LESIONS AFFECTING THE PELVIS AS A WHOLE:

I. EXAMINATION. The examiner must not neglect to examine the spine in relation to pelvic lesion, as malpositions of this structure are almost sure to destroy spinal equilibrium and thus to affect spinal relations, sometimes to a serious extent. The most common of such results is swerving or curvature of the spine in response to the efforts of nature to adapt the spine to a crooked pelvis.

The pelvis as a whole may be *tipped forward or backward*; may be *turned to either side*; or may be *tilted*, throwing *one crest up* and the *other downward*. These malpositions may be combined in various ways. The *general symptoms* of such trouble are pelvic diseases, female disorders, backache, sciatica, lameness or paralysis of the lower limbs, etc. In case of lesion of the whole pelvis, the point of movement upon the spine is usually the lumbo-sacral articulation, but the fifth lumbar vertebra may be carried with the pelvis, or the yielding point may include the whole lumbar region.

INSPECTION AND PALPATION aid each other in the examination.

(1.) Both *superior posterior iliac spines* are found equally too *prominent* in case of backward luxation of the pelvis, or

(2) They are alike found to have *receded anteriorly* in forward luxation, or

(3) *One is prominent* and the *other has receded anteriorly* in twisting of the pelvis sidewise or,

(4) *One stands higher* than the other in case of tilting of the pelvis laterally. In the latter case comparison shows *inequality in the length of the limbs*, and *tenderness* is often found in the tissues upon the iliac crest of the low side owing to greater tension upon them. At the same time the *waist line is deepened* upon the high side and filled out upon the low side.

Examination and comparison of the posterior superior spines is best made upon the bared back, with the patient sitting sidewise upon the table. The practitioner sits upon a low stool directly behind the patient, placing a hand upon each spine, examining and comparing them carefully. Care must be taken that careless posture of the patient does not cause an apparent inequality, or, on the other hand, that an assumed position does not mask the lesion.

With the patient sitting or lying on the side, careful palpation is made of the superficial and deep soft tissues in the sacro-iliac and posterior sacral regions. These are commonly sensitive to pressure, but are always tensed, congested and strained over the sacro-iliac articulation and the posterior sacral foramina. These ligamentous lesions alone cause much ill by obstructing nerve action. The hand is also passed along the crests of the ilia making deep pressure in the tissues, to discover tenderness in them.

Tilting of the pelvis may be ascertained also by measurements between the coracoid process of the scapula and the anterior superior spine of the ilium upon each side. A better method is to have the patient hold the tape between his teeth in the mid-line of the body, from which point measurement is made to the inner maleolus of the tibia on each side. Tilting of the pelvis cannot be ascertained by measurements unless a fixed point above the pelvis is used as the starting point.

II. TREATMENT.

In the treatment of all the lesions above described, a preliminary step may usually be made with advantage by thorough relaxation of the soft tissues in the sacro-iliac regions as already described. (Chap. II, divs. III, XIII, XIV, XIX.)

All the lesions described may be treated with the patient sitting upon the stool, his pelvis fixed by an'assistant, who stands in front or behind and grasps the iliac crests, one with each hand.

(1) For *backward tipping*, the assistant stands in front and draws the pelvis forward, while the practitioner stands behind, grasps the patient beneath the axillae, and raises and draws the trunk backward. His work is aided by pressure of his knee against the sacrum. During this treatment, slight rotation of the body from one side to the other during the lifting process helps the reduction of the lesion.

(2) For *tilting upward on one side* or for *turning to either side*, this same treatment may be applied with variations to suit the condition.

(3) For *tipping forward*, the assistant stands behind and draws the pelvis backward, while the practitioner manipulates the trunk from in front, in a similar manner as before, gradually working and drawing it forward.

(4) For *tipping forward*, the patient may lie upon his side. the practitioner stands behind the pelvis, making a fixed point with one palm against the lower portions of the innominates and sacrum. He now draws backward, with the other hand, upon the uppermost iliac crest and anterior superior spine. The patient lies upon the other side and the motion is repeated.

(5) For *tipping backward*, the patient lies upon his side, the practitioner stands behind and presses the flat of his knee against the upper portion of the sacrum. He now grasps the uppermost limb with one hand, the uppermost shoulder with the other, and draws the body backward, while forcing the pelvis carefully forward.

(6)   For *tilting upward* of the pelvis, one may adapt to the reduction of this lesion the treatment described in Chap. VII, A, Downward Displacements of Lower Ribs, for the stretching of the quadrati lumborum muscles.

(7)   For *turning of the pelvis to one side*, one may adapt to the reduction of this lesion the treatment as described in Chap. II. div. XVIII. third treatment.

B.—Lesions Affecting Parts of the Pelvis.

We deal here chiefly with lesions of the innominate bones. They are more frequent than lesions of the pelvis as a whole, and are realatively more important.

The *general indications* of innominate lesion, which would lead one to examine for such displacement are back-ache, sciatica, pain or lameness in the limbs, limping or unequal gait, pelvic disease, female disorders, etc.

The *lesions* of the innominates commonly met with are:

I. The innominate displaced *forward or backward*.

II. The innominate displaced *upward or downward*.

III. *Combinations of the above*, which are the rule. It is rare that the simple lesion I. or II. is found. Frequently the displacement is *downward and backward* at the same time, lengthening the leg. This lesion is, on the whole, the most common, but the opposite luxation, *forward and upward*, is frequent. Generally if the lesion is backward, it is at the same time downward; if it is forward, it is at the same time upward. In the latter case, the leg is shortened. Yet it cannot be stated as the invariable rule that the backward lesion is combined with the downward one, and that the upward and forward positions always combine. The luxation may be back and up, or *vice-versa*. Yet, whatever the combined lesion be, a lengthened limb indicates a downward displacement of the innominate, while a shortened limb shows the reverse.

The reason why the downward lesion usually complicates the backward one is found in the beveled edge of the sacrum where it articulates with the ilium. This bevel is wedge-shaped, with its broad end up. Moreover, its posterior margin is longer, and rises higher than its anterior edge. Thus the beveled auricular surface of the sacrum, which bone is broader in front and tilts forward so that the posterior margin of its base stands higher, directs the ilium either downward and backward, or upward and forward, according to the direction of the forces causing the lesion.

IV. *Each innominate* may suffer from lesion at the same time, which may be alike upon both sides, or different.

Examination: Palpation, aided by Inspection, is used in the examination.

I. *The length of the limbs is compared*, and is one of the first and most reliable methods of examining for lesion of the innominate. The patient is laid upon his back; care is taken that he shall lie perfectly straight; the limbs are flexed and rotated to relax muscles and ligaments, and to prevent any unnatural tension in these structures from causing merely apparent difference in length. The limbs are now drawn down and compared at the heels. It is best to have the patient keep the shoes on, but care must be taken to notice that the heels of the shoes do not differ in thickness, and that they are pushed back snugly against the patient's heel.

This examination is for confirmation only, and while it is a clear indication that one innominate is luxated, further examination is necessary to determine whether one leg is too long, or the other too short.

II. *Tenderness* in the sacro-iliac ligaments upon deep pressure, and tenderness in the tissues along the crest of the ilium indicate that the lesion is upon the side upon which such tenderness occurs. The sacro-iliac ligaments are found tensed upon the side of lesion.

While this tenderness and tension will usually indicate unilateral lesion it is not an invariable sign, as the strain thrown upon the opposite side often causes like effects.

Tenderness at the public symphysis is often present in these cases.

The *position of the posterior superior iliac spines* is the best indication of lesion, receding anteriorly, prominent posteriorly, up, or down, down and back, forward and up, etc., indicating the corresponding malposition in the bone. Comparison of the spine of the luxated bone with that of the normal bone is made. This examination must be made upon the bared back with the patient sitting. The practitioner sits directly behind the patient, palpation of both spines alike is made at the same time, one hand upon each. This facilitates comparison.

IV. The *waist line* is frequently changed in each case. Usually that upon the side of lesion is deeper through the patient's favoring that side; bending toward it. For the same reason the muscles about the hip, pelvis and lower spine upon the opposite side may be hypertrophied,

V. The *spine* adjacent to the pelvis must be examined for curvature, swerving to one side, hypertrophy or tension of tissues, etc., secondary to pelvic lesion.

VI. *Measurements* may be made between coracoids and anterior superior spines, also from the mid-line of the teeth to the inner maleolus of each tibia.

TREATMENT: Preliminary relaxation of all surrounding tissues is first done by methods already described.

I. BACKWARD LUXATIONS and their combinations:

a. Patient lies upon his back; practitioner stands at the side and places the clenched hand as a fixed point beneath the posterior superior spine of the luxated bone; the knee is flexed against the throax and is rotated outward strongly enough to raise the weight of the patient and throw it upon the clenched hand. In this way the weight of the body is made to force the bone forward.

b. Patient lies upon his side; practitioner stands in front of the pelvis, slips one hand between the thighs and grasps the tuberosity of the ischium, the other hand is upon the posterior crest. He now draws forward upon the latter point while he pushes backward upon the tuberosity, by pulling forward on the tuberosity and pushing backward on the crest, the *anterior* displacement of the bone may be set.

Commonly one alternately pushes and pulls to thoroughly loosen the bone, ending by the appropriate motion to set it.

c. Patient lies upon his sound side; practitioner stands behind the pelvis ,making pressure with his hand upon the upper back part of the innominate, while at the same time he draws the uppermost thigh backward. This forces the bone forward.

II. FORWARD LUXATIONS and their combinations:

a. Patient lies on his side, lesion uppermost; the practitioner stands behind the sacrum and places his hand or the flat surface of his knee against the lower part of the sacrum, while he draws backward upon the anterior spine and crest of the luxated innominate.

b. See "b" above.

III. UPWARD LESION:

a. The patient sits upon a stool and an assistant stands in front and fixes the pelvis by firm pressure downward upon the crests of the ilia. The practitioner stands behind, grasps the patient's trunk beneath the axillae, and lifts; turns and springs the whole trunk away from the side of lesion.

This same motion may be applied to forcing the body down toward the side of lesion in *downward* luxations.

b. For reducing the upward lesion one may adopt the treatment described in chapter VII. A. for the stretching of of the quadratus lumborum muscle.

For *downward* luxation see "a" above.

The SACRUM and COCOYX have already been discussed. (Chap. I. divs. V., VI., VII ; Chap. II. divs. XIX., XX.) Anterior or posterior, upward or downward luxation of the sacrum may be overcome by combinations of the treatments described for the sacrum and for the innominate.

Spinal treatment must be given in conjunction with pelvic treatment as the case may require.

C.—GENERAL POINTS CONCERNING THE PELVIS.

The *pudic nerve and artery* may be located where they cross the spine of the ischium, and be reached by deep pressure. The patient lies upon his side, the practitioner stands in front and bends the uppermost thigh backward to loosen the muscles and tissues. Pressure is made down upon the spine at a point between the middle and lower two thirds of a line drawn from the posterior superior spine of the ilium to the outer side of the tuber ischii.

The *gluteal arteries* may be impinged in the same way by deep pressure at a point between the upper and middle two thirds of a line drawn from the posterior superior spine of the ilium to the outer side of the great trochanter when the thigh has been rotated forward.

Deep manipulation may be made over the course of the *iliac blood-vessels*, beginning at a point about two inches below the umbilicus and thence diagonally outward to the point where the femoral vessel leaves the pelvis beneath Poupart's ligament. The internal iliac artery runs diagonally downward into the pelvis from about the mid-point of the line of the first manipulation.

The *spermatic* or *ovarian* vessels may be manipulated by deep pressure along a line beginning at the level of the umbilicus one inch external thereto, and running down to enter the pelvis at a point one and one half inches internal to the anterior superior spine of the ilium.

In case of these vessels one aids the venous flow by centripetal progress along the lines defined. As an aid in relieving or restoring blood-flow in various pelvic diseases the treatments are of value.

The *Hypogastric plexus* is reached by deep pressure at a point about two inches below the umbilicus. The plexus lies between the common iliac arteries, just below the bifurcation of the aorta.

The *pelvic plexuses* are reached a little lower and outward from the mid-line, where they lie deep in the pelvis each side of the rectum.

D.—OSTEOPATHIC WORK PER RECTUM.

The *index finger* is generally used in rectal work as its use is less interfered with by the knuckles. Proper precautions for cleanliness and to guard against infection must be employed. The patient lies upon the right side or stands bent over a table. The examining finger, lubricated with vaseline or soap-suds is inserted, palm down, into the rectum. It *notes* malposition of sacrum or coccyx; weakness, folding or prolapsing of the rectal walls; whether the grasp of the external sphincter is normal; enlargement of the prostate gland in the male; protrusion of the cervix or fundus of the uterus against the rectum in the female; the presence of tumor or other growth; hæmorrhoids, protruding or internal.

The prostate gland lies below the anterior wall of the rectum and is felt in that position about one and one-half inches from the anus. Either lateral lobe, or the central lobe may be enlarged. In the latter case, stricture of the urethra is threatened, as the gland surrounds its first position.

Treatment:—In prolapsed and weakened walls the finger should smooth out the walls and press them upward as far as possible. This aids reposition, tones nerve and blood force, and helps to establish normal tone to the muscular walls.

A weakened sphincter is much stimulated by the simple insertion of the finger. It may be dilated by introducing two or three fingers held in wedge-shape, spreading them apart upon withdrawal.

For an enlarged prostate gland, the finger makes pressure upon it and is swept laterally over it to aid in freeing the blood-flow from it. Care must be taken not to irritate it.

In hæmorrhoids, all the surrounding tissues are gently manipulated for relaxation and to remove interference with free circulation, after which pressure is made directly upon the distended vessels to empty them of blood, and to gently force them back into place if external.

Rectal treatments should not usually be given oftener than once a week or ten days. Great care should always be exercised to cause as little irritation as may be. As a rule these treatments are but secondary to the removal of pelvic or spinal lesion.

E.—Osteopathic Work per Vaginam.

This examination is made with the index finger for the same reasons as in the case of rectal treatment. The same precautions as to cleanliness, etc., should be observed.

As a rule local treatment is secondary to that done upon spinal or pelvic lesion, which is usually the real cause of those conditions which require local treatment.

It is proposed here to review this subject only in a general way, giving the main points in connection with the examination and treatment of this region as a part of the body, leaving detailed consideration to the portions of the course dealing specially with the specific diseases of these organs.

I. Local Examination:—The patient lies on her back or on her side. In the latter case the practitioner stands behind. The index finger anointed with vaseline is introduced, passing from the region of the fourchette forward. The guiding hand is placed upon the abdomen, and by deep pressure may aid in locating the organ and in diagnosing its position. External pressure over the region of the broad ligaments will sometimes reveal tenderness in them in cases of prolapsus uteri. In case the tenderness is unilateral it is usually in the ligament suffering from the most tension because of the organ having fallen toward the opposite side.

The examining finger should first note the condition of the *vaginal walls*, which may be weak and flabby, or prolapsed and contorted by the malposition of the uterus. The presence of *enlargement or tumor* of surrounding organs is to be noticed. At the upper extremity of the vaginal canal is felt the *cervix* protruding into the canal.

The external *os uteri* opens *transversely* at the lower end of the cervix. In women who have borne children the external os inclines to be circular, but by careful examination the transverse axis may be distinguished. This is made more certain by the shape of the cervix, which is somewhat flattened antero-posteriorly. By these two points, the transverseness of the os and the position of the cervix, the main diagnosis of the position of the uterus is made. If the transverse os (or the longer transverse diameter of the cervix) has assumed an oblique direction in the pelvis, it indicates a corresponding turn in the position of the organ. This turning to one side is usually combined with the prolapsus of the organ in one direction or another.

If the cervix points forward and upward, the fundus has gone down and back, and may be against the rectum.   In such case the fundus is often felt through the posterior vaginal wall.   Or the uterus may have turned in falling backward, so that the fundus lies down toward either sacro-iliac region. If the cervix points backward and upward, it indicates that the cervix has descended anteriorly upon the bladder.   It may often be felt through the anterior vaginal wall.   There are all degrees of prolapsus, some may be so slight that the cervix and fundus have deviated but little from normal position.   By noting the direction of the os, the direction of the cervix, and (if possible) the position of the fundus, no difficulty is usually experienced in discovering the form of prolapsus from which the patient is suffering.

The different forms of flexion are more difficult, but may be made out by the relative position of the cervix and fundus.   For example, if the cervix remains near normal position while the fundus is found backward, retroflexion is diagnosed.

II.   LOCAL TREATMENT:—The patient may lie upon the back, upon the side, or kneel upon the table with the trunk inclined forward and the chest touching the table.

In the first or second position, the patient may, while the operating finger still supports the organ, slip off of the table and stand upon the floor, bending forward to remove the weight of the viscera above, while the finger presses the organ back toward its position.   In any case, the idea of the treatment is to so manipulate the cervix, by pressure or traction, as to cause the cervix, thus the fundus, to assume its natural position.

The knee-chest position is the best for the treatment of such cases. It allows the force of gravitation to act to draw the intestines from the pelvis, which permits easy reposition of the organ.   At the same time the vagina may be dilated, and atmospheric pressure aids materially in forcing the uterus high up to its position.   Moreover, when the patient has changed her position first onto the side, then onto the feet, the intestines fall back around the organ and help support it.

The treatment described in Chap. VIII, div. III, may be applied to the external treatment of pelvic disorders.

The *round ligaments* of the uterus may be located and may be stimulated by pressure upon the upper margin of the pubic arch, about a half an inch externally from the symphysis.

Inspection of the *female perineum* sometimes reveals a downward bulging of it in place of the natural slight arch of the healthy perineum. Such a condition indicates prolupsus of the pelvic viscera.

In child-birth, strain upon the perineum may be relieved by grasping both tubers ischii from below with one hand, while the other hand presses the tissues over the pubic crest in front down toward the perineum.   The first hand, meanwhile is tending to spring the tuberosities toward each other.

CHAPTER X.

THE LIMBS.

I. SHOULDER DISLOCATIONS. The head of the humerus may be dislocated downward into the axilla; forward beneath the clavicle; backward upon the scapula; or forward beneath the coracoid process.

With the patient sitting, and the trunk fixed by an assistant, the practitioner stands at the side, rests his foot upon the stool and places his knee in the patient's axilla. Traction is now made directly downward upon the arm, overcoming the tension of the muscles and drawing the head back into the glenoid fossa. This treatment will answer for any of the dislocations.

The same object may be accomplished by placing the patient upon his back, while the practitioner stands at the side, places his stockinged foot in the axilla, and exerts strong traction upon the arm.

II. ELBOW DISLOCATIONS. The radius and ulna may be both displaced backward, externally or internally; the ulna backward; the radius forward or backward.

The patient sits, and the practitioner satnds at the side with his foot resting upon the stool and his knee in the bend of the elbow. The upper arm is fixed and traction is made strongly upon the forearm. This will be sufficient for the first four dislocations. When the radius is backward, direct pressure upon it is sufficient to reduce it. When the radius is forward the hand is supinated, it is bent upon the wrist away from the radius, thus bringing traction upon it, while pressure is made upon the head of the bone above.

III. WRIST DISLOCATIONS. The radius and ulna may both be forward, backward, or outward. Simple traction will reduce them.

IV. RADIO-ULNAR DISLOCATIONS. The radius is regarded as the fixed bone, the ulna being displaced forward or backward. Direct pressure upon it will force it to its place.

V. CARPO-METACARPAL dislocations are more frequent in case of the thumb. Direct pressure will reduce them.

VI. Dislocations of CARPAL bones are easily reduced by pressure.

VII. METACARPO PHALANGEAL dislocations in case of the thumb are most frequent. For the *backward* one, continued strong hyper extension, followed by flexion are used. If this treatment does not succeed, the metacarpal is rotated and pressure is made upon its head. In the *forward* displacement traction and pressure are employed, or strong flexion is followed by direct pressure.

In case of the fingers, simple traction and pressure are sufficient, as is also the case in PHALANGEAL dislocations.

These remarks apply to all cases of recent dislocation as described. It more often comes within the Osteopath's province to work upon old dislocations, so frequently given over as incurable. As far as possible he applies the usual motions for the reduction of them, but prepares the joint for reduction by a course of treatment directed to relaxing surrounding muscles etc.; to restoration of free circulation about the part and the upbuilding of the tissues. Often a persistent course of treatment restores a bone to position when it had been given up as hopeless. These remarks apply especially to old dislocations of the hip joint.

GENERAL TREATMENT FOR THE UPPER LIMB. In treatment for various conditions the arm is manipulated in special ways.

I. The *shoulder-joint* may be sprung to allow of free blood-flow and to remove tension in the ligaments. The clenched hand is placed in the axilla, care being taken not to press the knuckles against the axillary lymphatics, or against the nerves and vessels on the inner side of the arm. It is best to turn the hand sidewise. The patient's arm is now forced against his side, springing the head of the humerus outward.

II. The *elbow* may be sprung by flexing the fore-arm over the hand placed upon the arm just above the bend of the elbow. Or the fore-arm may be flexed to a right angle, and the treating hands draw it away from the lower end of the humerus. They may follow along down the fore-arm, working deeply between radius and ulna to relax the interosseous tissues.

III. The branches of the *brachial plexus* and the *axillary* artery may be impinged against the inner side of the humerus just below the axilla. Transverse friction reaches all these nerves and may be used to tone them.

IV. Catching of the anterior fibres of the deltoid muscle under the *coracoid process,* and attendant slight forward luxation of the *head of the humerus* may be remedied by grasping the arm just above the elbow and drawing it directly back and up to the level of the shoulder. Now the arm is carried forward at the same level, and the movement is finished with a slight upward turn.

V. The *biceps muscle* and *its long head* may be strongly stretched by drawing the extended fore-arm directly backward and upward.

GENERAL TREATMENT FOR THE LOWER LIMB.

I. Strong flexion of the thigh on the thorax and the leg upon the thigh stretches the quadriceps extensor muscle.

II. Hyper-extension of the thigh stretches the anterior structures, including the femoral vessels and anterior crural nerve.

III. Hyper-extension of the foot stretches the anterior muscles of the leg. Strong flexion of the foot stretches the calf muscles.

IV. Adductor muscles of the thigh are stretched by forced abduction. The patient lies upon his back, the practitioner presses against one leg which remains upon the table, at the same time keeping the other leg straight and abducting it to the extreme. He may stand between the legs. The same object is accomplished by flexion combined with external circumduction.

V.   The muscles of external rotation for the thigh are stretched by flexion combined with internal circumduction.

VI.   The extensor muscles of the thigh are stretched by raising the straightened limb to or beyond right angles with the trunk. This may be accomplished with the patient on his back. The limb, still straight, may be supported at right angles while the foot is strongly flexed on the leg. This *stretches the sciatic nerve*. This nerve is also stretched by motion I. Motion V. stretches the pyriformis, gemelli, and obturator muscles, and aids in removing irritation from the sciatic nerve. All of the motions for stretching this nerve act partly through relaxation of tissues about it.

VII.   Pressure at the mid-line of *Scarpa's triangle*, about two inches below the middle of Poupart's ligament, impinges the femoral vessels and the anterior crural nerve.

VIII.   The popliteal nerve and vessels are reached at the popliteal space. The patient lies upon his back. The limb is drawn over the edge of the table and the foot is supported between the practitioner's knees. Manipulation is now made deeply just below the knee behind.

IX.   Forced flexion, extension, inversion and eversion of the foot may be made for the purpose of relaxing all the ligaments of the ankle.

All of the treatments described for the upper and lower limbs are given in a general way. They may be used in the treatment of specific cases of disease in various ways. One should not forget that they are used as aids in the reduction of special lesions or as secondary thereto.

X.   In treatment upon the *feet* one notes the two natural arches, the transverse and the longitudual. Springing these arches by pressure upon the arch above and traction at the same time upon the ends, aids in relaxing ligaments and other tissues, reducing bony luxations, removing pressure from nerves and blood-vessels. The treatment may be made more effective by springing the arch both ways, i. e., first applying pressure such as to increase the concavity of the arch, then to lessen it.

XI.   In treatment for the *toes* the blood-vessels, which lie upon the sides, are stretched, and the tissues about them relaxed, by bending them laterally. The lateral movements, combined with extension flexion, and traction, free the joint and its nerves, vessels, and tissues.

XII.   The *saphenous opening* an inch and a half below the inner end of Pouparts' ligament, is often in an occluded condition such as to seriously impede the flow from the long femoral vein. The muscles and tissues about it may be stretched by external rotation of the flexed knee. Following this movement by internal rotation of the extended limb relaxes the tissues still further and allows of direct manipulation upon the opening.

XIII.   With the patient lying upon the back one notes the angle of deviation of the toes, i. e., the angle between the feet. If one foot rotates outward too much or too little, it reveals tenseness or laxness of the rotattors of the thigh, and may lead one to the discovery of abnormal pelvic or hip conditions.

Concerning *dislocations* of the lower limbs, one must bear in mind that many of the cases presented to the Osteopath are old dislocations. The success of Osteopathy in the reduction of such has been marked. Again, many cases are met with in which gross dislocation is not present, but a slight luxation, or "slip," of a joint has occurred and has been overlooked by other practitioners. The number of cases in which such a slight displacement in the hip-joint has caused apparent disease in the knee, sciatica, lameness, etc., is remarkable. The fact that these things are commonly, or at least frequently, not discovered by others than Osteopaths indicates something of the need and importance of osteopathic methods. The practitioner must bear in mind the probability of such occurrences, and must be upon his guard to discover them. As a rule, in all old dislocations and chronic subluxations of this nature, the really important osteopathic work is the preparation of the parts for the restoration of normal relations. Relaxation of old contractures in muscles, softening ligaments, development of atrophied parts through the upbuilding of blood and nerve-supply are the preliminary steps taken by general osteopathic methods already described. In case of such luxations, gross dislocations excepted, the standpoint of the Osteopath in diagnosis is a new one. This teaching leads him to look for such causes of disease, which are meaningless to other methods of practice.

I. DISLOCATIONS OF THE ANKLE. The displacement may be of both leg bones forward, backward, inward or outward. In either case, the patient lies upon his back; the leg is elevated to a right angle and fixed by an assistant, and strong traction is made upon the foot. The muscles draw the ankle into place.

II. DISLOCATIONS OF THE KNEE. The leg may be forward, backward, inward or outward. Strong traction restores it to place.

In cases of slight backward luxation, short of dislocation, a good method is to have the patient lie on his back, hang the leg, bent at the knee, over the edge of the table, while the foot is supported between the practitioner's knees and his hands work in the popliteal region. The hamstring muscles are grasped by the two hands and stretched away laterally from the condyles of the femur, while the tibia and fibula are drawn forward.

III. DISLOCATIONS OF THE HIP. In such cases, the head of the bone may be displaced as follows:

(1) Up and back onto the dorsum of the ilium, shortening the limb and turning the toes inward.

(2) Down and back onto or near the sciatic notch, somewhat shortening the limb, and turning the toes inward.

(3) Forward and down onto or near the obturator foramen (thyroid

dislocation), in which the knee is flexed, the toe points to the ground and rotates inward or outward.

(4) Forward and up onto the pubic crest. The toe invariably turns out.

In (2), as the patient sits up from a lying posture, the limb shortens; in (3) and (4) it lengthens.

In the *treatment* of such conditions, fresh dislocations are set at once, but as in our practice many old dislocations are presented, the success of the treatment lies largely in knowing how to thoroughly prepare parts for adjustment as above stated.   Much lies in our way of regarding disease, for even gross dislocations are often overlook. These, and the many luxations of lesser degree found in osteopathic diagnosis, could scarcely be overlook in our method of minutely scrutinizing the mechanical relations of all parts in examination of acase.

In (1) the knee in flexed and rotated a little inward to disengage the head of the femur, then, while pressure is made to force the head toward the acetabulum, the flexed knee is rotated well outward and extended. This draws the head into the acetabulum. The patient is lying on his back.

In (2) the manoeuver is the same, except that during outward rotation and extension the trochanter is grasped and forced forward toward the acetabulum. In the inward rotation the head has been disengaged from the notch.

In (3) the flexed knee is rotated far inward, freeing the head from the obturator foramen, while the "Y" ligament acts as a fulcrum. As the inward relation is carried downward to extension the head is forced toward the cotyloid notch.

In (4) the patient lies upon his sound side, the dislocated thigh is hyper-extended by being strongly drawn backward. This stretches all the muscles about the head, which, after slight flexion of the thigh, is lifted over the crest of the pubes.

In (1) and (2) the patient may sit upon a stool, the dislocated limb is crossed above the other knee, the pelvis is fixed by an assistant, the trochanter is pressed by one hand toward the acetabulum, while the other hand draws the limb well across its fellow and extends it to place the foot on the floor.

In (1) and (2) the patient may stand upon one foot, supporting his hands upon the back of a chair ; the thigh remains straight, and the knee is flexed to a right angle; the ankle is supported by the practitioner who stands at the side of and behind the patient. He new places one knee upon the popliteal region, allowing the weight of his body to come down upon it. This forces the head downward, while a swing of the ankle outward disengages it. Now a swing inward, while the weight is still applied, brings the head into the acetabulum.

These various motions may be applied to subluxaitons as well as to gross dislocations.

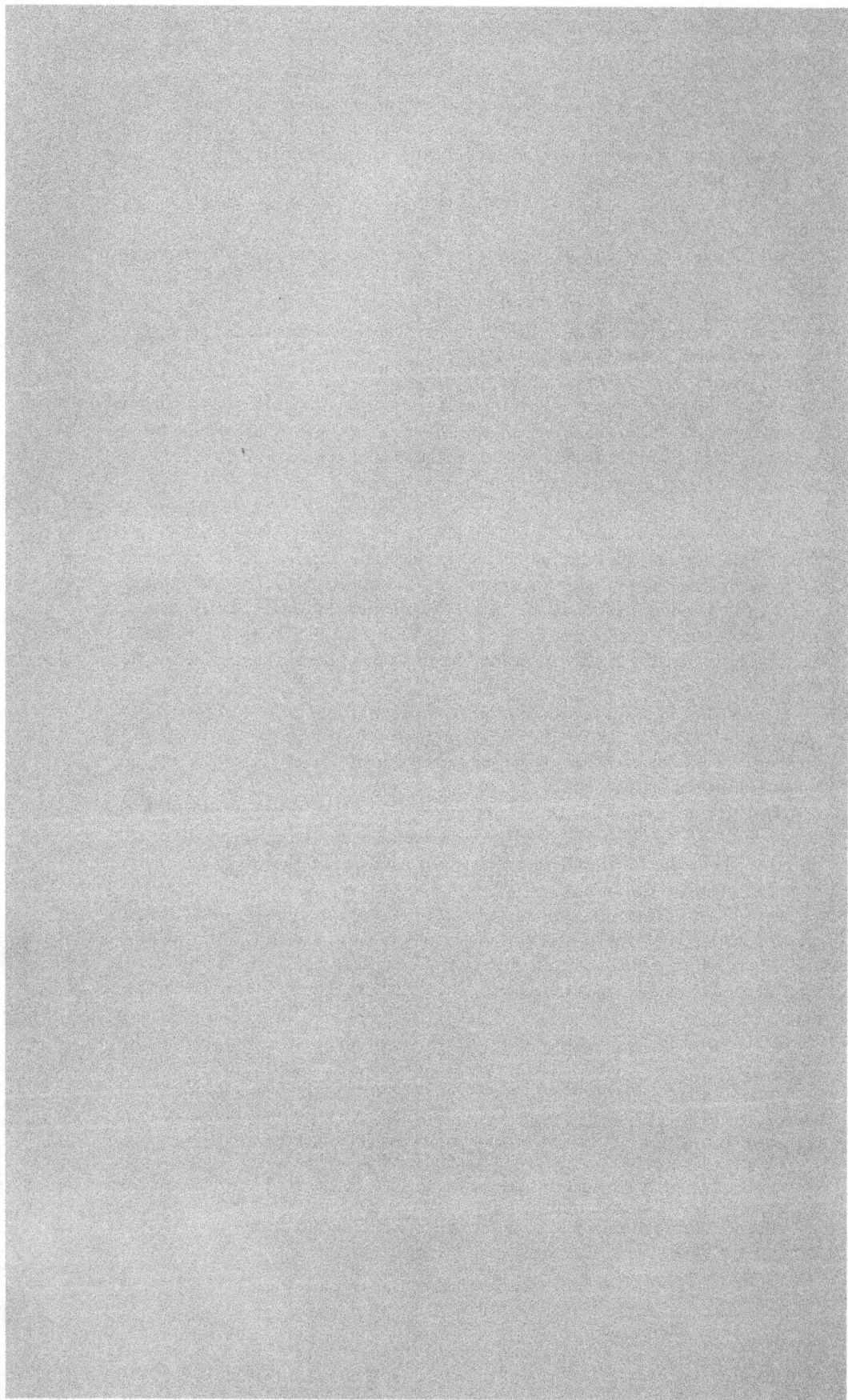

PART II.
DISEASES.

NOTE.—*It is the intention to deal here only with the osteopathic views, principles and methods in relation to the various diseases considered. Any standard medical text will supply the reader with these facts, theories, etc., which he may desire to know, and which it is unnecessary to reprint here.*

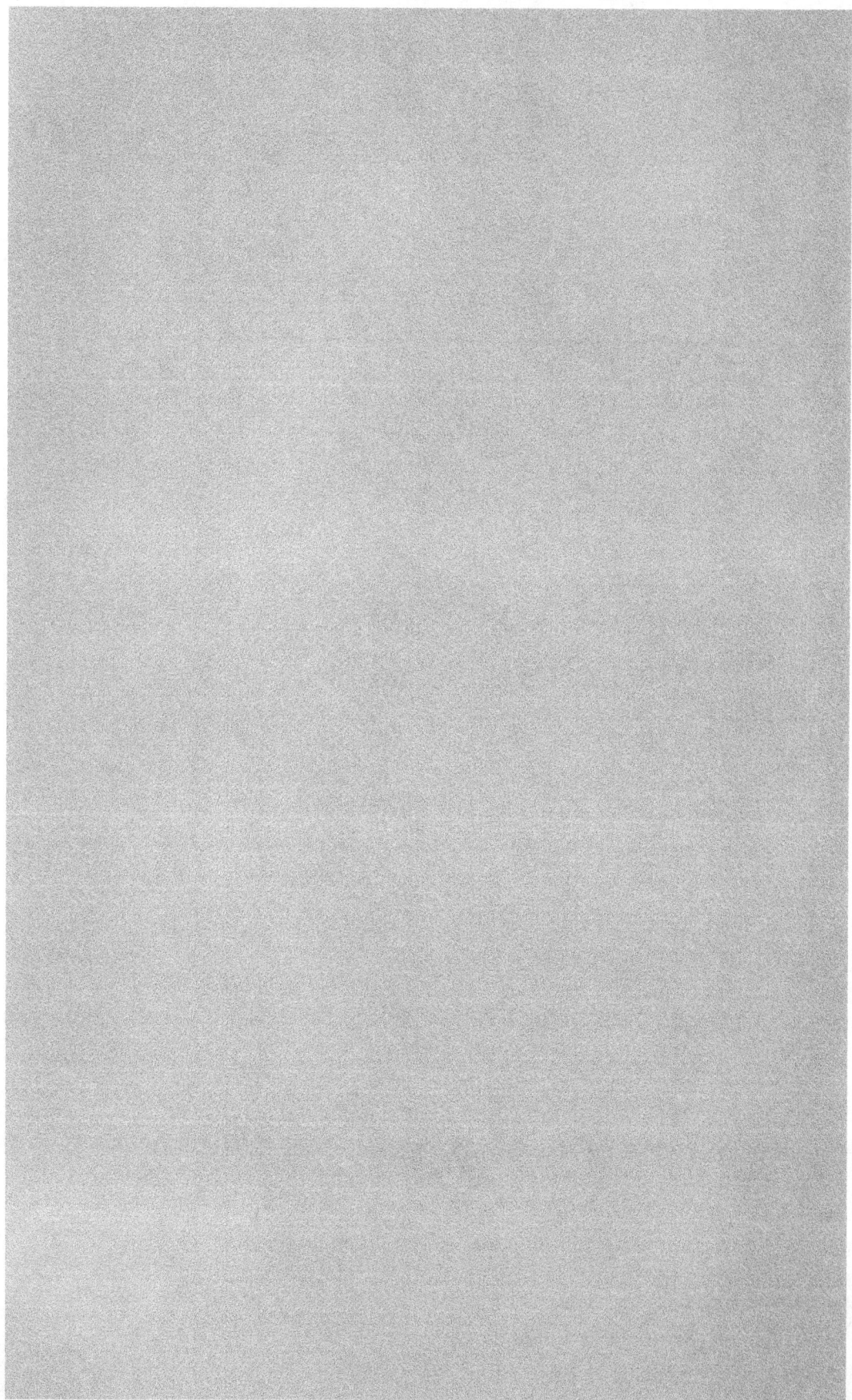

ASTHMA.

DEFINITION: Asthma is a disease of the bronchial tubes characterized by dyspnea. It is spasmodic in nature, the air tubes being narrowed by spasm of their muscular fibers or by swelling of the mucous membrane from hypermia.

CAUSE:—This disease always presents definite lesions, muscular and bony, of the upper dorsal spine and of the thorax. Secondary lesions usually occur in the cervical region. *The chief bony lesions affect the ribs from the second to the sixth on the right side.* (A. T. Still.) The majority of cases show lesions of this region, but they may occur higher up or lower down. Lesion is often found in the neck. (A. G. Hildreth.) The sternal ends of the ribs and the costal cartilages, as well as the spinal ends of the ribs may show the lesion. Lesions of the ribs from the second to the seventh on either side; of the corresponding dorsal vertebrae; of the anterior and posterior thoracic muscles; of the atlas, axis and hyoid bone, and of the cervical muscles are all active in producing the disease.

A review of the typical cases, reported from various sources, and in which cures were made by the removal of the specific lesion, shows a definite area in which such causes occur. (1) Luxation of first, second and third left ribs. (2) Fourth, fifth and sixth dorsal vertebrae anterior; the corresponding ribs lowered. Two treatments stopped the attacks, and patient was discharged as cured after three weeks' treatment. (3) Second dorsal vertebra lateral. (4) Fifth right rib down and much tenderness of tissues at the fifth dorsal vertebra. This case was of thirty years' standing, and is reported cured by two weeks' treatment. (5) The scaleni, mastoid and anterior and posterior thoracic muscles very tense. (6) Right fourth and fifth ribs, and left fifth and sixth ribs luxated. This case was also of thirty years' standing. One month's treatment cured it.

(7) The axis luxated to the right, cervical muscles contractured, all the ribs depressed. A case of twenty years' standing, cured in one month. (8) The left fifth and sixth ribs downward. (9) The first to the eighth ribs on both sides down; spinal muscles of the same region contractured; luxation of the atlas and axis; depression of the hyoid bone. (10) The second dorsal vertebra luxated laterally, involving the corresponding ribs; several ribs below down. (11) All the upper dorsal vertebrae anterior, carrying the ribs forward; closeness of the first rib to the clavicle.

One can but note how all of these lesions occur in those regions it which it is claimed the cause of asthma occurs. No other school of practice notices such causes of this disease. Their theories are various, many exciting causes are agreed upon, but Anders makes the statement in regard to the real and original causes that they are of an unknown nature.

The spinal area of motion is given by Dr. Still as extending from the fourth to the sixth dorsal vertebra. These lesions affect this area. They cause abnormal motor effects both in arousing spasmodic conditions of the muscles of the bronchial walls, and in the vaso-motor activity that produces the hyperemia of the mucous membranes.

There are good anatomical reasons why lesions in these regions affect the lungs. The American Text Book of Physiology states that stimulation of the vagus in the neck produces constriction of the pulmonary vessels, while stimulation of the sympathetics in the neck causes dilatation of them. Quain's anatomy says that the pneumogastrics convey motor fibers to the unstriped muscle fibers of the trachea, bronchi, and their subdivisions in the lungs. Vaso-constrictors for the lungs exist, in some animals, in the second to the seventh spinal nerves. (Quain.) The anterior pulmonary plexus is composed of the pneumogastrics and the sympathetics; the posterior, of the pneumogastrics and branches from the second, third, and fourth thoracic sympathetic ganglia. These regions of the spine, with their important nerve connections with the lungs, are naturally investigated by the Osteopath in relation to asthma. It is reasonable that obstruction to the nerves here should cause the disease. Anders gives among exciting causes "irritating lesions of the medulla." The Osteopath finds in lesions of atlas, axis and cervical tissues sufficient cause of such irritation of the medulla as well as of the pneumogastric, through their sympathetic and spinal nerve connections. In these ways, lesions to the cervical, dorsal and upper thoracic structures act as obstructors of these nerve mechanisms concerned in asthma, the pneumogastric nerve, pulmonary plexuses, sympathetic and vaso-motors, and cause the disease.

Exciting Causes of the paroxysm, such as bronchitis; the inhalation of irritants, such as dust, fog, smoke, chemical vapors, pollen of plants, odors of animals; reflex irritation from nose or stomach; the results of other diseases, etc., would not act to cause asthma did these anatomical lesions not exist. They are the real cause of the condition; existing in an individual, they obstruct the vital forces of the bronchi and deteriorate the vitality of their tissues, perhaps gradually during a term of years, and make it possible for these various exciting causes to act.

The PROGNOSIS is good under osteopathic treatment, though under medical treatment comparatively few cases recover. Very many cases, a large number of them apparently helpless, have been cured. The fact that most of these cases coming under osteopathic treatment are of long standing and have usually tried every known remedy seems to make little difference in gaining results upon them. Some cases the most severe and longest standing yield quickest.

EXAMINATION AND TREATMENT are carried out according to the methods described in Part I, (Chapters I, II, III, IV, VI, VII.) Any of the lesions that may affect the bony parts in the regions mentioned may produce the disease. Displacements of ribs, vertebrae, etc., need not take place in a particular direction. Rib and thoracic vertebral lesions are more likely to act as causes.   Lesions in the neck alone seem quite unlikely to cause it. Those of the fourth and fifth ribs upon the right side are most frequently the cause.   It is unnecessary to name the various probable causes of the an-atomical derangements or lesions named, as that subject has been fully dealt with elsewhere, as well as the theory of the exact way in which such lesions as the Osteopath finds act to cause disease.

Treatment must always depend for its success   upon removing the causative lesion, but treatment *during the attack* must look more particularly to immediate relief of the patient, for as a rule these lesions can be removed only by a course of treatment.   At this time great relief is given and the spasm usually quieted by thorough relaxation of the spinal muscles (Chap. II, div. I. p. 8), followed by raising of all the ribs (Chap. VII) and clavicles to allow free thoracic and lung action, and by relaxation of the muscles and other soft tissues of the neck.   Loosen the clothing about the neck.

The best time to treat for removal of the lesion is between attacks, it being located and treated, according to its kind, by methods already de-scribed.   Attention should be given the sternal ends and cartilages of the ribs, and to the intercostal tissues, as well as to the heads of the ribs and the vertebrae.   The scapular muscles should be relaxed (pp. 10, 11), the clavicles raised (p 34), the tissues of the neck thoroughly relaxed (p 20), the spinal column relaxed (p. 8, II; p. 9, III, IV, V), and the ribs raised at their angles.   If the patient finds it difficult to take a full breath raising or correcting the fifth rib will sometimes give relief.   Pressure upon the phre-nic nerve aids the work by relaxing the diaphragm, which is sometimes ele-vated (p. 16, VIII.)

Treatment once a week or ten days is often enough in most cases. Fre-quent treatment may undo the results accomplished and keep up constant irritation.   Many severe cases have been cured by a few treatments at long intervals, or by a single treatment.

Under this course of treatment the patient usually feels relief at once. As a rule the spasms and the various attendant symptoms terminate abruptly.

Care of patient should include the wearing of loose clothing, living out of doors in pure air if possible, or in large, well ventilated rooms.   The di-et should be light and easily digested to avoid danger of stomach reflexes, and the patient should avoid dust and other exciting causes.

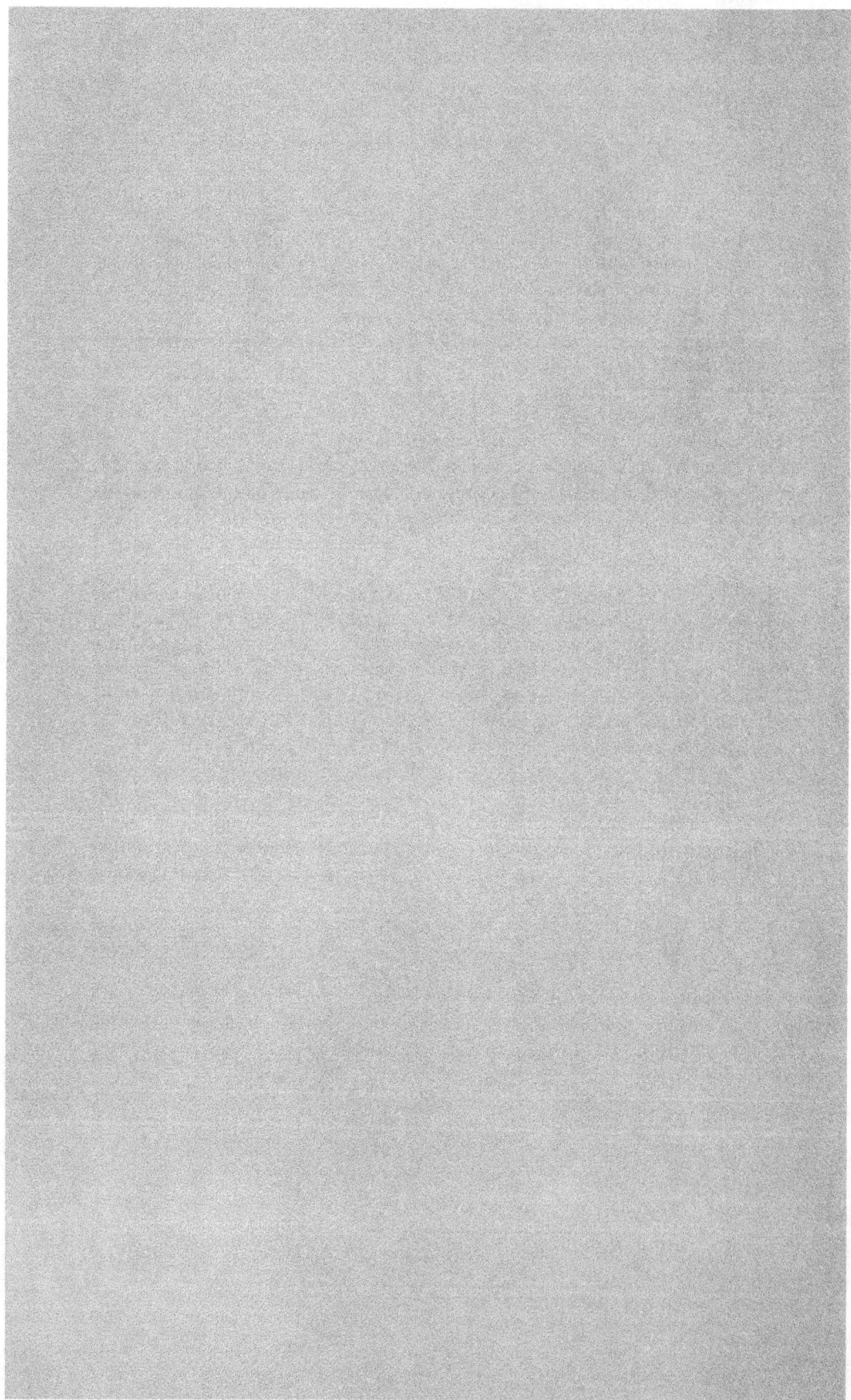

BRONCHITIS.

DEFINITION: Bronchitis is an acute or chronic inflammation of the mucous membrane of the large and middle sized air tubes. It is attended by increased secretions and cough, and is caused by a vaso-motor disturbance of the vessels of those membranes due to specific lesions in the upper spinal, anterior and posterior thoracic, and cervical regions. These lesions may be bony displacements, muscular contractures, ligamentous derangement, etc.

CAUSE: These various specific lesions cause the condition by obstructing peripheral nerves or centers connecting with the vaso-motor innervation of the bronchi. They usually occur high up in the thorax, and in the neck, in close relation to the vaso-motor areas for the bronchi.

Lesions found causing bronchitis are as follows: (1) Luxation of atlas and axis, depression of hyoid bone, lowering of upper eight ribs, congestion of spinal muscles. (2) Third cervical vertebra anterior, muscular tension from the second to the sixth dorsal vertebra, second left rib much depressed. (3) Fourth dorsal vertebra lateral. (4) Luxation of clavicle and first rib anteriorly. (5) Anterior and posterior intercostal spaces as low as the fourth or fifth either changed by misplacement of rib or the seat of irritation to the intercostal structures by contracture. (6) Lesion to the vagus nerve by cervical luxation and contracture, also luxation of the four upper dorsal vertebrae. (7) Luxation of the first, second and third ribs. (8) Displacement of the anterior ends of the first, second and third ribs, and derangement of these cartilages. (9) Bilateral contracture of cervical and spinal muscles as low as the sixth dorsal. (10) Second to fourth dorsal vertebrae lateral. (11) Luxation between manubrium and gladiolus of the sternum.

The *anatomical relations* between these lesions and the seat of the disease are clear. While generally located higher than in the case of asthma, they still fall within the vaso-motor area to the lungs. As to lesion of the atlas, axis, and other cervical tissues, in relation to the vagus and cervical sympathetics, as well as of the upper dorsal vertebrae, ribs, and muscles to the vaso-motor innervation of the bronchi, the same remarks apply as in case of asthma, q. v. Noting from the above lesions that they, being higher, are more concentrated upon the vaso-motor centers of the bronchi, (2nd, 3rd, 4th dorsal), may explain in part the reason for a more intense vaso-motor effect necessary to produce the inflammation of the membranes. Luxations of the clavicle and first rib anteriorly are anatomically related to the disease as causing contracture of the anterior deep cervical tissues and thus obstructing both phrenic and pneumogastric nerves, concerned in innervation of the lungs, retarding the circulation in the cervical vessels, and collaterally obstructing circulation in the lungs. The general dilatation of the air tubes, often seen in chronic cases, is likely caused by those lesions especially affecting the vagus, which innervates the involuntary muscles regulating the calibre of the bronchi. Lessened action of the nerve allows a dilatation of the tubes through loss of tonicity of those muscle fibres. The same explanation probably accounts for local thinning and dilatation of the walls of the tubes.

Osler's statement that the cause of the disease is probably microbic is a confession that the real cause is not known. We hold the true cause to be anatomical lesions as described. The fact that the disease is often a sequel of catching cold is suggestive from an osteopathic view point. The contraction of muscles and tissues from exposure may be sufficient lesion, or may produce actual bony luxations by drawing parts out of place. The further fact that the subjects of spinal curvature are prone to the disease is a confirmation of the osteopathic idea of making bony lesions the cause.

The PROGNOSIS is good for both acute and chronic cases. Many of the latter are cured in a comparatively short time, varying usually from one month or less to three months. In the former the first treatment gives great relief, and, if the case is seen early enough, may abort the attack. A few treatments usually start the patient well on the way to recovery, and as a rule he is well in about one half of the time these cases usually run, which is stated to be two or two and a half weeks.

In the TREATMENT of the case the specific lesions should be at once sought and treated. Often relief can be given only in this way. A thorough treatment should be given the spine, thorax and neck to relax all contracted tissues. Easing of the tension in this way gives great relief, as the constriction of the chest and neck causes much of the comfort from which the patient suffers. This is aided by raising all the   T   tment of the neck corrects the vagus and aids in dispelling th. inflammation by its participation in the vaso-motor control. In the same way relaxation of all the tissues of the dorsal region about the second, third, and fourth vertebrae particularly, also correction of these vertebrae themselves, tends to the same end. The clavicle should be raised and the first rib lowered to free irritation to the phrenic, vagus, and cervical vessels. Thorough treatment of the spine from the second to the seventh dorsal vertebra (vaso-motor area) aids in equalizing bronchial circulation, the work on the left side as low as the sixth aiding this result by strengthening the pulse beat. This initial portion of the treatment should be brisk and energetic enough to arouse good reaction. It relieves the patient at once of the constriction, langor, and aching pain in the back. It frees the lungs and starts perspiration.

The patient should be laid on his back and the upper anterior ribs, cartilages and intercostal structures thoroughly treated. Strong manipulation of the tissues upon the anterior chest and along the sternum reddens them and acts as a mustard plaster would. These treatments, together with treatment directly along the trachea in the neck will relieve the cough The pain along the sternum is relieved by raising the ribs and by the above treatments along the anterior chest. The fever is taken down by the equalization of circulation wrought by the general treatment, and by pressure in the superior cervical region. The blood flow may be diverted from the bronchi to the abdomen by a slow, deep, inhibitive treatment over it, including pressure over the solar and hypgastric plexuses. By the process of raising the ribs and treating the spine the engorged azygós major vein is emptied. The restoration of free thoracic play by these treatments is an important consideration in the eqalizing of the circulation throughout the lungs.

An acute case should be treated daily at least once, and oftener in case of need. One thorough general treatment daily may be sufficient of the kind. Some special treatment being given for cough or fever at other times. In chronic cases the treatment should be given two or three times a week. In case of local or general dilatation of the bronchi, and in the thinning of the walls, close attention to the vagus nerve should be given for reasons already explained.

Good care should be taken of the paient, particularly as to guarding against exposure which may lead to complications. Treatment should be given bowels and kidneys to keep them active.

HAY-FEVER.

DEFINITION:—Hay-Fever or Autumnal Catarrh, is a disease of the upper respiratory tract, styled by some writers a form of asthma. It is caused by specific lesions in the upper dorsal, thoracic and cervical regions, which deteriorate the vitality of the membranes of this tract and lay them liable to the effect of certain irritants, such as the pollen of various plants, leading to an inflammatory or catarrhal condition.

LESIONS:—The anatomical causes for this condition are, from the osteopathic point of view, held to be derangements, in the regions mentioned, of bones or other tissues, which act as lesions upon the motor, vaso-motor and sensory innervation, also upon the blood-vessels of the upper respiratory tract.

In one case, complicated with asthma and bronchitis, the scaleni, sterno-mastoid, and anterior and posterior thoracic muscles were contractured. In another, lesions were found affecting the inferior cervical and upper thoracic regions.

In other cases lesions were found as follows: Right fifth rib; contracture of muscles from the 1st to 10th dorsal vertebra, with ribs in this region drawn down; second cervical vertebra to the right and posterior; second cervical vertebra right, cervical muscles contractured, upper three or four dorsal vertebra to the right. In addition to these, lesions of the atlas, of the phrenic nerve, of the clavicles and upper three ribs (especially the first) and of the dorsal vertebrae as far as the fifth are all found.

The fact that this disease is often found complicated with asthma and bronchitis is readily explained by noting that lesions for all of these conditions occur at the same area of the spine. In all, as well, vaso-motor lesion seems a more potent cause than motor lesion. In the case of hay-fever, as with the other two, upper cervical lesion is less important than lower cervical lesion. The latter kind, with those affecting the first few dorsal vertebrae, the clavicle, and the first and second ribs, are always expected in cases of hay-fever. Purely muscular lesions are relatively less important than other kinds, as they are more likely to be secondary lesions.

The *anatomical relation* of lesion to disease in this case seems clear. The lesions mentioned affect the vagus, cervical sympathetic, and vaso-motor nerves as already explained. They also affect the fifth cranial nerve through the cervical sympathetic, including the superior cervical ganglion. This is the nerve which causes the swollen and painful face, the running eyes and nose, and the sneezing, all of which are so noticeable in hay-fever.

The fifth nerve and the vagus are intimately related in function, both of the respiratory and of the digestive tract, and are closely connected by the floor of the fourth ventrical, the superior cervical ganglia, and the cervical sympathetic. Lesions to the vagus in the region of the clavicle and first rib, to the sympathetic in the cervical region, and in the upper thoracic region of the spine, may affect one or both of these nerves. According to Howell's American Text Book of Physiology, vaso-dilator fibres for the face and mouth leave the cord at the 2d to 5th dorsal, pass up the cervical sympathetic to the superior cervical ganglion, thence to the Gasserian ganglion of the fifth and to the regions mentioned. Thus a low lesion, affecting nerves which ascend to supply the parts, may be the sufficient cause of hay-fever. At the same time the close association of this disease with asthma is shown, since the vaso-motors to the lungs occupy this same region of the upper thoracic spine·

While the common form of irritant producing the attack is supposed to be dust or pollen in the atmosphere, the fact that emotional excitement, a deflected nasal septum, the presence of a nasal polypus, hypertrophied mucous membranes, etc., may produce attacks, shows that there are other causes, some of them anatomical, accounting for an irritable nasal mucous membrane or acting as an irritant upon it. It is as reasonable for an Osteopath to maintain that lesions acting as obstructions to natural nerve and blood supply to these membranes, weakens them and lays them liable to the action of various irritants, thus being the real cause of the disease. Immunity from attack in certain climates or altitudes is but alleviation. The patient has gone away from the special irritant which produces the attack in him. The real causes of the disease still exist, and it generally returns upon his again exposing himself to the same irritant. Although a patient is more liable to attacks in rural districts, more city people contract the disease, showing that a locality in which much pollen occurs has nothing to do, *per se*, with the matter. Osler states that three elements are necessary to the production of the disease; "a nervous constitution, an irritable nasal mucosa, and the stimulus." Yet nervous people, with colds or catarrhal in-. flammation of the nasal membranes, may be with impunity in districts filled with the common irritants which excite attacks in hay-fever subjects. Evidently some further etiological factor is necessary, and is found in the specific anatomical abnormality pointed out by the Osteopath, the removal of which has, in great numbers of cases, cured the disease. The most severe cases yield quickly, often, upon the removal of the specific lesion. The length of standing of the case seems to have but little relation to the length of time necessary to cure. A case of fourteen years' standing was cured in three weeks; one of twenty-four years, in three months; one of five years in one and one half months. This rehersal might detail great numbers of cases, but the few mentioned illustrate the whole matter, In view of these facts it seems incontrovertible that the specific lesions found by the Osteopath, and held by him to be the cause of disease, are the actual causes of the disease.

The *diagnosis* of this condition is easily made according to the manifestations of the disease described in standard medical texts.

The PROGNOSIS, under osteopathic treatment, is good. A large percentage of the cases are cured. The most severe and oldest cases may be safely encouraged to take the treatment. Of medical prognosis in hay-fever, Anders says that permanent cure is a rare event.

THE EXAMINATION AND TREATMENT, made by methods already given, (See Part I) consist in the location and removal of the particular anatomical derangement that is causing the condition. The removal of lesion is the first consideration. It may, occurring in the fegion described, be any one of the mal-adjustments of tissue considered in the general chapters relative to the examination and treatment of the parts. An immediate effort should be made for its removal. In addition special treatment is given to alleviate the condition. All the upper spinal, thoracic and neck muscles, and deep tissues should be thoroughly relaxed for freedom of circulation and to release tension upon nerves. The ribs and clavicles, apart from correction of displacement, should be raised. Attention should be given to releasing and toning the vagus nerve, and the vaso-motor nerves from the 2d to the 7th dorsal. For the lachrymation, itching of the eyes, swelling and pain in the face, and rhinorrhœa, special treatment should be given the fifth nerve. This may be aided by deep manipulation and pressure in the sub-occipital fossae for the superior cervical ganglion, but is done especially by relaxation and quiet, deep inhibitive treatment to the facial branches of the fifth nerve (p. 23). Treatment is given along the sides of the nose (p. 23) to free its blood-vessels, nerves, and to reduce the swelling and irritation in the mucous membranes. Strong pressure is made with the palm upon the forehead (p. 23) to open the nostrils. Cervical treatment, inhibition at the superior cervical region, and opening the mouth against resistance (II, Chap IV), all relieve the congested circulation about the head and face and give much relief.

For the sneezing one may make inhibition of the phrenic nerve (p 16, VIII), may press upon the palatine branches of the fifth nerve where they run over the hard palate, or may grasp the head as in (4) p. 21, and raise it from the spine.

Treatment is ordinarily given three times per week. The patient should be kept from exposure to the particular irritant that excites his attacks.

PNEUMONIA.

DEFINITION: Lobar Pneumonia, or Lung Fever is an acute inflammation of the parenchyma of the lungs caused by specific lesions; bony, muscular, or ligamentous, in the upper spinal, thoracic, and cervical regions. In other forms of pneumonia the same lesions are found. Lobular or Catarrhal Pneumonia is an inflammation of the capillary air tubes, which extends also to the lung tissue proper. Chronic Interstitial Pneumonia is characterized by increase of the interstitial connective tissues.

CAUSES: Anatomical lesion in the form of displaced bony parts, ligaments, etc., and of contractured or tensed muscles and other soft tissues are found affecting the spine as low as the eighth or ninth dorsal; the ribs in the corresponding region, but more generally the 1st, 2d, 3d, 4th and 5th; the intercostal tissues, including nerves and vessels; the cervical vertebrae and tissues, the clavicle and first rib. More specifically, lesions have been found affecting the 2d to 5th dorsal vertebrae; contracture of intercostal, cervical and spinal muscles; thoracic muscles; 4th and 5th ribs; 8th and 9th ribs; the vaso-motor area, the 2d to 7th dorsal; neck lesions to the vagi; the recurrent laryngeal nerves at the 1st and 2d ribs.

The *anatomical relations* of such lesions to the lungs have been explained. It is to be noted that the neck lesions assume greater importance in these cases than in asthama or bronchitis, though there is considerable concentration of lesion about the portion of the spine in which is located the most important vaso-motor area for the lungs, the region as low as the fourth dorsal. In regard to neck lesion, important considerations are pointed out by McConnell in regard to the vagi and the recurrent laryngeal nerves. Such obstructions to the vagi, which are motor nerves to the lung, cause loss of motor power in them and favor the stasis and engorgement present. Obstruction to the recurrent laryngeal nerves by luxation of the 1st and 2d rib, or by engorgement of the aorta or sub-clavian artery where they are in relation to them, causes catarrhal inflammation of the air tubes. Lesions of the 8th and 9th ribs, affecting fibres to the lower lobes of the lungs, are more usual in cases in which the disease occurs in the lower lung.

The fact that more men than women are attacked by the disease; that a debilitated system is more susceptible; that exposure, winter season, and trauma are exciting causes, favors the theory that such anatomical lesions cause the disease. The result may be caused directly by them, or they may make the anatomical weak points that lead to deterioration of the lung tissues and lay them liable to invasion. The specific microbes found in such cases could not live and grow in tissues whose vitality had not been weakened by such causes.

If the case be seen before it has passed the stage of engorgement, the fever may be gotten under control at once, and a few treatments may abort the case. This is the experience of our practitioners, although Osler says that the disease can neither be aborted nor cut short by any means (medical) at command. The means at the Osteopath's command to control vasomotor action are sufficient to relieve the engorgement. In the stages of red and gray hepatization it is natural that slower results must be expected as the treatment has more work to accomplish. Yet vaso-motor correction must lessen the inflammatory process, allow of less solidification, and hasten the process of resolution.

In the first stage there is better opportunity to correct the specific lesion, as the patient's strength will allow of such treatment. The work is also aided by the fact that the alveoli are still open, and lung action, stimulated by treatment, may become a valuable aid in dispelling the engorgement. In view of these facts, and as experience shows, every symptom of the case can be lessened because the pathological processes are modified. Less poison is generated and the patient's general condition remains better. In one case the treatment was applied in the first stage; the fever was under control from the first and the temperature became normal in three days. In another it disappeared in four days; in another in five days. A case in which the temperature was 104½ degrees when first seen showed three degrees less fever the next morning. It had been treated in the evening. In a case in which the temperature was 103 degrees, the temperature, pulse, and respiration became normal in five days. It is true that cases vary naturally, yet in view of the fact that Osler states that the fever persists for from five to ten days, and that after its fastigium is reached (usually within a few hours) it remains remarkably constant, it is evident that osteopathic work is successful to a marked degree in bettering the case.

The *diagnosis* is made according to directions given in standard texts, and by the location of specific lesions.

The *prognosis* is good under osteopathic treatment.

EXAMINATION AND TREATMENT for the location and removal of lesion are made according to methods considered in Part I. In beginning the treatment, as the patient finds it easy to lie on the sound side, the muscles and deep tissues are gently but thoroughly relaxed along the length of the spine, particularly upon the affected side. This starts vaso-motion and brings a sense of relief from the constriction that so distresses the patient. During this treatment upon the side, treatment is given the centers for bowels, kidneys, and superficial fascia (2d dorsal and 5th lumbar) to rouse them to action and to aid in the elimination of poison from the system.

This initial treatment has thus prepared for the more specific treatment for the fever, itself being part of the process. The next step consists in turning the patient gently upon his back and thoroughly relaxing the cervical tissues, the tissues behind the clavicle and first rib, raising the clavicle and depressing the first rib, after relaxation of the scaleni muscles. Treatment should also be applied to the course of the vagi, and to the recurrent laryngeal nerves at the lower inner parts of the sterno-mastoid muscles. In these ways motor power to the lungs is increased, and vaso-motion is corrected. The treatment for fever is now completed by steady pressure in the sub-occipital fossae in the usual way. The fever is not likely to go down at once, but is gradually reduced after the treatment, for some hours. This is because of the freedom given to the vaso-motors in the course of the treatment, and to the gradual change now being wrought in the patient's system by the recuperated forces.

The treatment for fever may be aided by the deep inhibitive treatment to the abdomen, before described, to dilate the immense abdominal veins and aid in calling away the blood from the engorged lung.

Further treatment is given the lungs, with the patient on the back, by gently elevating the ribs from the second to the seventh on both sides. This stimulates the vaso-motor centers to the lungs. Elevation of all the ribs gives much relief from tension, and is the specific method of relieving the pain in the side.

Stimulation of the accelerators of the heart, second to fifth dorsal on the left side, aids in circulation through the lungs, and stimulates the heart against failure.

For the cough, the treatment should be close and deep along the trachea from the larnyx to the root of the neck, also relaxation of the anterior tissues of the chest, including the upper intercostal tissues. The middle and inferior cervical regions should be treated for the lymphatics to the lungs. (McConnell.)

The amount and strength of the treatment must be regulated by the patient's condition. Strong treatments are not allowed on account of weakness. The general treatment should be given, thoroughly but gently, once a day at least. The patient should be seen three or four times per day, but the whole treatment outlined need not be given each time. A little treatment for the fever, to release tension over the lungs, to relieve pain in the side, etc., may be enough at a time.

Hygienic precautions, the use of hot applications, foot baths, rectal injections, etc., may be employed according to direction of the standard texts, as necessary. The patient should have plenty of water to drink, and should be kept upon a liquid diet.

ACUTE NASAL CATARRH, OR CORYZA, AND COLDS.

DEFINITION:—Acute Nasal Catarrh is an inflammation of the nasal mucous membranes, accompanied by an increased secretion of mucous and by various general symptoms, and is caused by specific lesions, in the cervical region chiefly, which may be secondary to contractures of muscles and soft tissues by exposure. After repeated attacks the disease becomes *chronic*, upon account of the confirmed condition of the lesions.

A "cold in the head" is an acute attack of this disease. Yet "colds" may settle in any part of the body, as a rule, in "the weakest part," and then probably assumes the form of congestion instead of inflammation as in the case of coryza. Its manifestations are various, one of the chief ones being the disturbed vaso-motor reflexes of the body. These weak places liable to such congestion are commouly due to lesion of the part, which acts to deteriorate its vitality and lessen its resistance power.

CAUSES:—The specific *lesions* causiug such disease are, as a rule, high up in the cervical region, effecting especially the 1st to 3d cervical vertebrae, but they may occur as low as the sixth dorsal. One of the chief forms of lesion is that of contracture of the cervical muscles and deep soft tissues. These contractures, due primarily to exposure, gradually act to warp, or draw, the cervical vertebrae and intervertebral discs out of shape and out of their normal anatomical relations. The result is obstruction to blood and nerve supply, causing chronic catarrh. The deeper anatomical lesions due to contracture, and to other causes as well, produce catarrh, and not some other disease, because of affecting certain areas of nerve connections and certain centers. Thus lesion of the upper three cervical vertebrae act upon the superior cervical ganglion, in ways already discussed, and disturb the fifth nerve through its very intimate connections with the ganglion in question. In the same way, lesion to the inferior cervical or upper dorsal bony parts may affect those sympathetic fibers (or the area of the cord giving origin to them) which ascend in the cervical sympathetic chain, finally to reach the fifth nerve, which thus supplies secretory fibers to the parts in question. The very numerous vaso-motor, secretory and trophic fibers for all parts of the head and face; for salivary glands, eye, ear, tongue, face, mouth, etc., etc., passing to their points of distribution through various of the cranial nerves, quite generally arise in the upper dorsal and cervical cord, having also numerous connections with the cervical sympathetics. This matter has been fully discussed in another place.* This explains the importauce of cervical and upper dorsal lesions. Thus lesions low down act upon the ascending fibers of nerve supply and affect a part much above, as in the case of dorsal lesion here.

The fifth nerve bears special mention in these cases as the one concerned in the headache, lachrymation, sneezing, secretion of mucous, and inflammation of membranes. This nerve is also in part concerned in the loss or alteration of the functions of taste and smell, caused by pressure of the injected membranes upon the fine nerve terminals.

The PROGNOSIS is good for all forms of the disease. In acute cases it is particularly so, as one or a few treatments usually end the symptoms. In chronic catarrh good results are generally easily attained, and many times a cure is effected. Unfavorable climates do much to prevent cure as the patient is constantly exposed.

The EXAMINATION AND TREATMENT for the *specific lesion* is made according to directions in Chaps. I to VII. The specific lesion should be treated, and removed at once if possible. This applies to both acute and chronic cases. In acute cases one of the first steps is to relax all the upper dorsal and cervical tissues. A thorough spinal treatment tones all the vaso-constrictors (2d dorsal to 2d lumbar), and all the vaso-dilators (all along the spine), thus aiding to equalize circulation, and reduce congestion of parts concerned.

This effect is aided in an important way by raising all the ribs, and particularly treating all the 2d to 7th dorsal region on both sides, in this way increasing the activities of heart and lungs. The anterior thoracic region is treated to relax tissues and replace ribs; the clavicle is raised, and separated from the first rib to relax the deep anterior cervical tissues, free circulation through the carotid arteries and jugiar veins, and to free the pneumogastric nerves. All the cervical muscles are thoroughly relaxed, the ligaments released by deep treatments, and the vertebrae of the whole region manipulated. This frees the connections of the sympathetics, the venous flow from the head, and tones vaso-motion in the affected parts. It is an important step in remedying the congestion of the parts of the head. Inhibitive treatment should be given the superior cervical ganglion to dilate blood-vessels and allow the congestion to be swept out. The superior and inferior hyoid muscles are relaxed, and the work is carried down along the trachea to the root of the neck. The mouth is opened against resistance; the tissues beneath the angles of the jaws are relaxed. This releases the internal jugular veins, stimulates circulation through the carotid arteries, and corrects circulation.

Particular attention is devoted to the treatment of the fifth nerve for reasons already given. It is reached at points upon the face already described, and all the tissues over them are relaxed. Treatment of this nerve thus directly is a most important adjunct to that given its sympathetic connections. It is most important as a means of relieving the inflammation, secretion, lachrymation, and stopping of the nostrils. Manipulation along the sides of the nose frees the nasal ducts and relieves the congestion; strong pressure upon the root of the nose and upon the forehead frees the nostrils; tapping over the frontal sinus relieves congestion and pain in it. The headache is relieved by the treatment in the general cervical, superior cervical, and frontal regions; the cough is relieved by the treatment along the trachea; the chilly feeling by the brisk spinal treatment.   The soft palate may be treated by placing the finger gently upon it and sweeping it laterally across.   This treatment may be carried well up toward the opening of the eustachian tube.   The congestion of these parts is thus relieved.

The lungs must be kept well treated to prevent the cold from settling upon them.   The bowels and kidneys are treated to keep their action free. The treatment about the lower jaw and to the carotid arteries is efficient in reaching the eustachian tube, and in loosening the secretions that sometimes occlude it.

In chronic cases the treatment is devoted more particularly to the removal of the specific lesion, and the building up of the blood supply to the nasal membranes.   As these are often atrophied or hypertrophied a long course of treatment is generally necessary to their rehabliation.   The principal treatment is directed to the cervical tissues, where chronic contracture of the muscles exists

Daily treatments in severe acute cases, and three per week in chronic cases, are usually sufficient.

The patient should take care not to expose himself, but, on the other hand, should not keep the body tender and susceptible by dressing too warmly, sleeping under too many covers, or living in overheated quarters. One may contract a cold by going suddenly from an extremely hot to a very cold atmosphere, or *vice versa*.

*See "Principles of Osteopathy" Lectures XVI-XVIII.

EPISTAXIS,

DEFINITION:—Epistaxis is the term used to designate hemorrhage from the nose.   It is found in serious form in some people.   It may be caused by accident, as in fracture of the skull, or by local irritation, such as picking at the nose.   Cervical *lesion*, involving the atlas and the muscles, has been noted.   Other forms of cervical lesion, affecting the superior cervical ganglion or the cervical sympathetic may aid in causing it.

TREATMENT:— Holding of the facial artery where it crosses the inferior maxillary bone, and the nasal artery at the inner canthus, also pressure applied to the carotid arteries, slow the blood current and favor the formation of a clot.   In some cases, friction over the superior cervical region has been sufficient to arouse sufficient vaso-constriction to stop the flow.   The case may be helped by raising the arms high above the head.   It is frequently difficult to stop the hemorrhage at the time, but the treatment applied to the correction of the lesion and to the freedom of circulation through the neck will stop the recurrence of the hemorrhages.   In severe cases it may be necessary to resort to plugging of the posterior nares.   The application of ice or cold water to the superior cervical region, and the use of hot or cold injections into the nostrils are efficient domesiic remedies for the condition.

PLEURISY.

DEFINITION: An acute inflammation of a part or the whole of one or both pleurae, attended by cough and pain in the side, and caused by lesions affecting ribs, thoracic vertebrae intercostal and spinal muscles, nerves, etc.

CAUSES: The important lesions in these cases affect the ribs; cases are rare in which lesions of this kind are not the actual cause of the disease. Other lesions are consequent or subsidiary to rib lesions. They may affect the ribs of either side, as low as the 10th on the left and the 9th on the right, marking the lower limits of the pleurae. Secondary lesions in the cervical region, affecting pneumogastric, phrenic, or sympathetic nerves, concerned in the innervation of the pleurae, may occur. Lesion of the clavicle and first rib, impeding circulation through the subclavian and internal mammary arteries, are important. The cervical lesions mentioned, with lesions of the spinal muscles and dorsal vertebrae, affect the innervation, composed of branches from the pneumogastrics, phrenics, sympathetics, and pulmonary plexuses. Important derangement of circulation are thus caused by lesion to vaso-motors, aiding the process of inflammation, which is the active morbid process in the case. The drawing of spinal muscles, luxations of vertebrae, and the interference with spinal nerves also aid the causation of rib lesions. The latter sort is by far the most efficient one in causing pleurisy because of its relation to the intercostal vessels and nerves. These nerves and vessels all together total a vast area of blood and nerve supply to the pleurae, especially to the parietal portions. The nerves carry vaso-motor and secretory fibres to the parts supplied by them, hence to the pleurae. Hilton points out that the nerves innervating the linings of the body cavities supply also the skin and muscles of the walls of these cavities. This is well instanced in the case of the parietal pleurae, which are supplied by the intercostal nerves, they also supplying the intercostal muscles and the overlying skin. Such being the case, lesion by displacement of ribs, irritating intercostal nerves, disturbs the vaso-motor and secretory processes in the pleurae supplied by the same nerves. Hilton has also pointed out that a joint, the muscles moving the joint, and the skin overlying these muscles, are all supplied by branches of the same nerves. Hence vertebral lesion and lesions affecting the relations of the heads of the ribs may affect the nerves through their articular branches. In this way spinal lesion might be the origin of such disease. But further, since each intercostal nerve is connected by the rami communicantes with the sympathetic system, lesion of these nerves affects the sympathetics. These sympathetics in the dorsal region contain both vaso-dilator and vaso-constrictor fibres; they enter into the formation of the pulmonary plexus, which in part innervates the pleura. Hence intercostal lesion affects vaso-motor control of the parietal pleura directly, and of the visceral pleura indirectly. In another way does intercostal lesion act to set up the inflammatory process of pleurisy. Lesions of the clavicle, deranging circulation through the sub-clavian and internal mammary vessels, and of the other ribs, directly obstructing the intercostal vessels, and indirectly deranging the circulation through related vessels to the 'visceral pleurae, (bronchial, mediastinal, and diaphragmatic vessels) disturb the entire circulation to these parts.

In these ways may all the various lesions described work together to produce inflammation. The affected area is larger or smaller according to the nature and extent of the lesions. Lesion of a single rib has frequently been found responsible for an acute attack of pleurisy, either circumscribed and limited in extent, or spreading to involve cons'derable areas, The same sort of lesion may produce all the various kinds of pleurisy described in medical texts.

According to osteopathic theory, the bacteria present in this disease and ascribed by some writers as its cause,could not live and propogate their poisons in healthy tissues. The presence of the lesions described may weaken the tissues and allow the microbes to gain a foothold. It is significant that exposure to cold and wet, and mechanical injuries cause the disease, as the Osteopath looks for such causes to produce the displacements and other lesions to which he traces the disease

The *diagnosis* is made according to the symptoms and physical signs described in standard medical texts.

The PROGNOSIS is good. Cases generally recover without difficulty. Often all the pain and other manifestations disappear at once upon removal of lesion; the setting of a rib.

THE EXAMINATION AND TREATMENT for the specific lesion are carried on according to directions given for the examination and treatment of those regions. This lesion should be removed as soon as possible, and at once if the condition of the patient will allow. Treatment should be directed to the relaxation of all spinal, intercostal, and cervical tissues, and to the raising of the ribs, for the purpose of removing obstruction from and toning the circulation and innervation of the pleurae. The raising of the ribs and clavicle, including the repair of the particular luxation of ribs that is causing the trouble, are the most important steps. If the case is seen before the inflammation and exudation has progressed far, the process may be more easily stopped, as the necessary point is to gain control of circulation, which may be readily accomplished through nerves and vessels as already explained. In the stage of exudation, where quantities of the exudate occur in the pleural cavities, attention must be given to releasing the tension in parts due to contractures of muscles, etc., to raising the ribs to allow more free play of the lungs, and to the relief of the pain iu the side, and the distressing cough by carefully raising the ribs and manipulating the tissues at the seat of the pain. But the main point at this stage is, by the treatment to the circulation, to hasten the resorption of inflammatory products. This

may be done to a considerable extent.   Great care must be taken in handling the patient on account of the great pain.   By stimulating the process
of absorption, and by keeping the parts free from tension in the tissues,
also by keeping up, carefully, free motion of the ribs and parts, the adhesions of the pleurae, and the retraction of parts likely to occur as a result of
the inflammation, may be avoided.   This is during the convalescence of the
patient, when his condition must be carefully watched.   The point may be
reached in some cases where tapping might be necessary, but if the case is
seen in time the the process may be so controlled as to obviate this difficulty.   In cases of adhesions between the pleurae, if painful they should
be gradually broken up.   This is done in a course of treatment, carefully
giving the parts concerned the extremes of motion of which they are capable.   The process is aided by developing the circulation to in part absorb
the adhesive tissues.   This must frequently be done in the chronic case.
The treatment of such cases consists mainly in restoration of lesion, and in
maintaining free circulation for the absorption of pus, if present.

In treatment of pleurisy, stimulation of heart and lungs, of bowels,
kidneys and superficial fascia, for the removal of poisonous waste, and
attention to the general health of the patient are necessary.   Acute cases
should be kept upon a light, easily digested diet.   Exposure must be prevented.   One thorough treatment daily, with more treatment at times during the day for the relief of pain, etc., will usually be sufficient.   Chronic
cases should be treated three times per week.

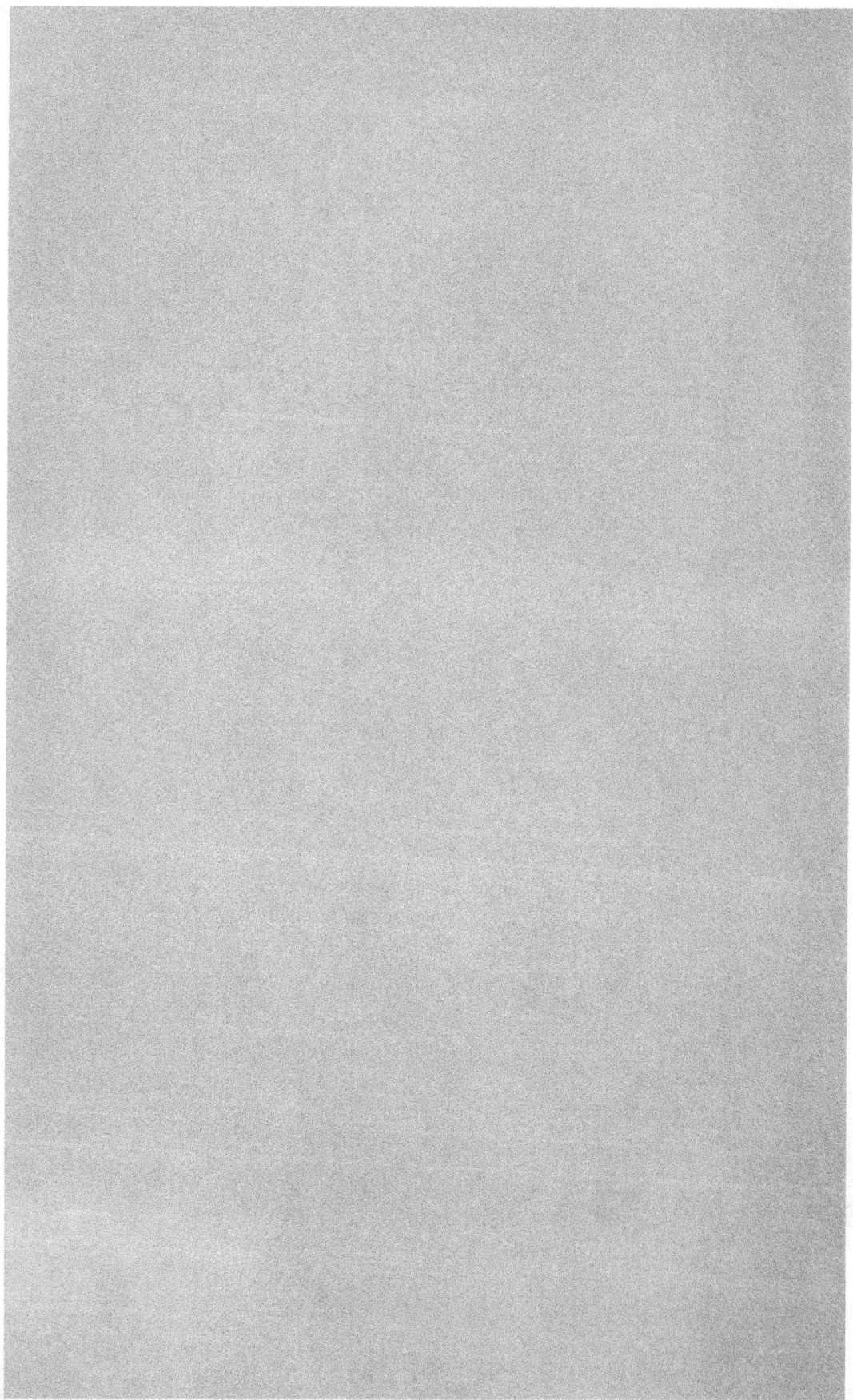

PULMONARY CONSUMPTION.

DEFINITION: Pulmonary Consumption, or Tuberculosis of the Lungs, is a destructive disease of the tissues of the lungs, characterized by the presence of the bacillus tuberculosis, and caused by specific lesions in the upper dorsal and thoracic regions.

CAUSES: "Cases; (1) In a case of "quick consumption," Acute Pneumonic Phthisis, the upper dorsal spine was swerved to the right; the 2nd dorsal vertebra was lateral; the 8th and 9th dorsal vertebrae lateral; the ribs down, narrowing the thoracic cavity. Reported cured in three months' treatment. (2) Second and third ribs luxated; marked lesion between the corresponding vertebrae and the tissues about them very tender. Three months' treatment so benefited the patient that recovery followed. (3) First, second and third left ribs down and in. Reported cured. (4) Left clavicle down; 1st to 8th dorsal vertebrae flat; 8th dorsal to 1st lumbar vertebrae posterior; 2nd right rib tilted; the spine and thorax flat. (5) The 4th dorsal vertebra sore; 3rd to 5th lumbar vertebrae tight and irregular; fifth and sixth left ribs close together; first rib on right luxated; all ribs down and irregular. Case benefited.

Lesions are often found of the 2nd, 3rd, and 4th ribs; of the 5th, 6th, 7th and 8th ribs (A. T. Still); 2nd and 3rd cervical vertebrae usually lateral, and lesions to the middle and inferior cervical sympathetic ganglia affecting the lymphatics of the lungs (McConnell); of the clavicle.

Anatomical relations. In these cases the neck lesion is not generally of prime importance, the dorsal lesion being the particular one, and of this variety, that more especially affecting the upper several ribs. Lesion of the spine, muscles, ligaments, or ribs, as low as the 10th may become the cause of the disease. In very many cases the lesion will be found to involve the second dorsal vertebra or the second rib.

There are important reasons why lesions of ribs lead to pulmonary tuberculosis, and why the flattened thorax, characteristic of the disease, is so closely related to the condition, either as primary lesion causing it, or as a lesion secondary to it. According to the American Text Book of Physiology, stimulation of intercostal nerves causes reflex constriction of pulmonary vessels. The intercostal nerves are all connected directly with the sympathetic system by *rami communicantes*, and the sympathetic vaso-dilator and vaso-constrictor fibres of the system are situated all along the thoracic spinal region. Luxations of ribs and a flattened thorax (dropped ribs) set up irritation in the intercostal nerves, leading to constriction of the pulmonary vessels. A vast area may be affected through the wide distribution of intercostal nerves. Very general, or localized, anemia of lung tissues follows upon pulmonary vascular constriction caused by this over stimulation of the intercostal nerves. This devitalizes the tissues of the lung, and gives a foot-hold to the pathogenic bacteria, held by medical authorities to be the sole cause of tuberculosis.

With regard to the microbic origin of this disease, the Osteopath does not deny the presence of such bacteria in the lung, nor their activity in destruction of lung tissue. He holds that there is necessary a lesion to the lung, in the form of an impediment to proper nerve and blood supply to the lung tissues, weakening them to an extent that allows the bacteria, which cannot grow in healthy tissues, to produce their kind and to form their toxins.

It has already been pointed out that the vaso-motor spinal area for the lungs (2nd to 7th dorsal), and particularly the region of the 2nd, 3rd, and 4th thoracic sympathetic ganglia, is most apt to suffer from lesion in diseases of the lungs. Rib, vertebral, intercostal or spinal muscular lesion, etc., is more likely to cause lung disease in this area than elsewhere. It is a well known fact that the apices of the lungs are most generally the seat of the disease. This fact is readily explained by the fact that upper rib and spinal lesions, most frequent in consumption of the lungs, affect this region of the lung generally, centering upon this important vaso-motor area. The further fact that the apex of the lung is not usually so well developed on account of lazy habits of breathing, makes lesion in this region more important. Anders states that special investigation has shown that the disease does not begin at the tip of the apex, but about one and one-half inches below, near the postero-external border. Posteriorly the first signs are discovered over the lower part of the supra spinous fossa; anteriorly, immediately below the middle of the clavicle, along a line about 1½ inches from the inner ends of the second and third intercostal spaces. The starting point may also be located at the first and second intercostal spaces below the outer third of the clavicle. These points of origin of this disease in the lung are thus in close relation with those upper ribs apparently most often luxated in this disease. In this way the osteopathic view that such lesion causes the disease is supported by the facts.

PROGNOSIS: Except in late and serious stages of the disease, the chances of limiting its progress are good. Some cases may be cured. The prognosis as to recovery, however, must be guarded. In many cases much may be done for the benefit of the patient's general health.

TREATMENT: The first consideration is the removal of the specific lesion causing the trouble. This is accomplished by methods already given. The removal of lesion has frequently been followed by recovery. On the whole a considerable number of cases have been cured. Thorough spinal treatment should be given for the correction and upbuilding of the vaso-motor activities. The spinal muscles and deep tissues should be relaxed, and the ribs should be raised to allow the greatest area of expansion possible. The vaso-motor area for the lungs should receive especial treatment. In all these ways the blood-supply to the lungs is upbuilt. This, next to the removal of lesion, is the main consideration in the treatment of the case. Phagocytic activity is said to constitute the natural power of resistance of of the system to the bascilli. By increasing blood supply to the tissues phagocytic activity is increased, the tissues are strengthened, and the encroachments of the bacteria are limited. As they cannot live and popogate in healthy tissues, and as pure blood is a germicide, the progress of the disease is checked as soon as pure blood and healthy tissue are opposed to to them in equal ratio. Thorough stimulation of the functions of heart and lungs materially aids this process. The very important nerve connections of the lungs, already pointed out in detail, afford the Osteopath the surest means of reaching this result. His is the natural method. Strong lungs remain immure to this disease because healthy tissues will not harbor the microbe. Consumptives have been cured by judicious exercise, fresh air, and careful regimen. In this way the tissues of the lung have been built up, the circulation to it has been increased, and the bacteria have been crowded out by the gain over them of the natural healthy processes thus aroused. Osteopathy removes the impediment to normal activities of the blood and nerve forces that make strong lung tissue. Its method does that which Nature unaided could not do,and further aids Nature to recover from the weakness caused by the disease. No other method would seem more sure of chances of success than this.

The clavicles should be raised, and the pneumogastric, phrenic, and cervical sympathetic nerves should be freed and toned for reasons already explained. Fresh air, judicious exercise, and nutritious diet are indispensable factors in the treatment. Antiseptic precautions in regard to the patient's sputum, linen, etc., should be observed as directed in medical texts. Bowels, kidneys, and skin should be stimulated to full activity. General circulation must be increased.

The *night sweats* generally soon yield to the spinal treatment. The *cough* may be relieved by treatment along the trachea and anterior thorax, but it, as well as the *expectoration, fever, and hemorrhages*, are relieved and checked by the favorable progress of the case. The greatest care must be taken for the patient's general condition and nutrition.

Treatment is given in the ordinary chronic case three times per week. In the acute form it should be given daily.

CONGESTION OF THE LUNGS.

DEFINITION:—A vaso-motor disturbance to the lungs, resulting in engorgement of the blood-vessels, and caused by lesions in the upper dorsal, thoracic, and cervical regions.

CAUSES:—The *lesions* producing this disease may be any of the lesions interfering with the innervation, especially vaso-motor, and with the blood supply to the lungs. These have been described in the discussion of the different diseases of the lungs already considered, q. v. With these lesions present and weakening the circulatory energy in the lungs, some direct exciting cause, such as exposure, over-exertion, and the like, may bring on the attack. In the passive forms of congestion, secondary to enfeebled heart action or to valvular disease, or coming on through stasis of blood due to a long continued dorsal position of the patient, also in the active form of pulmonary congestion, when the trouble may be symptomatic of pneumonia, pleurisy, etc., the lesion must be investigated with regard to the actual disease, and may be but in part responsible directly for this condition.

The Prognosis is good.

The Treatment must be directed at once to the removal of the specific lesion if possible. The main object of the treatment is to give vaso-motor control. As soon as the impeded circulation is released, and activity restored to the innervation of the vessels, further progress of the disease is prevented. As in the first stage of pneumonia the disease was aborted by gaining vaso-motor control of the parts, so here the whole matter rests upon the correction of the circulation. The accelerators of the heart, 2d to 5th dorsal on the left, and the vaso-motors of the lungs, 2d to the 7th dorsal, should be stimulated at once, and the treatment gives immediate relief from the dyspnea. Often the patient is sitting up in the effort to get air, and the practitioner may easily stand behind and thoroughly treat the upper dorsal region, releasing contractured muscles, stimulating the centers mentioned, and raising the ribs. Pressure with the knee upon the back, while the arms are both raised high above the head, expands the chest, draws the air into the lungs, and aids in restoring circulation. This work also aids the process by increasing activity in intercostal vessels and nerves. The latter should be thoroughly treated along the spine, intercostal spaces, and over the chest anteriorly, as stimulation of the intercostal nerves has been shown to cause reflex constriction of the pulmonary vessels. Treatment should be given the pneumogastric nerves, and any cervical lesion to them removed, on account of their participation in the pulmonary plexus. Treatment at the superior cervical region for general vaso-motor effect, and in the abdominal region to call the blood away from the lungs, will aid the case. In cases of hypostatic congestion the patient's position in bed must be changed so as to drain the blood from the parts affected, usually the postero-inferior.

Patients are usually relieved immediately upon treatment. The dyspnea being most easily relieved. The cough and bloody expectoration gradually subside with the betterment of the case, which quickly yields to treatment.

LARYNGITIS.

DEFINITION:—An acute inflammation of the mucous membrane lining the larynx. In acute and chronic catarrhal forms the inflammation is a catarrhal condition. In the spasmodic form (laryngismus stridulus), the condition is a nervous one. In the edematous form the inflammation is accompanied by exudation and infiltration of the tissues.

CAUSES:—Lesions to the innervation and blood-supply of the larynx are present. The chief ones are to the pneumogastrics and cervical sympathetics, and occur at the atlas, axis and third cervical vertebra, where they affect the superior cervical ganglion, and through it the nerves in question. Cervical lesion may also affect the other cervical sympathetics concerned in the innervation of the larynx. These lesions affect circulation of the larynx through the innervation. Direct lesion to the blood vessels may occur at the clavicle and first rib, at the deep anterior cervical tissues, and in the muscles along the neck anteriorly and about the throat. They may obstruct the circulation in the carotid arteries and the thyroid axis, or may impede the venous return through the small veins and the innominates and internal jugulars. Local weakness of the glottis, or of the laryngeal muscles, may occur primarily or secondary to other lesion. The edematous form is especially likely to be caused by obstruction to the internal jugular veins. Traumatism may be the sole cause, or cold, exposure, and irritation, etc , may act secondarily to cervical lesion to cause the disease.

The PROGNOSIS is good. Immediate relief is obtained from the treatment, and recovery soon follows.

In dangerous cases of edematous laryngitis great care must be taken. Tracheotomy may become necessary in some cases, but ordinarily this can be avoided by the treatment if the case be seen in time.

The TREATMENT must be directed as far as possible to the immediate removal of the specific lesion. This releases circulation and nerve supply as shown above. The tissues of the neck, particularly of the throat, must be thoroughly relaxed; the clavicle is raised, and the deep anterior muscles and tissues of the root of the neck are treated. These treatments free the circulation in the vessels as shown above. The circulation in the carotids is further aided by opening the mouth against resistance. The vagi are treated along the course of the sterno-mastoid muscle, and at the superior cervical region. Its superior laryngeal branch is treated behind the superior cornua of the thyroid cartilage. Its recurrent laryngeal branch is reached at the inner side of the lower portion of the sterno-mastoid muscle at about the level of the cricoid cartilage.

Deep treatment is made along the course of the larynx and trachea, from the hyoid bone and muscles to the root of the neck. Care must be taken to apply the fingers of the operating hand close along the sides of the trachea. This is excellent treatment for the huskiness and the spasm. The latter, however, is apt to depend upon some special lesion. In spasmodic laryngitis the epiglottis is sometimes caught in the rima, and must be released by introducing the index finger into the throat. Treatment of the phrenics and the diaphragm aid in lessening the spasm by quieting the action of the diaphragm. A warm bath is recommended to break up the spasm.

The vagi and cervical sympathetics are treated at the superior cervical region and along the posterior region.

Cases of aphonia, due to the changes in the vocal cords, or to weakness of the epiglottis, may be cured by this treatment.

TONSILLITIS.

DEFINITION:—Tonsillitis is an inflammation of the tonsils, accompanied by enlargement of the gland, fever and various constitutional symptoms. It is caused by lesions in the cervical region.

CAUSES: The lesion in the case may affect the general cervical region, but usually occurs high up, affecting the atlas, axis, or third vertebra. The lower vertebrae are often found luxated, and contracture of the posterior and lateral cervical tissues often acts as the primary lesion. Contracture of the upper hyoid muscles is always present, frequently as secondary lesion. Luxation of the clavicle and first rib, and tension in the deep anterior cervical tissues about them are sometimes found.

Lesions of the atlas, axis, and third vertebra probably act through affecting the fifth nerve through its connections with the superior cervical ganglion. Lesions of the lower cervical vertebrae, and or the posterior muscles of the throat, of the deep anterior cervical tissues, and of the first rib and clavicle have an important effect by obstructing the circulation through the carotid arteries and the external jugular vein.

In persons subject to tonsillitis through the presence of these specific lesions, acute attacks are frequently aroused by exposure to cold and wet, by bad hygenic surroundings, and by various nervous disturbances.

The PROGNSIS is good in the acute follicular and acute suppurative forms and in ordinary chronic enlargement of the glands. One or a few treatments may cure the case in the acute forms. Great relief is almost invariably given immediately by the treatment. The chronic enlargement requires long continued treatment. In the chronic form, described also as naso-pharyngeal obstruction, or mouth breathing, the prognosis for cure is not good. Much relief can be given, and long continued treatment aids the retarded mental and bodily development.

In the TREATMENT of acute tonsillitis, due attention must be given the general constitutional condition. Liver, bowels, kidneys and skin must be kept active. Thorough spinal treatment should be given for tonic effect. The treatment should be directed at once to the reduction of the spinal lesion. Treatment is given the upper three cervical vertebrae to affect the superior cergical ganglion. All the muscles and tissues of the neck are gently but thoroughly relaxed. Careful treatment is made over the supra-hyoid muscles and over the region of the tonsils. The extreme tenderness will allow of but gentle treatment, but by exercising care in applying the treatment at first, a deep and thorough treatment may be given after pre-liminary relaxation of the tissues. All the cervical vertebrae and posterior tissues should be thoroughly treated for the sympathetic connections of the fifth, (XIII, p. 21.) The treatment over the throat as described is to relieve the inflammation by freeing the circulation in the substance of the gland and in the carotid and external jugular veins. As the large arterial supply is from branches of the external carotids, particular treatment is made along them by relaxing the muscles and tissues over them and by open-ing the mouth against resistance as already described. This work over the throat is carried well down to the root of the neck over the carotid arteries and external jugular veins.

Manipulation over the tonsil aids the flow of the blood through the tonsillar plexus of veins into the external jugular. This vein is freed by raising the clavicle and relaxing the anterior cervical tissues about it and the first rib. In the same way the carotid artery is stimulated in action. Circulation in the substance of the gland is aided by internal treatment in the throat, made by sweeping and pressing the index finger over the gland, fauces and surrounding tissues. This treatment gives much relief. All the treatment directed to the throat and anterior cervical region is the most important part of the treatment. The large blood supply of the gland, and our ability to reach it directly more than through the innervation, make this part of the treatment important. It is readily efficient. Treatment to the first rib and over the upper anterior chest aids circulation.

The tonsils should be kept free from accumulations of secretions, which persist in chronic cases. The fever is treated in the usual way, being af-fected by the superior cervical and spinal work. The spinal and general treatment relieves the chilly feelings, aches, etc. The neck and throat treatments relieve the sore throat. Careful treatment will prevent suppura-tion in the suppurative form. The general tonic treatment must be persist-ent in these cases because of the severe general symptoms.

Acute cases should be treated daily one or more times as necessary. A few treatments are generally sufficient. The chronic enlargements (hyper-trophy) and the chronic naso-pharyngeal obstruction should be treated three times per week. In the latter local treatment upon the gland from within the throat is very helpful. Long continued treatment should be urged in all chronic cases to prevent, or to aid, retarded mental and physical development.

PAROTITIS.

DEFINITION:—Parotitis or, mumps is an acute inflammation of the parotid glands.

CAUSES:—The lesions in such cases affect the upper cervical region, mainly the atlas, axis and third vertebra. Other cervical vertebrae may be luxated, and the cervical muscles are contractured. The deep anterior cervical tissues may be tensed, and the clavicle luxated. Secondary contracture occurs in the muscles and tissues over the region of the gland.

Lesions of the upper three cervical vertebrae and to the tissues affect the superior cervical ganglion, and thus the carotid plexus through its ascending branch; the fifth nerve through this ganglion and through its sympathetic connections, and thus its auriculo-temporal branch; the second cervical nerve, and thus its auricular branch; while lesions to the muscles in this region may affect the facial nerve directly, and these and other lesions affect it through the sympathetic connections. Contraction of the tissues over the course of the external carotid arteries and the external jugular veins affect the flow of the blood to and from the gland. Luxation of the clavicle and its tissues affects the external jugular vein.

The PROGNOSIS is good. Treatment is rapidly effective and the course of the disease is shortened from the usual course, seven to ten days, to three or four days. Some cases may become obstinate and require longer treatment.

The TREATMENT is in most particulars identical with that given for tonsillitis, q. v., the lesions to vertebrae, tissues, and clavicle, etc., being practically the same.

The tissues over and about the gland may be more readily relaxed as the condition is less painful. The swelling is more persistent, and requires more treatment. The fever is treated as before, and a thorough spinal and general treatment is given for the constitutional symptoms. This should include treatment to the blood and nerve supply of the breasts, ovaries, and testacles to prevent metastasis. This point must not be neglected, as the inflammation may be driven by the treatment to these parts. By thorough treatment of them the danger of metastasis is much lessened. Thorough general treatment prevents the serious sequelae that sometimes follow parotitis. Careful nursing and care of the patient are necessary to prevent relapse. The patient should remain in bed during the acute attack

---

ACUTE AND CHRONIC GASTRITIS.

DEFINITION:—The acute form is an acute catarrhal inflammation of the mucosa of the stomach; acute indigestion. The chronic form, chronic dyspepsia, is associated with structural changes in the mucosa, and with change in the secretions and muscular activity of the stomach.

CAUSES:—Lesions have been noted in various cases as follows: (1) 2d to 6th cervical vertebrae to the right; 2d cervical anterior; 8th to 10th dorsal vertebrae separated; break at the fifth lumbar. (2) Luxation of the 8th rib; tenderness at the 8th dorsal vertebrae. (3) cervical and dorsal curvatures of spine, and luxation of the ribs. Lesions at the atlas, axis and third cervical affect the vagus nerve through its connection with the superior cervical ganglion. It may be obstructed along its course in the neck. Lesions to the cervical region and to the pneumogastric nerves in the neck are of secondary importance in causing stomach disease. The main lesions occur in the spine, affecting the splanchnic area, and may be of the ribs and their cartilages, of the vertebrae, or of the spinal and intercostal muscles and other tissues mentioned. Lesions to these structures occur mainly between the fourth and tenth dorsal region, but may occur either a little above or below these limits. The pneumogastrics and the splanchnics both contribute to the solar plexus, which has charge of the functional activities of the organ. The wide area of origin of the splanchnics along the spine, and their importance in the innervation of the stomach, accounts for the fact lesions to this area are most potent in producing derangement. At the same time this region is so readily accessible to the Osteopath's work that results are generally easily attained in the treatment of such troubles.

Lesions to ribs and cartilages act in part through interference iwth the intercostal nerves, which are in direct sympathetic connection with the solar plexus through the splanchnics. Luxation of the ribs may also interfere with spinal nerves by derangement of the tissues about the head of the rib. Lesions of spinal muscles, ligaments, and vertebrae act mainly through interference with the spinal nerves and thus upon the connected splanchnics. Muscular lesion may often be secondary to stomach disease, but in such case indicates the point of treatment, and may point to other spinal lesion at that place. The vagi nerves carry sensory, motor and secretory fibers to the stomach. The splanchnics contain vaso-motor and vaso-inhibititory fibers for the stomach. But as the influence of the abdominal brain is, according to Robinson, supreme over visceral circulation, and controls as well visceral secretion and nutrition, the results of our treatment upon the pneumogastrics and the splanchnics must affect the stomach mainly through the solar plexus. As the splanchnics contain these vaso-motors for the stomach, the main treatment for gastritis, a vaso-motor disturbturbance, must be through them. Lesions to the splanchnic area are likely to cause gastritis upon account of their being the vaso-motors.

McConnell states that lesion of the eighth and ninth costal cartilages may cause gastritis.

The mechanical irritation of coarse, poorly masticated food, the fermentation of over-ripe fruit in the stomach, and the effects of constant overloading of the stomach and of indiscretion in diet, may irritate the mucosa and cause gastritis in the absence of specific lesion. But in such cases secondary lesions are generally produced by the trouble. In the ordinary case of gastritis some causes beyond these must be sought, as the disease so frequently occurs without such indiscretions.

The PROGNOSIS for recovery is good in both acute and chronic cases. The ordinary acute case is relieved immediately by a treatment. More than one treatment may not be necessary. In chronic cases, even when severe and of very long standing, relief is soon given, and a cure can usually be made.

The TREATMENT must be directed to the specific lesion, generally of the splanchnic area, that is causing the trouble. Its main object must be to correct the circulation, and thus ts take down the inflamed condition of the mucosa and restore normal secretion. The splanchnics and solar plexus, having charge of the circulation and secretion, afford a most convenient means of doing this. The correction of lesion here, and the treatment given the splanchnics and solar plexus in conjunction with the removal of lesion constitute the main treatment in such cases.

With the patient lying upon his side or upon his face, the muscles and deep tissues of the splanchnic area are thoroughly treated and relaxed. The patient now lies upon his side, or sits up, and treatment is given the spinal vertebrae and ribs of this region. The former are thoroughly treated and sprung, to relax all their related tissues and remove obstructions to the nerves. The latter are raised, and adjusted in case of lesion, to aid in this process. Vaso-motor activity is thus aroused and corrected. This important process is aided by by deep treatment of the solar plexus from the abdominal aspect. (VI. p 36) As this plexus has the main control of visceral circulation and secretion, treatment of it rouses and normalizes its functions. Mechanical pressure of displaced ribs upon the stomach may be found. The upper abdominal treatment aids circulation in the stomach. (V, p 36). Attention is given the upper cervical region for lesions affecting the vagus. It may be treated in the neck as a means of aiding the general treatment. Inhibition by pressure upon the left vagus relaxes the pylorus. This pressure may be made in the neck directly upon the nerve, or may be made at the third or fourth intercostal space near the spine. This latter treatment is much used to relieve nausea and vomiting. Its effect is probably through the sympathetic connections with the vagus. In some cases pressure at this intercostal space has caused vomiting. In some cases abdominal manipulation induces vomiting. This should be encouraged to relieve the stomach of its irritating contents. Excessive vomiting should be checked A thorough treatment along the spine (splanchnic area) will aid in this. After inhibition of the left vagus to relax the pylorus, the patient may be placed upon his right side and deep pressure te made over or beneath the left hypochondrium, from the cardiac toward the pyloric end, to aid in the passage of the stomach contents into the intestine.

McConnell states that inhibition at the 8th and 9th dorsal relaxes the pylorus; inhibition at the 6th and 7th dorsal relaxes the cardiac orifice. He has found that correction of lesion in the lower left ribs aids in the absorption of gas. Deep pressure over the solar plexus also aids this process.

Liver, bowels, and kidneys must be kept in active condition by treatment. The patient should be abstemious in diet. It should be light and easily digested, and may be according to prescribed dietaries.

Acute cases should be treated frequently, chronic cases three times per week.

DISEASES OF THE STOMACH (Continued.)

CASES.— (1) Strain from heavy lifting, followed by severe lameness at the time, which gradually disappeared. In a few months severe stomach disease followed; no food could be retained, and rectal feeding was resorted to. He came under treatment too weak to walk or talk. Muscular contractures under the right shoulder and a slightly displaced rib were the lesions found. They were corrected and the case was cured.

(2) Ulceration of the stomach and a complication of troubles, due to spinal curvature. Correction of curvature gave great relief.

(3) Ascidity of the stomach and diarrhœa, caused by abnormal tension in the spinal tissues. Cured.

(4) Gastralgia; attacks so severe that they induced spasm in abdominal and neck muscles at the same time. The spasm was always stopped at once by inhibition of the solar plexus and of the posterior cervical nerves. Attacks grew less frequent under treatment.

(5) Gastralgia; agonizing pain followed taking even small quantities of food as long as it remained in the stomach. 6th, 7th, and 8th right ribs were down. These being replaced at the second treatment the trouble disappeared.

(6) Gastralgia of several years' duration. Lesions at 5th and 6th dorsal and 2d lumbar vertebrae. Luxation of the 8th right rib. Case cured by four months' treatment.

(7) Tenderness over the stomach (hyperæsthesia); 8th dorsal vertebra very tender and 8th rib luxated; cured by two weeks' treatment.

(8) Gastralgia; three years' standing; attacks after nearly every meal. Lesion, a lateral twist of the 6th dorsal vertebra. Cured in one years' treatment.

(9) Gastralgia; incessant pain in left side, stomach, and bowels; 4th and 5th right and left ribs drawn together; 8th left rib under 7th; spinal muscles tense. Great relief was given by one months' treatment.

(10) Dilatation of the stomach and a complication of diseases. The spine was straight and flat; thorax flat; 2d and 3d cervical vertebrae lateral; left cervical muscles tense; slight lateral curvature to left between the 5th dorsal and 3d lumbar; spinal muscles tense.

(11) Gastralgia. Seventh dorsal vertebra right; great tension at the 12th dorsal.

(12) Gastralgia. Lesions at atlas and 4th dorsal.

(13) Gastralgia. Luxation of the 11th rib.

LESIONS: In all the above cases the splanchnic area was affected; neck lesion was rare, and apparently of secondary importance; lesions to the spine, including vertebrae and muscles were important, occurring in ten of the cases; rib lesions were the most important and specific, occurring in seven of the cases. Lesions of the 5th to 8th ribs (area of greater splanchnic) occur most frequently.

Lesions to the splanchnic area, through rib or spinal lesion, apparently occur in all cases of stomach disease. We are not yet able to specialize as to lesion, and say that one particular style of lesion, or lesion of some individual rib or vertebra causes a certain kind of stomach disease.

It is probable that in the future compilation of lesions may show considerable specilization of them in the etiology of stomach disease. But it is also likely that such tabulation will indicate the probabilities only, for it is a matter of experience that a given lesion will produce in one patient one form of stomach disease, and in another a different form, depending upon individual peculiarities, and upon various attendant conditions. Hence one must be upon the lookout for any various lesion in the splanchnic area in all stomach diseases. They may cause a predominance of sensory, motor, secretory, or motor derangements, and complications thereof, and according to the predominating difficulty it may be that special lesion will be suspected, or that special areas will be treated in conjunction with the removal of specific lesion in the case.

The practitioner's simple duty in stomach disease is mostly thorough examination of the splanchnic region of the spine, just above and just below, and of the thoracic parts in relation thereto. When he has done this he has located the trouble, almost invariably, and his treatment of this, region, removing the lesion, almost as generally cures or benefits the case. Lesion outside of this area is of minor importance, and treatment directed elsewhere (abdomen and neck) is either secondary or for alleviation merely.

Special lesions have been noted as follows: in ascidity, the lesser splanchnics and the 4th and 5th dorsal (A. T. Still); in gastralgia, frequent luxation of the 8th and 9th ribs anteriorly (McConnell), also of the 5th, 6th and 7th dorsal; for gas on the stomach, the lesser splanchnics and the 11th and 12th dorsal; for gastric ulcer, frequent lesion of the 8th and 9th ribs anteriorly, and of the 5th to 8th ribs posteriorly (McConnell.)

Secondary lesion in the form of contracturing of spinal muscles, particularly along the splanchnic area, is of very frequent occurrence in stomach disease. Although in this case the result, and not the cause, of stomach disease, it is of much importance osteopathically. (1) It indicates the point of treatment, for it is an indication upon the surface of the body of what special nerve fibers or areas are suffering derangement by the particular form of disease present. There is a direct path between the diseased stomach and the contractured muscle, over which the abnormal impulses, generated in the stomach, pass out. It is Nature's landmark of a special diseased condition, or of a phase thereof. Experience shows that in the absence of any other lesion whatsoever, treatment at the point of contracture may cure the condition. It is evident that the nerve era thus indicated was the one needing treatment.

(2) These contractures do not always occur at the same location, nor always affect the spinal muscles over the splanchnic area generally. They may occur upon the one side of the spine only, high up in the splanchnic area or above it. They must therefore indicate lesion in different nerve areas or fibers, according to some condition present and determining which fibres shall thus suffer and produce contracture. It is possible that they indicate seat of lesion in the spine not otherwise discoverable. In such case this weak point would be the determining condition in the location of the situation of the contracture. Thorough treatment at this point may restore conditions and thus correct lesion which is important in the causation of the stomach disease. Contracture and soreness in the cervical or lumbar regions may follow stomach disease, and possibly indicate important relations, by lesion or otherwise, between these parts.

Anatomical Relations: Robinson states that the solar plexus is supreme over visceral circulation, that it controls also secretion and nutrition. The important lesions noted in stomach trouble affect its spinal connections, the splanchnics, and may therefore cause circulatory, secretory, or nutritional disturbances in its connected organs. Likewise they may cause sensory and motor troubles, as the same authority states that this plexus receives sensation and sends out motion. According to Quain, the terminal branches of the pneumogastric unite with the gastric plexus of the sympathetic, and carry motor and sensory fibers to the stomach. Flint shows that the pneumogastrics have much to do with gastric secretions, as secertion of them leads to almost complete cessation of stomach secretions. It is considered probable by investigatosr that its motor function in the stomach is derived from its sympathetic connections. Osteopathic work seems to influence it more largely through its sympathetic connections. It is treated also in the neck directly. It is important in sensory and motor diseases. The splanchnics contain vaso and viscero-motor fibres. Stimulation of the splanchnics lessens peristalsis; of the pneumogastrics increases it. Thus important control is gained in various conditions. Quain states that sensory nerves for the stomach pass from the dorsal nerves from the 6th to the 9th; the 6th and 7th supplying the cardia, the 8th and 9th to the pyloric end.

The PROGNOSIS in stomach diseases as a class is extremely good. Many severe cases of long standing have been cured. As a rule relief is immediately given, and cure follows.

The TREATMENT of stomach diseases as a class is very simple. It consists mainly in corrective treatment in the splanchnic area, together with a certain amount of neck and abdominal work. This is supplemented by certain special treatments for various purposes in the treatment of special diseases. Through the pneumogastrics and the sympathetic connections, the solar plexus and the splanchnics, control is had, to a marked degree, over the processes regulated by them; sensation, motion, nutrition, secretion, circulation. Few diseases can remain after correction of these functions by removal of the lesion disarranging them.

The treatment of the solar plexus, the spine (splanchnics), the pneumogastrics, and the removal of the various lesions likely to occur in these regions have already been discussed.

The various motor, secretory, and sensory neuroses, described under the general name of *nervous dyspepsia*, are treated by the removal of special lesion and by the work for the control of various functions as discussed. In cases of supermotility, peristaltic unrest, and nervous eructation, special treatment may be given to stimulate the splanchnics and solar plexus to lessen peristalsis. In nervous vomiting, the work should be directed to the cerebral centers, by treatment in the superior cervical region, and to the solar plexus.

In spasm of the cardia, inhibition should be made at the end of the 6th and 7th dorsal for fibers controlling it, while in spasm of the pylorus the inhibition should be upon the 8th and 9th dorsal and upon the left vagus (p. 84). In atony of the stomach, thorough stimulation should be given the vagi, splanchnics and solar plexus, to increase muscular tone and to develop circulation. Local manipulation over the region of the stomach would aid in toning the muscular walls (p. 84). In insufficiency of the cardia stimulation should be given the 6th and 7th dorsal, while in pyloric insufficiency the 8th and 9th dorsal and the left vagus must be looked to. Local stimulation, by brisk work over the abdomen, aids the operation.

In secretory disturbances, hyper-ascidity, super-secretion, and sub-ascidity, work upon the vagus and solar plexus, through the splanchnics, corrects circulation and rights secretion. Stimulation of the lesser splanchnics and of the 4th and 5th dorsal is important.

In sensory disorder attention must be given the sensory innervation. Hyperaesthesia needs a general stimulation. Gastralgia needs deep inhibition at the solar plexus, splanchnics, and vagi. Special inhibition should be made from the 6th to 9th dorsal, 8th and 9th ribs anteriorly, and the 5th, 6th, and 7th dorsal vertebrae. All of which points seem concerned in the sensory innervation of the stomach. For the abnormal sensations of hunger, lack of appetite, etc., general correction of secretions and sensation will be efficient.

For *dilatation* of the stomach, rapid cutaneous stimulation over the region of the stomach aids in contracting its muscular fibers. Treatment should be given for the stimulation of the vagi, and accumulated food must be kept worked out of the stomach. (p. 84.)

In *peptic ulcer* attention should be given to perfect freedom of circulation. The condition of the 8th and 9th ribs anteriorly, and of the 5th to 8th ribs posteriorly must be looked to.

In *hemorrhage* from the stomach, inhibit the splanchnics, and the solar plexus carefully, to lessen the blood pressure by vaso-dilatation. Also inhibit the superior cervical region for the general vaso-motor center, and make deep inhibitive treatment of the abdomen to dilate the great abdominal veins and call the blood away from the stomach.

In *cancer* of the stomach general corrective work and particular attention to freedom of circulation must be relied upon.

Look for lesion to any of the special points mentioned in relation to the various diseases. The bowels, kidneys and liver must be kept in free action. The diet should in all cases be limited and easily digested.

CONSTIPATION.

DEFINITION: "Infrequent or incomplete alvine evacuation, leading to retention of feces" (Quain). "A neurosis of the fecal reservoir" (Byron Robinson). Osteopathically it is regarded as a neurosis due to obstructed action of the nerves supplying the bowel with secretion, motion, and circulation. It may be symptomatic of other disease, or a complication. It is very frequently idiopathic, due to specific lesion to bowel innervation.

CASES have presented various *lesions*; (1) Contraction of the sigmoid flexure. (2) Spinal lesions, mostly in the lumbar, causing spinal cord disease and partial paralysis of limbs and bowel (3) A posterior prominence of the whole lumbar region. (3) Lesion at 5th and 6th dorsal, 2nd lumbar, and 8th right rib. (5) At 3rd and 4th dorsal, 9th dorsal, 5th lumbar. (6) Intense contraction of the external sphincter ani. (7) Slight parting of 1st and 2nd lumbar. (8) Prolopsus of the sigmoid. (9) Retroversion of the uterus against the rectum. (10) Right curve of spinal column; 3rd to 6th dorsal vertebrae posterior; 7th to 10th dorsal vertebrae anterior and flat; 11th and 12th dorsal and 1st lumbar posterior; 12th dorsal and 1st lumbar the seat of pain; 12th rib down; 2nd and 3rd lumbar close; 5th lumbar sore and anterior. (11) 2nd and 3rd dorsal separated, 3rd and 4th together, 3rd to 5th flat, 6th to the left, 11th dorsal to 2nd lumbar posterior. (12) 6th and 7th dorsal posterior, 9th to 12th flat, ribs irregular and prominent on the left. (13) Coccyx badly bent, lesion of 5th lumbar. (14) Separation between vertebrae from 8th to 10th dorsal, and between 5th lumbar and sacrum. (15) 2nd to 5th dorsal approximated and to the right, separations between vertebrae from 8th dorsal to 3rd lumbar, the right innominate up and back.

An examination of cases shows a wide distribution of lesion, ranging from the upper dorsal to the coccyx, and affecting ribs, vertebrae, spinal muscles and other tissues, innominates, coccyx, etc. The most important lesions in these cases appear in the region of the lower two or three dorsal, and in the lumbar region. It is in this portion of the spine that origin is given to the sympathetic nerves supplying the bowel. Particular attention should be given the 11th and 12th dorsal and the 1st and 2nd lumbar, as the sympathetic branches from these points supply the inferior mesenteric ganglion and the rectum with motor fibres, and the abdominal vessels with constrictor fibres. Sympathetic distribution for the small intestine is from just above the first lumbar; for the large intestine from the 1st to 4th lumbar. Hence the importance of the lower dorsal and lumbar lesion in constipation, as it may interfere with the functions of motion, secretion, and circulation by obstructing the spinal connections of these important sympathetics.

Lesions of the lower two ribs are important causes of constipation, not only by spinal interference with the sympathetics mentioned, but by direct mechanical pressure upon the bowel, sometimes. In yet another important manner they may cause bowel trouble by lesion to the diaphragm as already mentioned. The whole subject of change in the diaphragm is an important one in relation to bowel disease. It is reasonable to consider that certain spinal and rib lesions affect the diaphragm. They may cause it as a whole to weaken and sag, may cause contracture of the whole muscular structure, or may contracture or strain certain portions of it. Thus impingement is brought upon the important structure passing through the diaphragm, and having much to do with abdominal activities. The aorta, ascending cava, thoracic duct, pneumogastrics, phrenics, and splanchnics—may be interfered with. Or the sagging of the diaphragm may set up ptosis of the abdominal organs, thus causing constipation mechanically or otherwise. This subject has been discussed at length elsewhere.

Lesion to the fourth sacral nerve may cause contracture of the external sphincter, which it innervates. Lesion to the lower dorsal and the lumbar nerves may lead to loss of energy of the muscles of the abdominal walls, as may other causes, and lead to constipation. Robinson states that such a condition favors constipation by allowing congestion of blood and secretions. Lesions to the liver and pancreas, usually from the 8th to 12th dorsal, or through the splanchnics or solar plexus, aid constipation by lessening the secretions of these organs, necessary to stimulation of peristalsis. McConnell states that contractured muscles are generally found in constipation on the right side of the spine over the region of the liver. Dr. Still makes lesion of the 5th dorsal important in these cases.

The coccyx may be so misplaced as to act as a mechanical obstruction to the passage of the stool. Lesion at this point may cause contracture of the sacral tissues and interfere with the fourth sacral, or it may interfere in a similar manner with the sympathetic distribution to the rectum and cause atony or contracture of its walls. A prolapsed uterus, hernia, adhesions, or the presence of foreign bodies, fruit stones, etc., may mechanically obstruct the bowel.

Various lesions, as of the diaphragm, the weight of a loaded colon, of the spinal regions, etc., producing ptosis of the abdominal organs, or of the colon itself, cause a kinking of the flexures by their dragging upon their ligaments at those points. The same causes allow of a sinking of the caecum and sigmoid into their respective iliac fossae, allowing also the sigmoid to fold upon itself. In these ways obstruction to the passage of fecal matter along the bowel is caused. In enteroptosis the pressure of organs upon each other limits motion, peristalsis, and circulation. The elongated omenta and ligaments, in which the blood vessels and nerves run to the bowels, stretch these structures and abridge their function. These become important causes of constipation.

The *anatomical relations* have been described in detail in considering diarrhoea, q. v.

Various lesions, acting to weaken circulation and nutrition, lead to atony of the bowel muscles, and lead to constipation. Any lessening of circulation acts to cause it, as the circulation of blood about the nerve terminals in the bowel wall is necessary to their activity.

The PROGNOSIS is good. Most cases are cured in a reasonable length of time. The ordinary acute form, occasional constipation, is cured in one or a few treatments. Very quick results are often obtained. Cases which have been most obstinate, and those that have been from birth, have been readily cured. Many cases are obstinate under treatment, and require time and patience to effect a cure.

The TREATMENT for constipation, from the nature of the case, must look to the correction of the lesion that is obstructing circulation, peristalsis, or secretion in the bowel, or to the removal of the mechanical stoppage that sometimes causes the disease. Some one or more of the special lesions described is found, and may be removed by the appropriate methods. The main treatment is for nerve supply, as practically all of the lesions, except mechanical causes, act in one way or another through the innervation. The main treatment upon the spine is in the lower dorsal and lumbar regions, the seat of the chief lesions. The removal of the lesion is often all the treatment necessary, but various points must be considered. The treatment must, by the removal of lesion or otherwise, tone the splanchnics, spinal sympathetics, and solar plexus, as well as Auerbach and Meissner's plexuses, controlling the motor, secretory, and other functions of the bowels. Special attention must be given to lesion at the points mentioned as liable to them in this trouble.

Abdominal treatment should be a deep, slow, relaxing treatment carried along the course of the bowel. It relaxes all the tissues, and frees local circulation, affecting also the local nerve distribution. It dwells particularly upon those portions in which are felt the aggregations of fecal matter, releasing the tissues about them, softening and passing them along. This is the special method of removing obstruction by foreign bodies, such as fruit stones, etc. This treatment should be given especially to the caecal and sigmoid portions, as they are generally full. Attention must be given to raising and straightening them when necessary. This may be done in the treatments described in III and IV, p. 36. Likewise the colon as a whole should be raised and straightened to relieve kinking at its flexures and the evil results to nerves and blood vessels accuring from the stretching of its omenta in ptosis. Spinal work and the correction of lesion tones these omenta to hold in position the replaced organs.

The liver should be thoroughly treated to stimulate the flow of bile. By the removal of lesion, by treatment to its spinal connections through the splanchnics, and by raising the 8th to 12th right ribs, this is in part accomplished. It is treated at the abdomen, as are the gall bladder and bile duct. (V. p. 36, IX. p. 37).

The inferior mesenteric ganglion is the center for the fecal reservoir, and should be treated at the location already described. The vagi may be treated in the neck to aid in the general process. The coccyx should be straightened as the case requires. (XX, p. 13.) A contractured sphincter should be dilated. (p. 44). Or it may be released by strong inhibition over the fourth sacral nerves. They may be located at the fourth sacral foramina, just to the side of and below the bony prominences that mark the termination of the sacral canal, and which may be easily felt beneath the skin.

Peritoneal adhesions may be broken up gradually by deep and careful work upon the bowel at their site. In the absence of pain, or as it disappears, the treatment may be made strong, care being taken not to set up inflammation.

Obstruction from volvulus may be sometimes overcome by manipulation at the seat of the obstruction directed to the straightening the bowel. This requires long treatment at a time, and much care and patience.

Symptomatic cases must de treated in conjunction with the primary disease.

The use of cold and hot drinks before breakfast, rectal injections, cereal foods, fruits, regularity in habit, and exercise are all helpful.

CARARRHAL ENTERITIS; DIARRHOEA,

DEFINITION:—An acute inflammation of the intestinal mucous membrane due to specific spinal lesions. Diarrhoea is often symptomatic of other diseases.

CASES: Lesions were found as follows: (1) Tension of the spinal tissues from the 3rd to 10th dorsal. (2) Lateral lesion of the 7th, 8th and 9th dorsal vertebrae. (3) 9th to 11th right ribs depressed. (4) Right 11th rib down onto the 12th; 4th and 5th lumbar anterior; spine weak.

Lesions may occur anywhere along the splanchnic area and along the spine as low as the coccyx. The most important lesions effect the region of the lower two dorsal and the lumbar vertebrae. The 11th and 12th ribs on

each side are sometimes found luxated, most often downwards. Lesion
may occur at the 2d lumbar, the 5th lumbar, to the innervation of the
small intestine above the first lumbar, to the innervation of the large intestine from the 1st to 4th lumbar, to the coccyx, or to the innonimates. Lesions
from the 8th to 12th dorsal and ribs may affect liver and pancreas to aid
the diseased condition.

Anatomical relations:—In intestinal diseases as in stomach diseases, the
importance of the splanchnics and solar plexus must be borne in mind.
The former contain vaso and viscero-motors to the intestines, these vaso-
motors being, according to Fliut, among the most important in the body,
innervating the immense area of abdominal vessels, which, when fully dilated, are said to be able to accomodate one-third of the total quantity of blood
in the body They contribute to the solar plexus, which rules sensation,
motion, secretion, nutrition, and circulation in all these viscera. Our correction of circulation in these cases is an important consideration. Robinson
shows that movements of the intestines are largely dependent upon the
amount of blood circulating in the intestinal walls. For these reasons lesions
anywhere along the splanchnic region may produce important disturbances
of intestinal secretions, circulation, or motion, all of which may be disturbed
in diarrhoea.

The whole abdominal sympathetic is important in these diseases.
Stimulation of it lessens peristalsis; stimulation of the pueumogastric increases peristalsis. We work not to directly stimulate or inhibit either of
these for the purpose of controlling peristalsis, but to remove lesion from
them as it produces through them abnormalities of motion.

Auerbach and Meissner's plexuses of nerves have to carry on gastro-
intestinal secretion. Auerbach's is a motor plexus. They lie in the intestinal walls, and may be directly influencel by work upon the abdomen, but
are corrected by us through the removal of lesions affecting them through
their sympathetic and spinal connections. Lesions to them, disturbing both
secretion and motion, are important causes of diarrhoea. Robinson states
that the inferior mesenteric ganglion, upon the inferior mesenteric artery,
located from externally a little below and to the left of the umbilicus, innervate the muscular walls of the fecal reservoir, i. e., the left half of the
transverse colon, the descending colon, and the sigmoid. Spinal lesion to
it, through its connected nerves, is active in production of diarrhoea.

The fact that afferent sympathetic fibres pass from the abdominal
viscera to the thoracic sympathetic cord may explain the occurence of
secondary lesions in the form of contractured muscles along the thoracic
spine. The presumption is that they are sensory in function, and if so, sensory fibres for the abdominal viscera may be associated with them. Quain
states that among the medullated fibres passing into the sympathetic system,
some derived from spinal nerves are sensory fibres. This may be the ex-

planation why inhibition of the splanchnic area will stop pain in the stomach or intestines.

All these various facts indicate the importance in diarrhoea, of spinal or lower rib lesion, from the 6th dorsal to the coccyx, which may interfere with the spinal connections of all these abdominal sympathetics and derange their functions.

Our most important treatment is given from the 10th dorsal down, in these cases. Lesions in this lower spinal region are of prime importance in causing diarrhoea. The importance of the lesion to 11th and 12th ribs and vertebrae, and to the upper two lumbar, is found in the fact that nerve branches from the lower dorsal and upper two lumbar pass to the inferior mesenteric ganglion, shown above to innervate the fecal reservoir. These branches are motor fibres for the circular, and inhibitory fibres for the longitudinal, muscle fibres of the rectum. At the same time these lower dorsal and upper two lumbar nerves send branches to the sympathetics and supply vaso-constrictor fibres to the abdominal vessels. The motor fibres to the longitudinal, and inhibitory fibres to the circular, muscle fibres of the rectum are sent from the sacral nerves. This explains why the lesion of the innominate or coccyx may cause a part of the trouble in diarrhoea, also why strong stimulation to the sacral nerves relieves tensmus.

Branches from the four lumbar ganglia go to the plexus upon the aorta, and to the hypogastric plexus. Lesion in the lumbar region may in this way further interfere with the bowel.

The various forms of enteritis and diarrhoea seem to have as their basis derangement of nerve or blood supply in the form of inflammation (catarrh); lack of proper vaso-innervation, leading to congestion and exudation: improper preparation of digestive fluids, due to deranged glandular activity; or increased peristalsis, accompanied by increased secretion and exudation.

The removal of lesion obstructing nerve and blood supply corrects these manifestations of such derangement.

The PROGNOSIS is good. Most cases of diarrhoea are checked at once by a single treatment, many needing no further treatment. Cases of years' standing have been in many instances cured in a short time. The ordinary acute diarrhoea needs but one or a few treatments. Acute enteritis needs careful treatment for several days while the acute pocess lasts.

TREATMENT for diarrhoea consists in the removal of lesion as found, affecting any of the special points named above as subject to lesion in this disease. The main treatment aside from this is very simple, and is often given as the sole measure of relief. It consists of very strong inhibition of the spine from the lower dorsal to the sacrum. It may be given with the patient on his side, as described in III, p. 9. The "breaking up" spinal treatment may be used for the same purpose. (XXII, p. 11). The former seems preferable. It may be applied to either side or to both sides of the spine.

Inhibition may be made at the 11th and 12th dorsal region by sitting the patient upon a stool, pressing the knee against the spine, first on one side then upon the other, and grasping the arms of the patient, raising them above his head, and bending the body backwards against the knee. This not only inhibits these nerves, but stretches all the anterior spinal parts and related tissues in the lower dorsal and upper lumbar regions. This result is more important than the mere inhibition. The 11th and 12th ribs are often displaced downward, and may then drag portions of the diaphragm in such a manner as to prevent free circulation of blood and lymph in the vessels perforating it. This result alone might cause diarrhoea.

Muscular contractures along the spine should be removed. Deep but careful manipulation should be made upon the abdomen over the intestines for the purpose of relaxing all their tissues, freeing circulation and correcting the activities of the Auerbach and Meissner's plexuses. One may treat to tone the solar plexus, splanchnics, and general abdominal circulation. The liver should be thoroughly treated, lesion to it be removed, and the secretion of bile corrected. Its presence in abnormal quantities may cause biarrhoea through increasing peristalsis. In other cases its presence in the bowel does not hinder the case. And it is said to allay irritation of the mucosa. Lesion of the 8th to 12th dorsal and ribs may derange either liver or pancreas, In fatty diarrhoea the latter must be looked to.

For tormina or griping, inhibition of the splanchnics is done. For tenesmus, or bearing down pains in the bowel, strong stimulation of the sacral nerves is made by thorough manipulation of the tissues over the sacrum.

It is said that in such cases the abdominal fascia is contracted and causes congestion mechanically. (Chas. Still) When contracted it should be relaxed by abdominal manipulation.

The vomiting and purging should not be checked if they are the evident means of getting rid of the irritating contents of the bowel. The ordinary case is seen after plenty of opportunity has been afforded nature to remove the irritant by these means, and calls for immediate checking.

In *acute entritis* the case must be seen several times daily. Gentle relaxing treatment should be made over the abdomen. The liver is to be lightly treated; spinal muscles relaxed; the spine gently sprung to release tension in its tissues. The lower ribs may be raised a little and the neck treated for relief of the head. Careful attention must be given to the diet of the patient It should be light and restricted, Meat broths, mucilaginous drinks, etc., may be given according to prescribed dietaries. Warm baths and rectual injections may be employed.

Cases of acute diarrhoea and enteritis should remain quietly in bed. The various measures described may be employed as necessary. Spinal inhibition alone may be sufficient. When diarrhoea is symptomatic of other disease it may be relieved by these treatments. Its cure depends upon the cure of the disease present.

AN OSTEOPATHIC STUDY OF THE DIAPHRAGM, ITS RELATION TO ABDOMINAL DISEASE.

(Prepared for "The American Osteopath," Dec. '99.)

"The diaphram, next to the heart," says McClellan, "is the most extraordinary muscular arrangement in the body." Standing as a partition wall, or barrier between the thoracic and abdominal cavities of the body; being practically an involuntary muscle, and, like the heart, in constant motion throughout life ; assisting in many important functions of life, such as breathing, laughing, coughing, sneezing, vomiting, defecation and parturition, yet at the same time being a subsidiary, and not always an indispensible agent in the performance of these functions, it takes its place at once as somewhat of a physiological anomaly among the organs of the body. Arising by fleshy digitations from the ensiform cartilage, from the inner surfaces of the lower six ribs on either side, from the ligamenta arcuata externa et interna, and by its crura from the bodies of the upper four lumbar vertebra ; sweeping upward as a broad arch to its insertion, by its interlacing fibres, its own club-shaped central tendon, it forms a musculo membraneous sheet without counterpart in the body, and which further bears out the claim of this remarkable structure to be an anomaly, anatomical as well as physilogical.

To the Osteopath, since Dr. Still's declaration that downward luxations or dislocations of any of the lower ribs might cause such an alteration in the arch of the diaphragm as to allow of a binding of its substance upon the aorta at its passage between the crura, thus obstructing the blood current and leading to irregular heart-action, the diaphragm has become an important object. A study of the diaphragm, therefore, in the light of Osteopathic experience with the musculature of the body, and its innervation and blood-supply, and an application of well-known Osteopathic principles to the subject, would seem to be in place.

In other parts of the body the Osteopath makes much of muscular contractures or atony, of their interference with blood vessels and nerves, of mechanical derangements or dislocations of organs and tissues. May he not, then, apply such reasoning to the diaphragm, which occupies an important position, aids in carrying on important functions, and is related mechanically to organs, vessels, and nerves whose functions are concerned with the most vital operations of the body ? The importance of this subject becomes at once apparent when it is recalled that upon one hand the diaphragm is contiguous to the heart and lungs, that upon the other it is related to the liver, stomach, pancreas, kidneys, spleen and intestines, while it transmits to and from the abdomen, such important structures as the aorta, inferior vena cava, oesophagus, thoracic duct, vena azygos major, vena azygos minor, pneumogastric nerves, phrenic nerves, splanchnic nerves, and small blood and lymphatic vessels. To all of these structures it bears, directly or indirectly, a mechanical relation.

Byron Robinson is authority for the statement that "traumatic muscular action of the psoas magnus on the sigmoid, and traumatic muscular action lower right limb of the diaphragm on the descending colon, which muscular action induces emigration of pathogenic microbes to the serosa" may cause peritonitis. Gowers is authority for the statement that violent contractions of muscles may have a traumatic action upon nerves passing through their substance or beneath or around them. If these things be true, it is reasonable to suppose that the diaphragm might, when abnormal in action, unfavorably affect the structures to which it is so closely related. If it be possible for the psoas magnus and the right crus to so act as to irritare or wound a contiguous structure so freely mobile and so well lubricated as is the sigmoid or the descending colon, it would also seem possible that conditions could arise under which the diaphragm would wound or irritate the thoracic duct, one of the azygos veins, the oesophagus, or the aorta, all of which are more closely related to the diaphragm than is the sigmoid to the psoas magnus, or the descending colon to the crus, as they are less mobile and lack lubrication. If, as Gowers says, it be possible for violent muscular action to wound nerves impinged upon by muscles, it would also seem possible that the diaphram, when in violent action, as in hiccough, might irritate the pneumogastrics phrenics, or the splanchnics.

It is a well-known fact one of much significance to the Osteopath, that the voluntary muscles of the body are capable of entering into a state of continued contraction technically known as tetanus, and that, as Kirke states, while this term is not applied to involuntary muscles, they likewise are often thrown into a condition of unduly protracted contraction, known as tonus. The causes of such conditions are various, the different authorities pointing out that they may arise as the results of, (a) constant irritation, affecting either nerve or center, (b) traumatism, the result of direct force upon the muscle, as a blow, strain, etc., (c) disease of the muscle, (d) loss of antagonism, or excess use. The Osteopath lays great stress upon the potency of such conditions to act as mechanical interferences and to cause disease of various kinds. Such reasoning applies as well to the diaphragm as to any other muscle. The motor nerves of the diaphragm are the phrenics and, according to McClellan, branches from the lower five or six intercostal nerves, which are reinforced by sympathetic fibres from the neighboring supra-renal plexuses. The phrenics or intercostals, as our daily experience shows, may be irritated by spinal lesion at their origins, such lesion acting upon the nerve either directly or indirectly, through its connected nerves, its blood-supply, or its center. The intercostals may also be irritated by crowding together of the ribs, and just as such irritation may cause intercostal neuralgia, when affecting the sensory function of the nerve; it may produce contracture of the diaphragm and other muscles when affecting the motor function.

Such a condition might be set up in the diaphragm, as in other muscles, by traumatism, or the result of force directed upon the diaphragm. As a blow or strain may contracture spinal muscles, so the direct traumatic effect of an enlarged liver or spleen, or of a distended stomach, or of an accumulation of pus or other fluid in the pleural cavity may so irritate the muscle directly as to result in tonus.

Loss of antagonism, too, would seem as potent in this situation as in any other, to cause contracture of the muscle. Just as a dislocated hip is held out of place through contracture of muscles, the normal antagonism to which has been destroyed by the displacement, so may tonus or contracture of the diaphragm follow loss of antagonism. Those muscles which raise and spread the ribs in inspiration, and maintain the full form of the thorax, particularly the levatores costarum and the intercostales, are the natural antagonists of the diaphragm. We are all familiar with the antero-posterior flattening of the chest in the paralytic or the neurasthenic, with the lateral flattening of the thorax in rachitis, and with the multitudes of cases in which all the ribs, or many of them, are dropped down and drawn close together. When for any reason this change in the position of the ribs and in the diameters of the thorax has taken place, then the agents which have held the ribs apart and raised them, thus keeping well separated the points of attachment of the diaphragm, have ceased, in greater or less measure, to operate, perfect antagonism to the action of the diaphragm no longer exists, and, following the rule that a muscle whose points of attachment have been approximated contracts to accommodate itself to the changed conditions, the diaphragm, it would seem, contracts to adjust itself to the limits set for it by the narrowed thorax, and is thus allowed to assume an unnatural condition of tonus which bodes ill to the free play of the many important structures passing through it.

If it be reasoned that the nature and function of the diaphragm would not admit of the existence of such a condition of its muscular substance, it being an involuntary muscle performing rhythmic motion continually which is well nigh indispensable as an aid to vital functions, and that these functions seem to be carried on without apparent embarrassment even when all the untoward conditions pointed out above seem to exist, let it be remembered that in other parts of the body we have important involuntary muscular organs, also in rhythmic action almost continually, and more indispensible than is the diaphragm to certain vital operations, which are well known to become the seat of tonus or contracture, even while still performing their functions. I refer to the intestines. Every Osteopath's experience with abdominal work will teach him that at times there are in the intestines more or less extensive areas of tonus, in which the walls of the bowel become so drawn as to be clearly perceptible to the touch. Such a spasmodic action of the muscles takes place in an acute form in colic. The functions of the intestines may still be carried on under such conditions, though it be with pain and difficulty.

In gross displacement of the ribs, as best seen in the enormous change in position that may affect the eleventh and twelfth ribs, it is likely that there is a dragging upon special fibres or portions of the diapragm. The central tendou is held in place by the attachment to the pericardium, and by the lateral bands extended downward from the deep cervical fascia. If, nows one or several lower ribs be displaced dowoward, the portions of the diaphragm attached thereto would be carried downward, causing traction upon them, and perhaps drawing them across an important structure, it might be the aorta, impeding its blood current, or the splanchnics, interfering with their function.

If these views are correct, it is apparent at a glance what harm might be caused by such interference with the structures passing through the diaphragm. In such case it seems that the inferior vena cava and the structures passing through the oesphageal opening would suffer least through impingement, since the former passes through a fibrous portion, which is naturally less yielding, and the shape of the aperture is maintained by attachment of the wall of the inferior vena cava to the central tendon, while the oesophagus and pneumogastric nerves, though surrounded by the upper part of the eight-spaped arrangment of the muscular crura, are protected by the yielding character of the oesophagus, which, when not occupied by the passage of food or drink, is merely a potential cavity, its walls lying in apposition.

The aorta, however, surrounded by the crura of the diaphragm upon both sides and anteriorly, and by the bony spinal column behind, would, together with the vena azygos major and the thoracic duct, be subject to serious pressure from contracture. This is on account of the muscular nature of the crura, the unyielding spine behind the aorta, and the fact that the aorta, to fulfil its function, must have walls resistent enough to maintain its form. Moreover, the walls of the aorta are supplied by delicate sympathetic nerve fibres which are very susceptible to irritation. The sympathetic and splanchnic nerves, and the vena azygos minor, transmitted by the crura, and the phrenic nerves, which perforate the substance of the diaphragm, would all likewise suffer from pressure and irritation through contracture or dragging of its fibres.

In the consideration of the pathology of the diaphragm there is another matter which invites our attention, namely: atony of its muscular fibers. If the diaphragm is like other muscular organs there can be no doubt that such a condition might occur. We are acquainted with the condition known as atony of the bowel, or of the stomach, and with the serious consequences of such a pathological change.

It is a well-known fact that section of a motor nerve is followed by loss of nutrition in the muscles supplied by such nerve. We are also familiar with the fact that pressure upon a motor nerve leads to wasting of the muscles supplied by that nerve. Hilton reports a case in which pressure upon the circumflex nerve by the head of a dislocated humerus caused atrophy of the deltoid muscle. Gowers says that a muscle remains small after lesion of its nerve. Such occurences are common enough in our practice. Now it is a reasonable supposition that the lower six ribs might be so crowded together as to impinge the intercostal nerves supplying the diaphragm, that pressure upon these nerves would be followed by wasting of the muscles supplied by them, and that lack of tone in the diaphragm would follow. It is also quite possible that derangement of cervical vertebrae would so interfere with the third, fourth and fifth cervical nerves, from which the phrenic nerves arise, as to contribute to, or produce, the same result. Add to these facts the possibilities of various interferences with the lower intercostal, internal mammary, and phrenic arteries, which supply blood to the diaphragm, and there would seem to be sufficient grounds for supposing that this muscle can not be immune to the various causes that would lead to atony of its muscular fibres.

Here is fruitful soil for evil. Very possibly hese is the origin of enteroptosis, the evil consequences of which have been so well portrayed by Byron Robinson. Enteroptosis is a neurotic disease; the neurasthenic is flat-chested; the lowered ribs in the flat-chested allow of an atonic diaphragm. To the under surface of the diaphragm, by the various omenta, are attached the liver, the stomach, the spleen, and the splenic flexure of the colon. Following atony of the diaphragm, these organs sink downward in the abdomen. They crowd the other organs, weight them, and cause them to gravitate downward. The colon kinks at its splenic and hepatic flexures, and the passage of its contents is impeded. The dragging of the various organs upon their omenta and ligaments causes them to elongate, and thus stretches the blood-vessels and nerves conveyed in them to the abdominal viscera, in short, the whole blood and nerve mechanism of the abdomen is deranged, and discord reigns in the family of abdominal organs.

Another ill result would arise from an atonic diaphragm. The ordinary quiet, abdominal breathing that carries on respiration generally, would suffer from lazy action of a weakened diaphram, leading to poor oxygenation of the blood and an accumulation of waste material in the system. The aspiration of the venous blood through the liver and other abdominal organs, which is effected by free diaphragmatic action would be weakened or lost, leading to sluggishness of these currents, and to abdominal congestion.

It would be well for the Osteopath, in all cases in which there is altered chest form, luxated lower ribs, irregular heart action, general nervousness, digestive disturbance, biliousness, constipation, and other abdominal troubles, etc., to consider well whether or not the diaphragm might be in such a condition as to cause or aggravate the symptoms.

The method of treating the diaphragm in such contingencies is simple enough, since it depends upon the application of the same principles as are used in our work upon any muscle or organ similarly affected; to stmiulate or inhibit, or to remove the special lesion which is causing the mischief. There are, generally speaking, two methods of relaxing or stimulating muscles; (a) through affecting their nerve connections, (b) through affecting the muscle directly. Either or both of these ways may be brought into play by removal of lesion. An example of the former, in relation to the diaphragm is seen in pressure made in the neck upon the phrenic nerve, releasing the spasm of hiccough. An example of the latter is seen in a method employed by one of my friends; in a case of hiccougs, after trying the usual method of stopping the spasm, he inserted the fingers beneath the lower ribs on either side, and by spreading them away from the median plane of the body, brought traction directly upon the diaphragm by separating its points of attachment, thus relaxing it and stopping the spasm. The same principle is involved in Dana's method of stopping hiccough. He lays the patient upon a table with the upper half of the body hanging over the edge. This arches the thorax, spreads the ribs and brings tension upon the diaphragm, inhibiting the spasm.

But, aside from hiccough, there are important considerations for the Osteopath in treatment of the diaphragm in conditions of contracture or atony as pointed out in this paper. This whole question was suggested to my mind by the remark of a friend that my lower costal treatment first stimulated the diaphragm, leading to clonicity, which was soon followed by fatigue of its muscular fibres, allowing of a complete relaxation and a consequent freedom of all structures passing through it. Of the correctness of this view there seems to be no doubt. Naturally, we propose to repair atony, contracture, or distortion of the diaphragm by removal of the lesion causing it. By correcting cervical or spinal lesion, by shaping a narrowed thorax, by raising and replacing dislocated or luxated ribs, and by separating rips when crowded together, we are to remove the active and original cause of such conditions. But, aside from these considerations, in cases in which it is desirable to affect the diaphragm either as adjurant to the removal of lesion or independently of it, in such cases as seem to need extra stimulation or relaxation of the diaphragm, there are important considerations for its treatment. There is no doubt that much abdominal and lower costal treatment goes much further that the operator supposes in effecting the body. The proposition may be stated as follows: Lower costal and abdominal treatment profoundly affects the diaphragm. (a) It stimulates and strengthens it when lacking energy, adding to it that force and tension so necessary to a perfect performance of its function. At the same time pneumogastrics and sympathetics, thoracic duct, and blood vessels are stimulated in their action. (b) It sets up clonicity of its muscular fibres, this leads to fatigue and relaxation of its fibres, relaxes the contractured condition of the whole organ and allows of perfect freedom in the action of all structures passing through it. Which one of these affects follows depends upon the condition of the diaphragm to begin with, and upon the method of treatment adopted by the operator.

If these views are correct, it does not need much penetration to see that such treatment must necessarily have a marked effect upon the health of the whole body.

To the examination of this proposition let us again apply well known principles used by us upon other parts of the body. Atony: In an atonic or lifeless condition of the bowels, allowing of sluggish performance, or non-performance, of duty, resulting in lessened, or lost, peristalsis, leading to constipation, etc., the most important part of our work (aside from removal of lesion, which is also left aside for the present, in the consideration of the diaphragm), is direct manipulations upon the intestines, stimulating their substance, and the blood vessels and nerves contained in their walls and about them. Increased vigor, peristalsis, follows. Contracture: In tormina and in all kinds of contracturing or drawing of the intestinal walls, our most important effects in relaxing the muscular walls are attained by direct inhibiting treatment upon the intestines (removal of lesion aside). The same principles apply to diaphragmatic treatment. With us it is an aphorism that muscles and nerves may be stimulated mechanically. Witness the production of the patellar reflex, or our abdominal treatment to increase peristalsis. This point must be supported by quotations at length from authorities, but I take it to be unnecessary to prove this point again to Osteopaths. Suffice it to quote from Howell's Text Book, "A sudden blow, pinch, twitch, or cut excites a nerve or muscle." Neuro-muscular contraction follows excitation of motor nerves. Idio-muscular contraction follows excitation of a muscle directly. Moreover, Gowers states that slow tonic contractions of a muscle occur when its points of attachment are suddenly approximated.

Now all of these conditions can be easily applied in treatment of the diaphragm. Both idio-muscular and neuro-muscular contractions may be set up in it. It may be directly stimulated mechanically by quick abdominal manipulations which thrust the liver, stomach, spleen and intestines up against its cura and vault. It may be stimulated through its intercostal nerves by the excitation given them in the lower costal treatment, which squeezes the ribs together and separates them, this motion as well stimulating these nerves through their spinal connections through the spring given to the ribs at their spinal ends by such manipulations. In addition to this, the costal and abdominal treatments, by approximating the ribs, narrowing the lower thorax, and raising the abdominal viscera, result in suddenly approximating all the points of attachment of the diaphragm, which must, in accordance with the law enunciated by Gowers, enter into slow tonic contractions.

Add to this, now, the fact that by removal of lesion the injured nerves may be restored, resulting in the muscle regaining its nutrition. Considering the above points, we have all that is necessary to affect the repair of the diaphragm in atony, or its stimulation in all cases where desirable.

We must now consider the removal of contracture in diaphragmatic treatment. As we remove abnormal tonicity in the intestinal walls by deep pressure and inhibition, directly applied, so we may remove it in the diaphragm by direct inhibition of its substance. This may be accomplished in several ways. It has already been pointed out that spreading of the ribs from the median plane of the body brings inhibition upon the fibers of the diaphragm. Here, also, deep pressure and inhibition may be directly applied by firm pressure of the abdominal contents upward against the diaphragm.

The law of muscular action and fatigue affords us another means of effecting this result. If we consider the nature of muscular action, we learn from Howell's Text Book that all normal physiological contractions of muscles are regarded as tetani. This means that the contraction of a muscle as a whole is not due to a single contraction of its substance, but to many succeeding contractions of its elements. Repeated excitations lead to a gradually increasing state of contraction, the "stair-case contractions" as shown by Bowditch upon the ventricle of frog's heart. Howell's Text Book shows that stimulations of a muscle once in about every two seconds leads to an incomplete tetanus of the muscle, while eight to thirteen excitations per second can cause voluntary tetani. But it also shows that, "rapidly repeated stimuli, though at first favorable to activity of a muscle, soon exert an unfavorable influence by causing the lessened irritability which is associated with fatigue." "Mechanical applications to nerve and muscle first increase and later lessen and destroy the irritability. Thus pressure, gradually applied, first increases and later reduces the power to respond to stimulants." Hence it seems that the Osteopath would be able to apply to the diaphragm mechanical stimulation frequently enough and continuously enough to first excite and contract it, and later fatigue it, leading to its relaxation and the consequent freedom of all structures penetrating it.

Careful attention to the condition of the diaphragm, both in diagnosis and in treatment, would well repay the Osteopath.

Extract from "Appendicitis" by G. R. Fowler. Edition 1...

In all 75 specimens examined the presence of some form of obstruction to the blood current in the mese-appendix was demonstrated. xx Evidence of chronic irritation exists in some of the mese-appendix ... showing these lesions to ... of the nerve-fibres. The effects of these lesions upon the nerves, whether preceding or following infection of the tissues, is such as to produce the most profound ... disturbance ... of the organ ... with consequent lessened vital resistance, and finally localized necrosis. Another source of trouble is disturbance xxx ... hyperploid of the coats of the appendix. This is probably due to repeated ... or chronic stasis through interference with the return circulation in the mese-appendix, and results eventually in the ... the nervous lesions above alluded to.

APPENDICITIS,

DEFINITION.—An inflammation of the vermiform appendix, acute or chronic, caused by traumatisin, or by specific rib or spinal lesions, These lesions obstruct bowel action, limit its motion, deplete its nerve and blood-supply, leaving a weakened condition, allowing of aggregation of fecal matter, foreign bodies, etc. The vigor to pass these onward is lacking, and they are pressed into the appenpix, which itself is suffering from a weaken-ed state due to these causes. Or direct irritation of lesion may affect nerve and blood mechanism, derange vaso-motion, and set up the inflammation. Or the direct mechanical irritation of a displaced lower rib may set up the inflammation.

CASES:—(1) Three attacks had occured, another one was threatening. Operation had been advised, but osteopathic treatment relieved at once and cured the condition in two weeks. (2) In a case in which operation had been advised, one month's treatment cured the condition and chronic con-stipation as well. (3) Case showed a history of constipation; cured by the treatment. (4) Lesions; 2 l lumbar lateral, with heat and pain about it; 11th right rib luxated. Treatment relieved at once, and the patient was cured in two weeks. Surgeon had been ready to operate. (5) 12th right rib down and inside of the crest of the ilium. Setting the rib cured the case in a few days (6) Recurring appendicitis; spine posterior in lower dorsal and upper lumbar; lateral curve at 6th to 9th dorsal; constipation chronic; cured by ten weeks' treatment. (7) Tenderness upon right side of spine from 6th dorsal to 2d lumbar, especially at the 6th to 10th dorsal and 1st and 2d lumbar. (8) Acute attack cured by the treatment. (9) Lesion at lower dorsal and upper lumbar; 10th and 11th ribs overlapping 12th, due to a fall. Operation had been advised, but two months' treatment cured the case.

Lesions and causes:—(1)There is usually a history of constipation in these cases. In some it follows diarrhoea. There can be no doubt that the lesions causing these diseases, q. v., are the real causes of appendicitis in many cases. Many apparently robust men suffer from this disease, but experience shows that many such have unhealthy bowels to begin with. Many show the specific spinal lesion. The ordinary case caused by a foreign body, seeds, shot, enteroliths, etc., would probaby not become victims of appendicitis but for weakened bowel condition due to such lesions as cause constipation. The fact that very often the body is a fecal concretion supports this view. The inflammation is a vaso-motor disturbance. Such disturbances, due to lesion, have been seen to be the causes of constipation, etc. The appendix must suffer with the rest of the bowel from these causes, and thus being weakened cannot further resist special causes of vaso-motor disturbance.

(2) Displacement, or dragging of the colon at the hepatic flexure pre-

vents the passage of fecal matter and forces the introduction of fecal masses into the appendix.

(3) The most important bony lesions seem to be displacements of the lower two ribs on the right side. They may add mechanical obstruction or irritation to deranged nerve connections at the spine.

(4) Lesions of the dorsal and lumbar regions are very important on account of the nerve connections with the bowel. From the 9th, 10th, 11th and 12th dorsal region sensory nerves pass through the sympathetics to supply the intestines down to the upper part of the rectum. For this reason strong inhibition to this portion of the spine is useful in controlling the pain in appendicitis. The sympathetic vaso-constrictor fibres for the abdominal vessels pass from the lower dorsal and upper two lumbar nerves, whiel branches from the lumbar ganglia pass to the plexus upon the aorta and to the hypogastric plexus. Thus lower dorsal and lumbar lesion has an important effect in disturbing the vaso-motor innervation necessary to the production of this inflammation.

The anatomical relations given for lesion in diarrhoea apply to those in appendicits.

The appendix has the same structure as the caecum, practically; is nourished by a branch of the ileo-colic artery, possesses innervation (Auerbach and Meissner's plexus?) causing in it peristalsis and secretion of abundant tough mucous from its numerous mucous glands. In health the free secretion of this mucous fills the caviy of the structure to the exclusion of foreign bodies, but upon lesion to the blood or nerve supply such as mentioned above, lessened secretian allows of room for the entrance of foreign bodies. Anemia may become a cause of the inflammation in it.

The *Prognosis* is favorable for recovery in nearly all cases. The experience with cases, even the most dangerous acute ones, has been very satisfactory. Many such are upon record, restored to health after operation had been advised as the last resort. If seen in time, very few cases need ever come to the knife. The point of surgical interference may, however, be reached. Osteopathic treatment prevents the case falling into the chronic forms so commonly met, and in which operation, to prevent an acute attack, is so often resorted to. The acute case is usually aborted by prompt treatment.

TREATMENT:—The first consideration is the removal of the lesion if posible in the patient's condition. This applies particularly to displacements of the 11th and 12th ribs. Here gentle manipulation and slight elevation may be sufficient to remove the irritation. Immediate attention should also be given to the relief of the constipation commonly present. If not soon affected by the treatment, rectal injection should be employed. This measure materially aids conditions by removing the pressure of bowel contents from tender points, by giving freedom of circulation in the bowel, and by aiding to remove foreign bodies.

An essential part of the treatment is local treatment of the tissues at or above the site of the inflammation. By care, little difficulty will be experienced in applying such treatment even in very painful cases. The relaxation of the tissues thus accomplished gives immediate relief to the patient. Not only the abdominal walls, but the deep tissues and circulation about the appendix are thus treated. The treatment must slow, deep, and inhibitive and given with great care. In the intervals of treatment, it may be necessary to apply the ice bag or hot fomentations at the seat of the inflammation.

It is not likely that in this contingency spinal work to increase peristalsis would be at all successful in removing the foreign body from the appendix. Local manipulation must be depended upon for this. The pain is relieved by spinal inhibition from the 9th to the 12th dorsal particularly. Nausea, vomiting, fever, and hiccough, aside from being relieved by the general treatment of the case, may be relieved by the usual methods before described.

The patient should go to bed at once upon the attack threatening. A restricted fluid diet, taken a little at a time, should be enforced. Attention should be given the kidneys and general condition. The patient should be seen several times daily until out of danger. Continued treatment should be given for a while after recovery to prevent recurrence or relapse.

The chronic case, possessing various degrees of chronic pain, tenderness of tissues, and inflammation in the right iliac fossa is a familiar object. The object of the work is to remove lesion, to restore perfect freedom of circulation, and by local treatment of the tissues to remove tenseness and pain. Thorough spinal and abdominal treatment, and attention to the general condition of the bowel are necessary. The disapperance of tenderness in the right iliac fossa does not remove the danger of acute attack, as extensive morphological changes have usually taken place in the tissues of the appendix which call for a course of treatment to so restore circulation as to enable it to repair them.

INTESTINAL OBSTRUCTION,

DEFINITION:—The occlusion of the bowel may be but partial, persisting as a chronic condition. In acute cases it may be wholly or partially obstructed.

CASES: (1) Fecal impaction. Severe radiating abdominal pains, griping, and some dysentery had been present for twenty-four hours. The impaction was located at the hepatic flexure. Treatment relieved the pain at once, and the manipulation removed the obstruction. Complete recovery followed.

(2) Volvulus was diagnosed, located near the ilio-caecal valve. The

surgeon was ready to operate. Persistent treatment straightened the bowel and a movement of the bowels was had. The recovery was complete.

(3) Impaction of the ileo-caecal valve. The attack came on violently at night. The family physician, after eighteen hours' work over the patient advised operation. Osteopathic treatment reduced pain and inflammation at once, and allowed a further examination. The impaction was located at the ileo-caecal valve, and manipulation removed it within a short time. The patient was asleep in thirty minutes.

LESIONS AND CAUSES: Only in rare cases would it be likely that some specific lesion would lead directly to this trouble, but in most of them it is probable that lesions would be present accounting for the bad condition of the bowel that resulted in some form of obstruction. In general one would expect such lesions as have already been described as interfering with the abdominal organs. Intussusception is sometimes due to irregular, limited, sudden, or severe peristalsis. In such cases special lesion to the splanchnics, or to the sympathetic connections of Auerbach's plexus, might result directly in the abnormal paristalsis producing the invagination. In such cases the outer layer, or receiving portion of the bowel involved, draws up by contraction of its longitudinal fibers. Such abnormal activity of these fibers might also be due to some special lesion to motor innervation.

In some cases McConnell suggests that special spinal lesion could cause paresis or paralysis of a bowel segment. Such a condition could allow of a pouching of the affected portion, and of accumulation of feces or foreign bodies. Specific lesion might also cause stricture by contraction of a segment.

The fact that obstructions often follow constipation or diarrhoea shows the importance of lesions producing a bad bowel condition. Volvulus is especially frequent at the sigmoid and at the caecum, enteroptosis being often the cause, through allowing the parts to prolapse and turn. The frequency of spinal lesions causing the weakened omental supports that allow of the ptosis shows the importance of spinal lesion as a factor in causing obstructions. Spinal or rib lesion may be looked to as the original cause of a large number of the various forms of obstruction. It may produce the tumor whose pressure obstructs the bowel; the peritonitis, following which adhesions cause strangulation; the ulceration in the bowel which gives place to cicatrization and stricture; or the inactive condition of bowel motion and secretion that allows of accumulation of old fecal matters, foreign bodies, etc. A healthy bowel, perfectly free from the effect of lesion of any kind, could only under rare conditions become the seat of one of the various forms of obstruction.

The importance of lesion producing unhealthy abdominal or internal conditions must be acknowledged in the etiology of most of these cases.

The *anatomical relations* of these various lesions have already been pointed out in the consideration of various intestinal diseases.

The PROGNOSIS must be guarded. Very many cases die, and surgical measures have generally been considered necessary after the third day of obstruction. Yet osteopathic treatment has been successful in a number of cases after the necessity for operation had been urged. Probably, as in the case of appendicitis, many lives could be saved by osteopathic means before surgery is resorted to.

In chronic cases the prognosis for recovery is very favorable. Most cases could be prevented from coming to the point of absolute obstruction. If they could be foreseen, most acute cases could no doubt be prevented by osteopathic treatment.

TREATMENT: In such cases as seem to depend upon a special lesion it should be removed. Generally the first consideration is the alleviation of the patient's condition. Strong inhibition of the splanchnic area, especially from the 9th to 12th dorsal, and of the lumbar region, aids in lessening the pain. This step may be necessary before abdominal manipulation can be borne. This solar plexus should now be inhibited. A slow, deep, but gentle inhibitive treatment should next be given over the bowel to relax the tissues, decrease the inflammation, and lessen the pain. This treatment may be used also to quiet abnormal peristalsis if present. After this preliminary treatment the practitioner may proceed by careful palpation to locate the seat of the obstruction if possible. This is often impossible, and in such cases one must work over the bowel generally. In some cases the obstruction is felt, or the seat of the pain is an indication of its position.

The main work must be done by abdominal manipulation. The parts of the intestine must be so managed as to be raised, straightened, and drawn away from each other. The caecum and sigmoid may be raised and straightened, (Chap VIII, divs. II, III, IV.) Deep treatment may be made in the right and left hypochondriac regions to free the hepatic and splenic plexuses. In intussusception the parts should be raised and drawn from each other toward the extremities of the cylindrical tumor, if it can be made out. In volvulus, raising and straightening the involved portions is relied upon.

The stricture and adhesions may be manipulated with the purpose of softening, relaxing, and breaking them down. Foreign bodies and fecal aggregations must be gradually loosened and worked along the bowel. They are more readily handled than other forms. It may be necessary to manipulate them after rectal injection, to aid in moving them. Copious injections sometimes aid in overcoming intussusception, volvulus, etc. During the abdominal treatment it is well for the patient to be placed in various positions; upon the back, sides, upon the abomen, etc., to get the aid of gravity in righting the parts. Some writers recommend thorough shaking of the patient. He is held by four men by the arms and legs, first with the abdomen upward, then downward, while the shaking is done.

There should be much persistence in the treatment. The practitioner should remain continuously with the case, and treat it as much as practicable, until relieved. In the intervals, hot applications over the seat of the pain may made.

In chronic cases the treatment may be carried on as usual, upon the plan given above for the treatment of acute cases. After removal of obstruction, a thorough course of general treatment should be undertaken for the removal of lesions that have originally impaired the bowel or have produced abnormal abdominal conditions.

ENTEROPTOSIS.

Enteroptosis is a disease in which various of the abdominal and pelvic viscera leave there natural positions, slipping downward into the abdominal and pelvic cavities. It is a common and distressing complaint, frequently overlooked or not recognized. It is sometimes regarded as a symptom group, but may, from the osteopathic point of view, be regarded as an idiopathic condition, due to specific lesion.

These cases are often treated for some one feature, as for nervous dyspepsia, constipation, operation for floating kidney, etc. It is a common error to overlook the essential condition of the disease. The Osteopath who gives close attention to a class of neurasthenic, flat-chested, constipated patients, who complain of lack of bodily and mental vigor, many and various indefinite nervous symptoms, abdominal pulsation, vaso-motor disturbance, etc., will find most interesting material. The multitude of symptoms may vary greatly in different cases, but the presence of neurasthenic conditions, altered thorax and spine, and unnatural abdominal condition, either of walls, viscera, or both, will usually afford an unmistakable sign of the disease. After a little experience with such cases one learns to recognize them at a glance when presented for examination. Once seen these cases can hardly be mistaken, and a few moments examination reveals a story of disease beginning imperceptibly, the growing conviction through many months or some years that something was the matter, the attempt to seem well because no decided disease seemed present, or a long course of treatment for various ills, none of which reached the true condition. This most common disease is still but seldom clearly recognized or intelligently handled.

LESIONS AND CAUSES: The common description of its aetiology is unsatisfactory. Tight lacing, traumatism, muscular strain, and repeated pegnancies are mentioned. The condition of relaxed abdominal walls and prominent viscera due to repeated pegnancies may probably be rightly regarded as a separate condition. It is due to a physiological act, and does not present those specific lesions nor the resulting symptoms found in neurasthenic enteroptosis. Tight lacing, traumatism, and muscular stran may produce those lesions found to be the causes of such conditions.

These cases commonly present spinal, rib, diaphragmmatic and abdominal lesions. Spinal lesions may be of any of the kinds found the spine ordinarily, and may occur anywhere along the splanchnic or lumbar region. Rib lesions may occur in any or all of the lower six ribs on either side.

Mobility of the tenth rib is regarded by a German physician, Dr. B. Stiller, (Phila. Med. Journal, Jan. 13, 1900,) as the pathognomonic cause of enteroptosis.* Undoubtedly it could interfere with the sympathetic connections of the abdominal viscera and become a factor in causing this condition. But, from an osteopathic view-point, lesions of other ribs, and of spinal vertebrae, etc., may be as potent in producing the "basal neuropathy" concerned in this disease as its fundamental pathological condition. Further, rib lesions may cause a condition of the diaphragm in which its normal tone is lost, and prolapse in it causes ptosis in the abdominal organs which it aids in supporting. (p. 100.) Spinal lesions may participate in causing the atonic condition of the diaphragm.

Spinal and rib lesion, aside from derangement of the diaphragm, acts to produce enteroptosis by interfering with the spinal sympathetic connections of the viscera and of their omental supports. Impeded circulation and nerve-supply, vaso-motor, motor, secretory, trophic and sensory, produces at the same time derangement of function in the organs and weakness in their mesenteric supports. These conditions work together to bring about the disordered function and the displacement of these organs. The displacement of itself furthers the present bad conditions by mechanically interfering with the activities of organs, stretching nerve-fibres and blood-vessels which are carried in the now elongated omenta, kinking the colon at various points, etc. The viscera, having sunk down into the abdominal cavity, cause prominence of the lower abdomen, leaving a hollow in the upper abdomen, thus giving to it the peculiar boat-shaped appearance described as "scaphoid abdomen."

Lower dorsal and lumbar lesion may interfere with the spinal innervation of the abdominal walls, cause them to loose their tone and to dilate. Intra-abdominal pressure is thus lessened and the organs are allowed to prolapse.

According to Byron Robinson, enteroptosis begins with a weakening of the abdominal sympathetic, which looses its normal power over circulation, secretion, assimilation and rhythm. That this weakness of the abdominal sympathetic and its consequent loss of function originates in spinal lesion to its origin in the splanchnic nerves has already been pointed out and fully discussed in considering the diseases of the stomach and intestines q. v. The *anatomical relations* of such lesions to parts affected was pointed out.

The PROGNOSIS in these cases is very favorable, but the progress of the cure is likely to be slow. Generally improvement begins immediately upon treatment and may progress to a cure in a few months. Other cases yield more slowly, though relief if soon given, and require an extended course of treatment to effect a cure.

The TREATMENT must be both constitutional and local. The latter consists in the removal of lesion and in abdominal treatment. Lesions anywhere to the splanchnic and lumbar regins, to the ribs, thorax and diaphragm, must be treated after their kind, according to directions given in Part I. With spine, ribs, and diaphragm restored to normal conditions, the underlying causes of the enteroptosis have been removed. Corrected nerve and blood-supply to the organs and their supports, aids in correcting their function and strengthens the supporting tissues to hold them in place when restored by abdominal manipulations.

Correction of spinal lesion also aids in restoring nutrition and tone to the relaxed and atrophied abdominal walls. This process is furthered by a thorough treatment upon the abdominal walls. This renders the use of the favorite abdominal bandage unnecessary, and it is gradually laid aside. Throughout the course of the case the restored abdominal walls act as the mechanical bandage has done to hold the organs to their places as replaced by the treatment. With corrected spine, free blood and nerve-supply to all the visceral supports, and a strengthened abdominal wall, no difficulty is found in getting the parts to gradually be retained in their normal positions. Thorough spinal stimulation over the splanchnic and lumbar areas is kept up for the purpose of increasing the blood and nerve-supply to the parts in question.

Abdominal work, aside from treatment of the walls, is directed to raising and replacing the viscera. This is readily accomplished by various treatments. (II, III, IV, Chap. VIII). This releases and renews circulation and nerve-supply at the same time, removes pressure of organs upon each other, gives freedom of motion, and aids in strengthening the omenta to hold the parts in place.

The diaphragm has been restored to normal position and tone by correction of those lesions originally deranging it.

The constitutional treatment must be thorough and general to restore the patient from the nervous, circulatory, nutritional, and other effects of the disease. A most thorough general spinal treatment must be given. Thorough stimulation or heart and lungs, treatment of the cervical sympathetic, and attention to kidneys, liver and skin accomplishes the desired object. The auto-intoxication usually present is overcome by this treatment of the excretory organs. The constipation, dyspepsia, and other functional disorder is corrected by the restoration of the organs concerned.

The patient should be much out of doors, free from worry, and careful not to become fatigued. Deep breathing exercises are beneficial.

NEUROSES OF THE INTESTINE.

The various lesions producing derangement of the intestinal innervation, sensory, circulatory, motor, secretory and trophic, have been described. Their anatomical relations to intestinal diseases have been fully discussed. Various of these lesions may occur and produce intestinal derangements by special interference with certain functional activities of the intestines, through acting as lesions to the particular portion of the innervation having those functions in charge. Thus the lesion may so act upon the sensory innervation as to cause sensory disease. Or the predominating disorder may affect particularly the secretory or the motor functions. Sensory, secretory, and motor neuroses of the intestine are common. The lesions producing them are not different in nature from the ordinary lesions found as the causes of gastro-intestinal disorders. For some reason, not well understood, certain of these lesions may produce, in a given case, certain special kinds of disturbance of function. In the diseases described below no special lesion has been as yet described as the special cause of each condition. One finds lesions already described producing them. As a rule, however, these special sensory, secretory, or motor neuroses are noted in cases of bad intestinal health, and frequently seem to be specialized pathological manifestations of this general bad condition. The sensory, secretory, or motor disturbance has gained the upper hand. In some cases the neuroses is itself the sole manifestation of the results of the lesion.

SECRETORY NEUROSES.

Membraneous Enteritis, or *Mucous Colitis*, is often met, frequently occurring in subjects of intestinal disease. The special lesions present and disturbing bowel innervation act particularly upon the secretory fibres. The result is over-action in the mucous secreting glands. The mucous membrane is not pathologically altered, and catarrh if present at all, is a secondary effect. It is a purely nervous manifestation. Special lesion is commonly found to be the active cause of irritation to the centers or fibres controlling this funcnion. Its results are apparent in the copious secretion of intestinal mucous, which passes away from the patient in conglomerate masses forming the whole or a separate part of the stool, in long ribbon-like strips, or in a complete cast of the intestinal canal of some inches in length.

It is not a serious condition, and removal of lesion, with thorough spinal and abdominal treatment, will at once begin to correct the over-action of the glands. Its cure may depend upon the restoration of a general healthy bowel condition. Relief is generally obtained at once from the treatment, but considerable treatment may be necessary to eradicate the chronic condition. Tenesmus, when present, is relieved by strong sacral stimulation. Colic is relieved by strong spinal inhibition and by local inhibitive treatment at the seat of the pain in the abdomen.

SENSORY NEUROSES.

These disturbances are due to irritation to the sensory nerves supplied by the splanchnics to the intestines.

Enteralgia, Colic, or *Intestinal Neuralgia*, is met with in neurotic and anemic subjects, and attacks are induced by exposure, gout, and local irritation to the sensory nerves of the intestine by inflamation, enteroliths, etc. Excepting mechanical irritants, lead poisoning, and like agencies, the actual cause that weakens the intestines and lays them liable to the action of such exciting causes, is spinal lesion irritating or weaking the sensory centers or fibres. Many cases occur spontaneously from spinal lesion. This spinal lesion may act by causing increased activity in the muscularis, leading to the ring-like contractions of the intestine present in colic. In many of these cases intestinal cramps cause localized contractions in portions of the intestines, which may be readily seen or felt through the intestinal walls. Here the most efficient treatment is by local manipulation over the seat of the contraction. Deep inhibitive treatment here quiets the nerves and releases the spasm. Such local work must be supplemented by corrective work upon the spine, which prevents further attacks. Strong spinal inhibition may be used to quiet the pain. Some one point is generally found along the splanchnic area at which inhibition is effective. This is often high up in the splanchnic region, but varies with the case, and is found by trial. Special lesion is to be removed, and stoppage of the pain may depend upon that.

Diminished Sensibility of the intestines is a common neuroses. It may be both sensory and motor, and leads to diminished peristalis, constipation and accumulation of the feces in a portion of the intestine, often in the rectum. It is likely to occur in diseases of the brain and cord in which the centers are effected. Special spinal lesion is often the direct cause, or causes the cord disease. Cure of this condition in such cases depends upon cure of the primary disease. In other cases, removal of lesion, and restoration of activity to the local nerve mechanism overcomes the paresis. Spinal and abdominal treatment, directed especially to the course of the intestine, to affect Auerbach's plexus, and to the solar plexus, will aid a cure. Specific lesion may cause a paretic condition of a bowel segment and be responsible for the trouble. A general weak condition of the nervous system, on account of which nervous shocks and other disturbances cause this condition, must be remedied by upbuilding it.

MOTOR NEUROSES.

Nervous Diarrhoea is a condition in which increased contractility of the muscularis of the bowel is aroused by purely nervous causes. It is an overaction of the bowel, not presenting the usual aspects of diarrhoea. The stools are softer than normal, and frequent, occuring two, three, four, or more times in twenty-four hours. The subject is as a rule a neurotic, being hysterical, neurasthenic, or of a very nervous temperament, but the characteristic lesions found in diarrhoea, q. v., are present and so act upon the nerve-mechanism of the bowel as to lessen its motor stability. Thus its abnormal activity made possible by the lesion becomes the special manifestation of the nervous condition. There must be some sufficient reason why the general nervous condition should be able to so center itself upon the bowel. The presence of such lesions as anatmically weaken the bowel affords a reasonable explanation of this phenomenon. These lesions, usually of the lower dorsal and lumbar regions, probably affect, through its connections with the 11th and 12th dorsal and the 1st and 2nd lumbar nerves, the inferior mesenteric ganglion ruling motor activity in the fecal reservoir.

The treatment commonly enployed for diarrhoea is efficient in checking this form. At the same time, thorough general spinal and neck treatment must be given to strengthen the nervous system. Spinal causes of the nervous condition must be sought and overcome. The case yields rapidly to treatment, but is very prone to setbacks due to nervous disturbance. For this reason the patient must be kept as free from exciting influences as possible. The condition is apt to recur until the nervousness has been lessened. Fortunately this latter condition yields readily to treatment.

Enteropasm is a neurosis of the intestine in which a spasmodic condition of portions of the intestinal walls occurs. It may result in temporary obstruction, but its most usual maniiestation is to cause the stools to be passed in separate, rounded masses, or in ribbon-shape. The latter is most frequent. While often a nervous phenomenon, special lesion is necessary to account for this peculiar manifestation of nervousness. Special lesion may affect the inferior mesenteric ganglion through its spinal connections, or the motor fibres of the circular muscles of the rectum, originating from the lower dorsal and upper one or two lumbar nerves, and passing thence through the inferior mesenteric ganglion to the rectum.

CHOLERA MORBUS.

DEFINITION: Cholera morbus is an acute catarrhal inflammation of the stomach and intestines, characterized by severe abdominal pain, colic, vomiting, purging, and muscular cramps.

CASES: (1) A young man in intense pain; had vomited blood several times, and continuous severe vomiting and purging were present, had a chill; severe griping in the epigastric and umbilical regions. Inhibition at the 4th and 5th dorsal vertebrae, on the right, stopped the vomiting. Inhition of the splanchnics stopped the purging. Cracked ice was allowed the patient, and a hot enema was administered After the first treatment no vomiting or purging occured, and rapid recovery followed. In his previous attacks he had usually remained in bed for three days, being incapacitated for a week. Morphine was usually necessary to stop the pain.

(2) Severe nausea, vomiting and cramps disappeared at once under the treatment.

LESIONS: Such lesions as described for enteritis, q. v., are present in these cases, weakening the bowel and rendering it susceptible to the agencies usually described as the exciting causes. The irritation of bad food, etc., may affect a healthy bowel in this manner, but there is often no such factor in the case. Simple chilling of the body may cause the attack, or slight indiscretion in diet may bring it on.

The PROGNOSIS is good. Treatment relieves the case at once, stopping the pain, vomiting, cramps, etc. The patient rapidly recovers.

TREATMENT: Correction of lesion protects the patient against further attacks. The severe abdominal pain and colic are removed by strong inhibition of the spine, especially over the splanchnic area, and from the 9th to the 12th dorsal. This quiets the sensory nerves of the viscera. Deep inhibitive treatment upon the abdomen, over the seat of the pain and about it, aids in relieving it. The vomiting is checked as before described. (p. 84), as is the diarrhoea. The cramps in the calves are relieved by strong inhibition over the sacrum and upon the popliteal nerve in the popliteal space. The system should be strengthened against collapse by stimulation of heart and lungs and by spinal and neck treatment for the general system.

HEMORRHOIDS.

DEFINITION: Varicose enlargements of the inferior hemorrhoidal veins or of the hemorrhoidal plexus.

CASES: (1) Protruding piles of fourteen years' standing cured in two months.

(2) Hemorrhoids of four years' duration cured in four treatments.

(3) Protruding piles of many years' standing, accompanied by constipation, cured in two months.

(4) Hemorrhoids and constipation. Lesion at 5th lumbar, coccyx badly bent. (5) 7th to 11th dorsal vertebrae posterior, coccyx anterior, innominate forward. Hemorrhoids were accompanied by indigestion and jaundice. (6) Internal hemorrhoids and constipation, no natural bowel motion for several years; cured in one month. (7) Protruding piles of several years' standing, constipation, prolapsed rectal walls. Lesion caused by strain from heavy lifting. A weakened lumbar region. Cured in one month.

(8) Constipation and piles of many years' standing caused by a bent coccyx. Four treatments gave great relief; case still under treatment.

LESIONS AND CAUSES: The common bony lesion present is a bent or dislocated coccyx, which acts as a local irritant and mechanical impediment of the venous return from the hemorrhoidal veins. Luxated coccyx, by local irritation and interference with the fourth sacral nerve, may cause obstinate contracture of the external sphincter, leading to constipation or straining at stool. Possibly coccygeal and innominate or sacral lesion, by direct interference or by dragging of tissues, derange the sacral nerves supplying motor fibers to the longitudinal muscle fibers of the rectal walls, weakening them. This result would probably be aided by the interference of these same lesions with the sympathetic (sacral) nerve-supply to the circulation through branches contributed to the lower hypogastric and hemorrhoidal plexuses. That of the coccyx seems to be the most important lesion in hemorrhoids.

Lumbar and lower dorsal lesion may be present and interfering with the innervation of the abdominal walls, relaxing them, lessening intra-abdominal pressure, and allowing of congestion of the abdominal circulation. By direct effect or by causing constipation, this condition may cause hemorrhoids. Lower dorsal and upper lumbar lesion to the nerve fibers which pass by way of the inferior mesenteric ganglion to supply motor fibers to the circular muscles of the rectal walls may become a factor by weakening the wall, relaxing its tone, and allowing of a congestion in its vessels. Lesion to the splanchnic and lumbar areas, affecting the sympathetic supply which, through the splanchnics, solar plexus, and other sympathetic vaso and viscero-motors originating along these areas, rules circulation and muscular tonus in the abdominal and pelvic viscera, may contribute in an important way to causation of hemorrhoids. Likewise those lesions to the spine and lower ribs, well known as causes of liver-derangement, become causes of hemorrhoids by producing obstructed portal circulation and constipation. The chief drainage of the hemorrhoidal plexus of veins is through the portal circulation by way of the superior hemorrhoidal vein. Lesions causing disease of heart and lungs, q. v., may secondarily become the causes of hemorrhoids through the impeded systemic circulation resulting. Lesions causing atomic diaphragm (p. 100), and other causes of enteroptosis, q. v., produce hemorrhoids by the mechanical obstruction of circulation, and by deranged nerve supply, etc.

The *anatomical relations* are pointed out above. The American Text Book of Surgery calls attention to the fact that these veins are unsupplied with valves and also that they tend to become congested by the natural upright position of the body. These facts aid in explaining the potency of the above lesions, and of any obstructive condition (pregnancy, over-eating, etc.) in causing this condition.

The EXAMINATION must be made by both inspection and palpation, the use of a proper speculum aiding a thorough inspection of the rectum.

The PROGNOSIS is very favorable. The usual medical treatment is palliative, or surgery is resorted to. The latter may often become necessary, but the success of osteopathic treatment prevents many operations.

Even the most severe cases have been successfully treated. The treatment generally begins to succeed immediately. Long standing cases are often cured in a few months. Some cases are slow and obstinate.

The TREATMENT is local, abdominal, spinal and constitutional.

Local treatment is first directed to correcting the coccyx if necessary. (XX, Chap. II.) The external sphincter should be well dilated. This may be accomplished by inserting two, or even three, fingers, well vaselined, and held together at the tips in wedge-shape. After being well inserted, they are spread apart and withdrawn carefully. The dilatation must be thorough. The rectal speculum may be used for this purpose. All the surrounding tissues, both externally and internally, are to be thoroughly but gently relaxed. Internally this operation should be carried as far up along the rectal walls as the index finger is able to work. Pressure is made upon the injected veins to empty them of blood and to stimulate their local nerve and muscle substance to proper tonus. In case of thrombi in straugulated veins, the manipulation about and upon them must be gently applied with the purpose of stimulating the circulation to a gradual absorption of them. They must not be broken up or detached, as there is danger of their being swept into the circulation as emboli.

After dilatation of the sphincter and relaxation of the tissues, protruding piles, first emptied if possible, must be gently pressed back beyond the sphincter. If the rectal walls are prolapsed, as is often the case in protruding piles, they must be replaced by the index finger directed to straightening out and pushing them up on all sides.

This local work removes irritation of the coccyx, frees the whole local circulation, tones the local musculature and other tissues, and stimulates the local sympathetics. It may be the sole and sufficient treatment in many bad cases. It should be given but once per week or ten days.

Abdominal treatment is for the purpose of increasing freedom of circulation and to aid in the venous return. The solar and hypogastric plexuses are stimulated and manipulation is made over the course of the inferior mesenteric and common and internal iliac arteries. Portal circulation is helped by deep abdominal work from the lower abdominal region upward to the liver. Lesions to the latter organ are removed, and thorough treatment given to the liver as in the treatment for constipation, q. v., which must be relieved, it being usually present. (V. Chap. VIII.)

The viscera are raised, and treatment is made deep in the iliac fossae to stimulate the pelvic sympathetic pexuses and to aid venous return from the hemorrhoidal, vescical, uterine, and other related flexuses of veins. (II, III, IV, Chap. VIII). If the patient is placed in the knee-chest position while abdominal treatment is performed with the ideas explained above, the force of gravitatation is made to assist in venous drainage of the parts.

Enteroptosis and diaphragmmatic lesion are repaired as before explained.

Thorough spinal treatment is given from the sixth dorsal down, stimulating splanchnics and other sympathetics, with all their contained vaso and viscero-motor, circulatory, and trophic fibres. This treatment is to strengthen circulation and to maintain its freedom. It is supplementary to the abdominal work. It also aids in restoring tone to the vessel walls, as well as to prolapsed rectal walls, and thus to maintain them in correct condition. Anatomical relations between the spinal work and abdominal and pelvic viscera have before been fully explained.

Correction of spinal, rib, or innominate lesion is made if necessary. In this way, and by work along the lower dorsal and upper lumbar regions, coupled with the local treatment upon the abdominal walls, the latter are built up and restored to normal tonus if relaxed.

The *constitutional* treatment consists in the general spinal treatment, and in special treatment for heart and lung disease if present and causing the hemorrhoids.

Light out-door exercise and absolute personal cleanliness should be enjoined upon the patient.

INTESTINAL TUMORS.

Intestinal Tumors of various kinds, both benign and malignant have been frequently treated osteopathically with sucsess. Medical treatment is but palliative, and the only means of removal has been by surgical operation. The fact that in numerous instances these cancers and tumors have been entirely removed by osteopathic treatment is in itself remarkable, and helps to sustain the claim often made, that the use of the knife is often obviated in the treatment of such conditions.

The TREATMENT is simple, and consists in the removal of spinal lesion, which may be of any of the kinds discribed as producing gastro-intestinal disease. At bottom the real cause of these growths is some obstruction or irritation to local blood and nerve-supply. It has already been shown how special lesion causes this obstruction, or lays the foundation of the condition which directly or indirectly produces the irritation. The treatment is therefore the removal of lesion and the restoration of normal nerve and blood supply. Spinal treatment, aided by abdominal work accomplishes this object. The latter is done, not upon the tumor itself, but upon the surrounding parts. It relaxes tensed tissues, opens arterial blood-supply and venous and lymphatic drainage, and restores normal condition. In this way the progress of the morbid process is stopped, healthy tissue is built, and the tumor disappears, probably by absorption. At least one case is upon record in which the tumor, a fibroid, was loosened by the treatment and passed per rectum. (Cosmopolitan Osteopath, Feby., 1900, p. 30.)

Attendant conditions, such as cotstipation, fecal impaction, colic, etc., are treateed as described elsewhere.

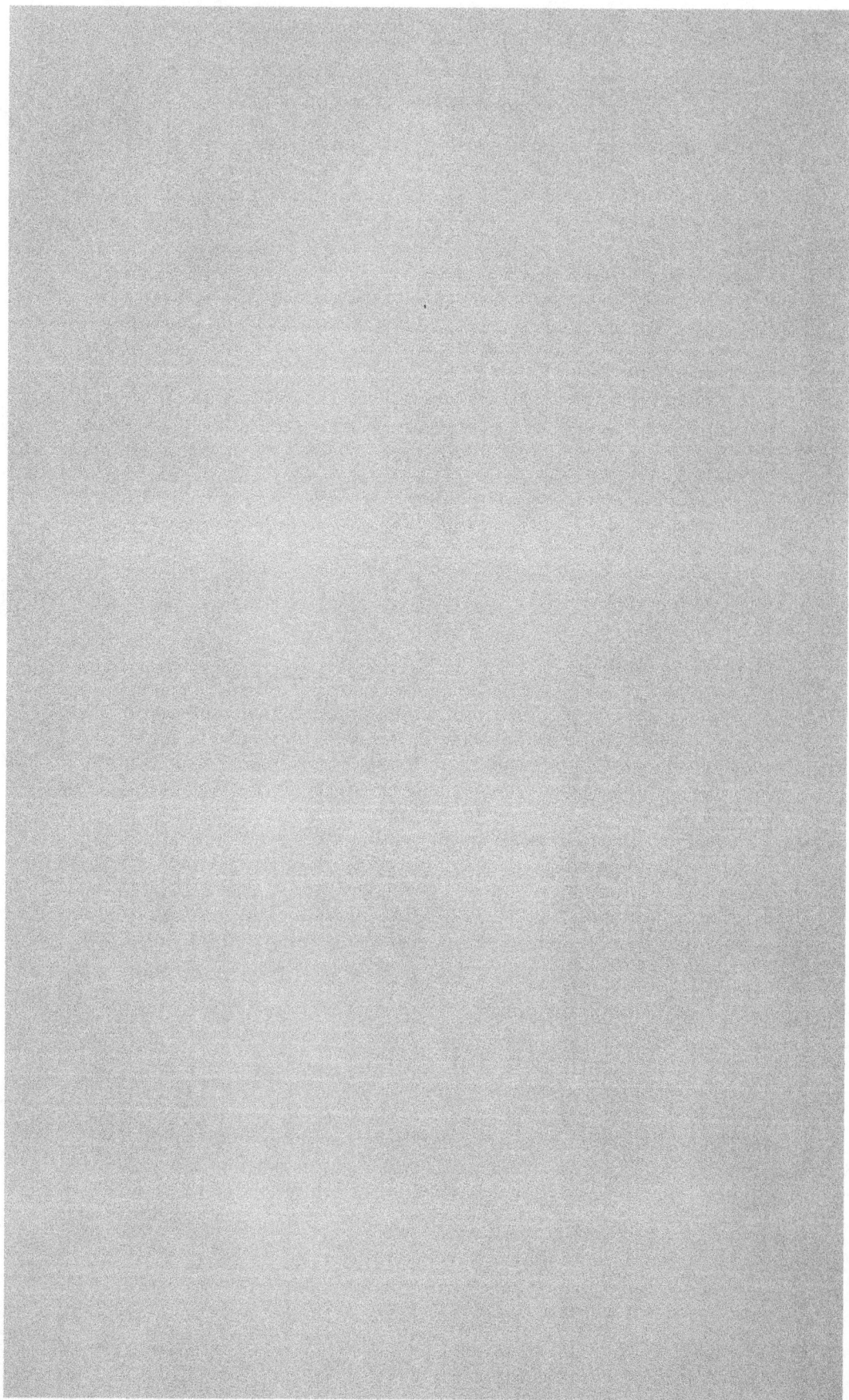

PERITONITIS.

DEFINITION: An acute or chronic inflammation of the peritoneum, localized or general.

CASES: (1) A case diagnosed as septic peritonitis, probably caused by appendicitis, under the care of celebrated Chicago physicians grew steadily worse until death was expected in a few hours. No hopes of recovery were entertained, and it was evident that the best medical treatment was of no avail. As a last resort an Osteopath was finally called, all medical treatment was discontinued, and the treatment began. Immediately, under the treatment, the great pain that had been present for hours at a time, was controlled, and during the next four weeks not two hours' pain in all was experienced. The other symptoms were also controlled, and the outcome was a cure. Spinal lesions were discovered upon examination, and led to inqiury concerning accident, which brought out the fact that the boy had had a serious fall a few weeks before. These were held to be the primary cause of the peritonitis, and treatment directed to them was the cardinal treatment. The fact that the child's life was saved at such a juncture, in disease of such a nature, by the removal of spinal lesion, is a convincing demonstration of the correctness of osteopathic theory and practice.

(2) A second case presenting the ordinary severe symptoms of the disease, and in a state of collapse when seen by the Osteopath, was cured in five days by the treatment.

The LESIONS expected in such cases are to the lower ribs, the lower dorsal and lumbar spine, and sometimes the pelvis. In such cases as are secondary to other disease, such as inflammation in the various abdominal organs, typhoid or diphtheritic ulcer, appendicitis, volvulus, etc., the active lesion in the case must be sought for as the cause of the primary disease. Such lesions may be various.

ANATOMICAL RELATIONS: The nerve-supply to the parietal peritoneum is from the lower intercostal and upper lumbar nerves, which supply also the muscles of the abdominal walls. The abdominal sympathetics also supply the peritoneum, being chiefly vaso-motors for the blood-vessels in the mesentery, but also having certain branches distributed directly to the substance of the peritoneum.

The blood-supply is from the coeliac axis through the hepatic and splenic arteries, and from the blood-supply of the parts with which the various portions of the mesentery are in relation.

The fact that the chief sympathetic supply to the peritoneum is to the blood-vessels in it is a significant one.

The inflammation of peritonitis is a vaso-motor disturbance. It has been before explained how spinal lesion deranges spinal sympathetic connections of the abdominal sympathetics and produces disease. Thus certain lesions among the lower ribs, and along the lower spine, result in derangement of the sympathetic, which, when affecting the peritoneum, becomes a chiefly vaso-motor disturbance because of these peritoneal sympathetics being mostly vaso-motors, and the inflammation results.

In another way, these lesions, affecting the lower intercostal and upper lumbar spinal nerves, may become the active cause of peritonitis. Hilton shows that these nerves, supplying the skin and muscles of the abdominal walls, as well as the parietal peritoneum, probably also supply the visceral peritoneum and send sensory branches through the sympathetic to the intestinal walls. Quain's anatomy shows that from the 9th, 10th, 11th and 12th dorsal nerves, sensory nerves pass through the sympathetic to the abdominal viscera. It also shows that from the thoracic sympathetic and from the lumbar sympathetic cord, vaso-motor fibres of the abdominal blood-vessels take origin. The intimate relation between the spinal and sympathetic nerves is well known. Hilton uses the facts he points out in regard to this connected nerve mechanism to explain why the abdominal walls become painful and contracted from the inward irritation of the inflammation. The connection of this nerve mechanism for all these related parts also explains how lower rib, lower dorsal, and upper lumbar spinal lesions may so interfere with the vaso-motor supply to the peritoneal vessels as to cause peritonitis. This immense abdominal nerve supply, both superficial and internal, spinal and sympathetic, offers the Osteopath, both through its surface distribution, its spinal connections, and its internal distribution, a vast and most readily accessible field for his work by superficial and deep abdominal and spinal treatment. This fact well explains his good results, even in desperate cases, in gaining control of the vaso-motor mechanism which is deranged in this inflammation.

Through the connection of this local vaso-motor mechanism with the vaso-motor system of the whole body, reflex irritation is set up which leads to a general vaso-constriction of the vessels of the whole body surface. Robison thus explains why the whole skin is waxy, pale and cold, saying that the patient, on this account, dies from circumference to center.

Robinson also shows that traumatic action of the left end of the diaphragmmatic muscle upon the gut wall, of the psoas magnus upon the sigmoid, and abrasion of the bowel mucosa at the splenic and sigmoid flexures, very frequently become the causes of peritonitis by allowing the migration and foot-hold of pathogenic bacteria. Spinal, or other specific osteopathic lesion, by causing bad bowel conditions which allow of the possibility of such traumatism may be present, and must be removed in the treatment for, or the prophylaxis of, this disease.

The Prognosis in these cases is fair. Considering that peritonitis patients usually die under medical treatment, in the acute form of the disease, and that operation must frequently be resorted to, the success Osteopathy has had with serious cases is marked.

The TREATMENT must aim at gaining vaso-motor control and thus reducing the inflammation. Lesion must be corrected as soon as possible. The treatment must be both spinal and abdominal. The first step should be thorough but careful relaxation of all spinal tissues. If the patient cannot be turned upon his side, he may continue to lie upon his back, and the operating hand may be slipped under him to work along the spine. Inhibition should be made along the splanchnic and upper lumbar regions, especially from the 9th to 12th dorsal, to quiet the pain through inhibition of the sensory fibres. After spinal relaxation and inhibition, the abdominal treatment will be better borne. Through this spinal treatment effect upon vaso-motor activities is gained by way of the sympathetic connections explained above. This aids in freeing the circulation. During the progress of the treatment of the case the inhibitive spinal treatment may be alternated with a thorough stimulation of the sympathetic connections of the parts involved, to check peristalsis. As soon as possible, thorough general spinal and neck treatment should be given to equalize the general circulation, and to overcome the intense vaso-constriction of all the superficial vessels, so noticeable a feature of the case. Heart and lungs should be stimulated, and inhibition of the superior cervical region be made.

· After spinal inhibition very light abdominal treatment is given. The walls are tense and painful, and much care is required in treating them. The treatment should be gentle, relaxing, and inhibitive, thus relaxing the contractured muscles, aiding general circulation, and decreasing pain. On account of the relation between the nerves of the abdominal walls and those of the inward parts involved, as pointed out above, work upon the abdominal walls has an important corrective effect upon the morbid conditions present internally. The theory that work upon nerve terminals affects parts supplied by connected nerves is well supported by fact. Thus restoration of a relaxed and natural condition of the abdominal walls it an important aid in restoring natural conditions in the parts supplied by these connected nerves. Gradually, deeper work may be done, affecting the abdominal sympathetic locally, increasing circulation and stimulating absorption of the inflammatory effusions and other products. Care must be taken in the treatment over the intestines, as their walls are intensely gorged with blood, and are friable.

The obstinate constipation present is due to pressure from congestion of the bowel walls, and by edema into them, checking peristalsis. As the circulation is restored this condition is corrected, and bowel action can be stimulated by the usual means. The liver, kidneys, and skin should be stimulated to aid in carrying off the effusions and the effete products of the disease. The hiccough is relieved by inhibition of the phrenic nerve (VIII, Chap. III). Treatment for the fever (p. 66), and for the vomiting and tympanites (p. 84) is applied as before directed. The treatment prevents the formation of adhesions, and takes down the thickening of the peritoneum. The patient should be kept quiet in bed, no food should be allowed as long the vomiting occurs. Later a restricted liquid diet is used in small amounts at a time. Cracked ice may be used to allay the thirst. Rectal injections may be necessary to relieve the constipation at first.

The treatment of the chronic case is directed to the gradual breaking down of adhesions; the restoration of circulation to absorb pus or effusion, and to remove the chronic inflammation, and to the relaxation of the abdominal tissues. Correction of the spinal lesion must not be neglected.

Cases of acute peritonitis secondary to other diseases must be treated in conjunction with them. Cases resulting from gunshot wounds and other traumatism are surgical cases. In the acute case the patient should be seen two or three times per day as long as the severe acute symptoms predominate.

JAUNDICE.

DEFINITION:—A condition in which bile is absorbed into the circulation and colors the tissues of the body and the secretions.

CASES: (1) Lesion from overexertion in the form of a "twist" between the 6th and 7th dorsal vertebrae. Jaundice followed immediately after its occurence. (2) 9th and 10th dorsal vertebrae anterior; intense congestion of the deep muscles of the right cervical region; looseness of the 7th cervical vertebra. (3) Catarrhal jaundice following difficult childbirth; extreme tenderness of the spine from the 10th dorsal to the 1st lumbar.

Lesions and causes:—Spinal lesion anywhere along the splanchnic area has been known to produce the disease. Lesion of the lower right ribs is common. Prolapsus of the transverse colon, due to various lesions (see Intestinal Obstruction and Enteroptosis), may obstruct the duct by compression. Various mechanical causes; stricture, gall-stones, parasites, tumors, etc., are well known as causes of obstructed bile-flow, leading to jaundice. The relation of lesion to these causes, osteopathically, is found in the agency of various lesions, whose nature and action are well undersood from discussions in the previous pages, in producing diseased conditions of the gastrointestinal tract leading to the presence of such obstructive agents.

ANATOMICAL RELATIONS:—The relation between spinal and other lesion and abnormal liver conditions have been discussed (see Cirrhosis and Gall-Stones). In catarrhal jaundice, the usual form presented for treatment as jaundice, lesion has occurred in the splanchnic area and is interfering with vaso-motor activity of the gastro-intestinal tract, producing, or allowing other causes to produce, an inflamed condition of the mucous membrane of the gastro-duodenal mucosa and of the mucous lining of the *ductus communis.*

The immediate appearance of jaundice after spinal lesion, as in case 1 cited above, as well as the presence of spinal lesion in other cases of jaundice, favors the probability of direct interference of such lesion with the in-nervation of the gall-bladder and duct. The presence in the sympathetic supply of the liver (hepatic and cystic plexuses. See Gall-Stones) of spinal fibres which, upon stimulation or inhibition of the *splanchnics*, cause con-striction or dilatation of the bladder and ducts; also the fact that stimula-tion of the pneumogastrics constricts the bladder while relaxing the sphinct-er of the opening of the common duct into the duodenum, make it probable that certain lesion to the splanchnic area or to the pneumogastric, directly or indirectly through its sympathetic connections, might so pervert the normal workings of this mechanism as to lead to retention of bile, i. e., a form of obstructive jaundice.

The *Prognosis* is good. The acute case yields immediately to treat-ment. The usual course (two to eight weeks) is materially shortened. In the chronic case, clearing of the tissues from the pigmentation is rather a slow process.

The TREATMENT must look at once to the removal as such active lesion as described above. Mechanical obstructions must be located if possible, and removed by work upon the duct, proceeding upon the lines laid down for the manipulative removal of gall-stones and of intestinal obstructions, q. v, Prolapsus of the intestines and pressure from surrounding organs must be relieved (see Enteroptosis).

In catarrhal jaundice the first step must be to gain vaso-motor control and relieve the inflammation. A peliminary inhibition of the splanchnic area of the spine may be necessary to relieve pain and to gain a degree of relaxation of abdominal tissues before local work is attempted. Next, slow, deep, inhibitive or relaxing treatment is directed to the upper intestinal region and ductus communis. This relieves the inflammation, aids in tak-ing down the swelling of the mucous membrane, and frees the secretion of mucous which may be obstructing the duct. At the same time, treatment of the splanchnics aids in correcting circulation in the parts.

After treatment for the inflammation and relaxation of the duct, the next step is the emptying of the gall-bladder and hepatic ducts. This is done by local manipulation which acts mechanically and by stimulation of the hepatic and cystic plexuses. The patient lies upon his back and the operator stands at the left side; he places the palm of the right hand be-neath the postero-lateral aspect of the lower four right ribs and, while rais-ing them, presses down upon their anterior portions with the right fore-arm. At the same time the left hand makes careful but deep pressure beneath the tip of ninth rib, against the fundus of the gall-bladder. This mechanic-ally empties the liver and ducts. It also stimulates the local cystic plexus to cause constriction of the bladder and ducts.

This same treatment, and the lower costal treatment (V. Chap. VIII). carefully applied, are given to regulate the circulation through the liver and to free it of accumulated bile. The splanchnics should also be thoroughly treated for the circulation. By these treatments the flow of bile is increased, and the system is cleared of it. Thorough stimulation of the kidneys and skin (2d dorsal, 5th lumbar) aids in freeing the blood of the bile acids. This allays the itching. The superior cervical region (medulla) should be inhibited to correct general vaso-motor action. This is for the itching and localized sweating. The bowels and stomach must be treated to relieve the constipation or diarrhoea, and the dyspepsia, as before directed. Other symptoms may be allayed by appropriate treatment.

The diet should be plain, avoiding pastry, starchy, fatty, and saccharine foods. Plenty of water should be drunk; lemonade and alkaline drinks are allowed,

CONGESTION OF THE LIVER,

DEFINITION:—An excess of blood in the vessels of the liver. In active congestion, or acute byperemia, an excess of arterial blood is circulating through it. In passive congestion the liver is engorged by retention of blood in its portal circulation.

The *lesions* already discussed in connection with liver diseases, i. e., these of the splanchnic area and of the lower ribs, interfering with the vaso-motor control of the organ, lead to the congestion. Heart and liver diseases are said to be almost always the causes of passive congestion. The lesions here must be sought according to the case, and treatment made as thus indicated.

The *Prognosis* is good. These cases are usually readily cured.

The TREATMENT is merely one to gain vaso-motor control. Thorough stimulation of the splanchnic area, and solar and hepatic plexuses are important means of accomplishing this. The lower costal and direct liver treatment indicated for jaundice, q. v., are used. Besides directly stimulating the local nerve-mechanism, these treatments, by squeezing the liver and mechanically forcing the blood into and out of it, cause the mechanical action of the blood upon the vessel walls to still further arouse vaso-motor activity. Local treatment should be made upon the liver to stimulate the flow of bile and prevent jaundice. A general spinal, neck, and abdominal treatment aids in correcting general circulation. Treatment for the abdominal vessels aids the work. Inhibiting the splanchnics, solar plexus, and abdominal vessels quiets active congestion by dilating the abdominal vessels and drawing the blood to them.

CIRRHOSIS OF THE LIVER.

DEFINITION: A chronic disease, characterized by an increase of connective tissue in or about the liver.

CASES: (1) Atrophic cirrhosis; a case brought on by social drinking, diagnosed and treated by physicians as such. The first tapping of the ab-domen brought eight and one-half quarts of fluid. The case now came un-der osteopathic treatment and it succeeded so well that a second tapping was delayed some days beyond the expected time. Later a third tapping beceme necessary, but after that none was required. Under the treatment the patient was apparently restored to perfect health.

(2) Diagnosis of cirrhosis; 6th and 7th dorsal vertebrae posterior, 9th to 12th flat; ribs irregular and prominent on left.

(3) Malarial cirrhosis; entire lumbar region bad. 11th rib on each side down.

(4) LESIONS AND CAUSES: The lesions commonly found in these cases affect the splanchnic area, the lower ribs on each side, or the lower right ribs. The latter may cause mechanical pressure and irritation upon the liver. The various lesions weaken the vaso-motor sympathetic supply and lay it liable to the action of special causes of the disease.

In those forms of cirrhosis in which ascites develops, the contraction of the connective tissue causes pressure upon the soft walls of the branches of the portal vein. Upon this account, and because of the low pressure of the blood in the portal system, obstruction soon follows, and ascites results.

The PROGNOSIS must be guarded in all cases. Various cases have been cured, among them even atrophic cirrhosis. In the latter case the prog-nosis is very unfavorable. It is probnble that other forms of the disease can be much benefitted or cured under the treatment in many instances.

The TREATMENT aims at gaining vaso-motor control and thus taking down the inflammatory or congestive process that is allowing of the in-crease in connective tissue. In those forms complicated with ascites as the main symptom, special attention must be given to it as being most immedi-ately dangerous to the patient's liie. (See Ascites.) It is doubtful if con-nective tissue, once formed, could be absorbed by the renewed blood-sup-ply. But the process of its formation could be stopped, the liver substance could be kept softened by thorough work locally over the organ, thus pre-venting hardening and contraction of it, and maintaining freedom of circu-lation through it. In this way danger of ascites could be avoided.

Vaso-motor control is gained by removal of lesion, by thorough stimu-lation of the splanchnic area of the spine, and by local abdominal work over the liver and over the course of the portal vein.

Local work may be done as described in V, Chap. VIII, workieg be-neath the right ribs, directly upon the liver, while the pressure from above upon the ribs, pressing them down upon the liver, alternating with that applied directly to the liver, is an efficient mode of stimulating the organ directly.

In atrophic cirrhosis attention must be given to relieving the conges-tion of the spleen, stomach and intestines present. This is done through treatment of the organs as described in considering diseases of them. In case of the spleen only slight treatment should be made over it locally on account of danger of rupture. Stimulation of the lower splanchnic area and raising the lower four left ribs, together with work upon the solar plexus and the abdominal circulation are sufficient for it. The constipation, gastric catarrh, nausea, vomiting, edema of the lower extremities, etc., are treated as before described.

In biliary cirrhosis, the chief object of treatment is to remove the obstruction to the duct and to empty the gall bladder. (IX, Chap. VIII.) The general corrective treatment for the liver as described is relied upon to soften the new tissue about the small ducts and to prevent its further formation.

In congestive and malarial cirrhosis the chief point is to remove and prevent the congestion. Otherwise the treatment is as indicated for the general case.

In all cases the general treatment outlined, with attention to the special symptoms manifested, should be applied.

In acute cases the patient should be seen daily.

GALL-STONES.

DEFINITION: Concretions in the gall bladder, chiefly of cholesterin due to a pathological process usually caused by spinal lesion to sympathetic nerves in charge of liver functions.

CASES: Very numerous cases of gall-stones, some of them noted, have been successfully treated. It is one of the most common things treated, and in no class of cases have more uniformly good, even striking, results been attained.

The LESIONS found in these cases are usually low down in the splanchnic area, affecting the lower four ribs upon either side, very frequently upon the left, for the spleen. Lesions of the 11th and 12th vertebrae may not be too low to cause it. However, any of those lesions to the ribs and splanchnic area, characteristic of bad gastro-intestinal conditions may, from the nature of the case, affect the liver to produce gall-stones. The liver is innervated from the same nerve supply, gastro-intestinal diseases are usually complicated with deranged liver function, and it is reasonable to find in the usual lesions deranging the activities of the former a sufficient cause for disease in the latter, which, owing to some particular form, degree, or concentration of lesion, results in cholelithiasis.

ANATOMICAL RELATIONS of lesion to disease: The liver is supplied by the splanchnics through the solar plexus, the secondary plexus, the hepatic, in the formation of which the left pneumogastric nerve participates, having special charge of the liver activities. Its branches ramify throughout the liver upon the branches of the portal vein and the hepatic artery, the chief supply being to the latter. The blood-supply from both of these sources is thought to be essential to the activities of the liver cells. The nutrient blood-supply (hepatic) is chiefly supplied by branches of the sympathetic. A cystic plexus of the sympathetic supply is spread upon the gall-bladder and bile-ducts. The American Text Book of Physiology states that special investigation has shown that these nerves are similar in function to vaso-constrictor and vaso dilator nerves, and that stimulation of the peripheral end of the cut splanchnics causes a contraction of the bile-ducts and gall-bladder, while stimulation of the cut end of the same nerve causes reflex di-latation. According to the same investigator, stimulation of the central end of the vagus nerve causes contraction of the gall-bladder and at the same time an inhibition of the sphincter muscle closing the opening of the common bile-duct into the duodenum.

These interesting and instructive facts cannot but be of much signifi cance to the Osteopath. Doubtless he could not avail himself of these de tailed facts to manipulate at will the activities of the biliary apparatus, but spinal and other lesions affecting the sympathetic connections of the organs must be efficient causes in producing abnormal function.

Osler states that any cause, such as tight-lacing, bending forward at a desk, enteroptosis, etc., which produce stagnation of bile favors cholelithia-sis. From an osteopathic standpoint, and in view of the above facts, it is a reasonable conclusion that certain spinal lesion, acting through this nerve-mechanism above described, may cause a stimulated, irritated, or over-ac-tive condition of the dilator fibers of the ducts and gall-bladder, thus maintaining a permanent dilated or sluggish condition of the apparatus, favoring stagnation of the bile and the formation of gall-stones. Likewise one must concede the possibility of lesion to the central end of the vagus nerve, cutting off the normal impulses through the nerve which contract the gall-bladder and relax the sphincter of the common duct, thus allowing of a lack of normal contraction of the bladder and opening of the duct; in other words, favoring a sluggish condition of the biliary apparatus leading to retention and stagnation of bile, thus to cholelithiasis. If any osteo-pathic spinal lesion can interfere with sympathetic viscereal supply, a point placed beyond controversy by demonstrated facts, it is a reasonable con-clusion that spinal lesion to the sympathetic supply to the liver can become the cause of gall-stones in this way.

According to the catarrhal theory of the formation of gall-stones, litho-genous catarrh of the mucosa of the bladder and duct modifies the chemical constitution of bile and favors the deposition of cholesterin about some nu-cleus, such as epithelial debris. Cholesterin and lime salts are produced by the inflamed mucous membrane to form the calculus. As shown above, both the hepatic and portal blood-supply is under control of the hepatic plexus, i. e., of the solar plexus and the splanchnics. According to the American Text-Book of Physiology, stimulation or inhibition (section) of the splanchnics produces at once vaso-constriction or vaso-dilatation of the blood-vessels of the liver.   Here, as in the case gastric or intestinal catarrh, spinal lesion to the splanchnics could disturb vaso-motor equilibrium in the liver and cause catarrh of the mucous membrane.

It is the practice of Osteopaths to give close attention to the condition of the spleen in case of gall-stones.   Important lesions to this organ are often found in such cases (8th to 12th left ribs, A. T. Still)   Removal of this lesion seems to prevent further formation of the calculi.   What influence the spleen naturally exerts upon the liver is not known.   The splenic and superior mesenteric veins unite to form the portal vein.   The abundant venous flow from the spleen is carried directly to the liver in the portal circulation.   The American Text-Book shows that there is little doubt that the materials actually utilized by the liver cells in forming their secretions are brought to them mainly by the portal vein.   The blood which has circulated through the spleen must compose an important part of the blood brought by the portal vein to the liver.   It may be that certain products of splenic activity are useful in maintaining the fluidity of the cholesterin and in preventing the formation of gall-stones.   The spleen is enlarged and tender in this case.

Sensory nerves pass through the sympathetic from the (6th?) 7th, 8th, 9th and 10th spinal nerves (Quain.)   This fact may explain the radiation of the pain in hepatic colic to the spine and right shoulder, and forms a good anatomical reason why inhibition over this spinal region will aid in stopping the pain.

The PROGNOSIS is good, even in serious cases in which operation has seemed advisable.   The case is frequently presented to the Osteopath as the last resort before operation, and results have been almost uniformly good.

TREATMENT: The success of the treatment seems to rest mainly upon the mechanical effect and upon the relaxation of all tissues concerned, gall-ducts included, gained by the use of osteopathic methods.   The main treatment in these cases is locally about the region of the liver; as much of the relaxing and inhibitive treatment, and the main work of removing the stone are done here.   Spinal work is important, as here inhibition for the pain of the colic is made, lesion is corrected, and circulation is stimulated. Nervous control is an important factor in the treatment.   It is gained by both spinal and abdominal work, perhaps alone by the removal of lesion.

The objects of the treatment are: (1) To remove the stone.   (2) To restore normal liver function and prevent further formation of stones.

The former is palliative treatment; the latter is the real cure.

In the acute case, if *colic* is present the first step is to make strong inhibition over the 7th to 10th spinal nerves. (Some say upon the right side.) This will lessen or stop the pain and allow of work upon the abdomen. This is deep, relaxing, inhibitive work upon the tensed abdominal walls, over the epigastric and lower anterior thoracic regions, and over the course of the duct (IX, Chap. VIII.) The pain is usually relieved in a few minutes.

The *stone* is removed by working it along the duct after the preliminary relaxing treatment. The patient should lie upon his back with knees flexed and shoulders slightly raised. The lower ribs are raised by inserting the fingers beneath their anterior edges, and manipulation is made deeply over the site of the fundus of the gall-bladder (tip of 9th rib) and down along the course of the duct. The latter may vary from its course on account of sagging of the intestines sometimes found. This treatment must be thorough and persistent. It should be firmly and deeply, but most carefully applied. Sometimes a few minute's work will pass the stone, but often continued treatment for three-quarters of an hour or an hour must be devoted to it. Only careful manipulation could be borne by the patient for this length of time. As long as the stone remains in the duct and causes the colic the attempt to remove it should be continued, though it may not be advisable to treat continuously all of the time. The stone may or may not be large enough to be felt in the duct. Stones are often passed without pain. Some stones are soft and may be carefully broken down by the treatment.

The *spleen* is treated by careful abdominal work over and beneath the lower left rib, anteriorly. It is chiefly affected by treatment to the splanchnics, raising the lower right ribs (8th to 12th), and removal of lower spinal and rib lesion.

The *janudice*, if intense, indicates impaction of the stone in the common duct. Its cure depends upon the removal of the stone. The kidneys should be kept active.

Fever, if present is allayed in the usual manner. Fatal *syncope* sometimes occurs. If imminent the patient should be fortified against it by thorough stimulation of the heart. For *obstruction of bowel* by calculi, see Intestinal Obstruction.

A *dilaled gall-bladder and duct* are treated locally by manipulation to remove the obstruction as for removal of the stone. Thorough treatment must be given the *liver* locally and thorough spinal treatment must be kept up for the purpose of circulation, etc.

According to Dr. A. T. Still the lesion of the 6th to 10 left ribs found in cases of gall-stones is obstructing pancreatic secretions. These, he says, dissolve gall-stones.

ASCITES.

DEFINITION:—A dropsical condition of the abdomen, due to an accumulation of serous fluid in the peritoneal sac.

The *Lesions* in these diseases are various, as it is commonly a condition secondary to some other disease, as of the heart, lungs, kidneys, liver, etc.

Lesions must be expected according to the nature of the primary disease. If it be due to a local condition, such as obstructed portal circulation (see Cirrhosis of the Liver), peritonitis, q. v., or abdominal tumor, the lesions expected are the ones usually found in these conditions. Lesions in the splanchnic area, the upper lumbar region, and among the lower ribs occur often in these cases as underlying causes, determining the local manifestation of the disease through interference with the sympathetic innervation of the abdominal vessels, as before explained.

The vast area and capacity of the abdominal veins, the ease with which they are dilated, and the relation of the portal circulation to the liver, together with the frequent presence of lesions in the splanchnic and upper lumbar regions of the spine, weakening vaso-motor control of these vessels are no doubt important anatomical factors in determining the dropsy to the abdominal region.

The *Prognosis* in these cases depend upon that for the condition producing the trouble. Generally speaking, it is good except in cases of atrophic cirrhosis of the liver,

The TREATMENT for ascites consists chiefly in the treatment of the disease to which it is secondary. Special lesion as found must be removed. Obstructed circulation must be opened, general abdominal circulation stimulated, and the collateral circulation through the superficial abdominal veins developed. This is accomplished by spinal correction and stimulation of the splanchnic and lumbar vaso-motor areas. The solar and other abdominal plexuses are stimulated, and deep abdominal manipulation is made from below upward along the course of the vena-cava and azygos veins, the portal vein, and the superficial abdominal veins. Thorough stimulation of the liver and portal circulation is the most important factor in the treatment of this condition. (See Cirrhosis of the Liver.) Treatment over the course of the superficial abdominal veins results, in the course of a few treatments, in considerable enlargement of them. As circulation is corrected the dropsical process is checked, and absorbption of fluid already effused begins to take place. Stimulation of kidneys, bowels, and skin aid the process. The distention of the abdomen may considerably hinder the treatment. By laying the patient upon his side, so that the fluid gravitates away from the uppermost side, the latter may be treated by deep manipulation. The patient may then be laid on the other side, and the process be repeated. On account of the accumulation of fluid paracentesis may have to be performed, but ordinarily under osteopathic treatment tapping does not become necessary, except in cases of atrophic cirrhosis of the liver. The lower limbs should be treated to increase circulation in them and to empty their dilated veins.

The patient should be treated daily.

DISEASES OF THE LIVER. Continued.

CASES: (1) Heptic abscess, complicated with gastric ulcer. Lesions at the 3rd cervical, and at the 4th, 5th, and 8th dorsal; rigid spinal muscles; 7th to 10th right ribs overlapped. The case was in a very serious condition, but began to improve after two weeks, and was finally cured by the treatment. (2) A case of hypertrophy of the liver; the organ was restored to normal size and function in one month's treatment. (3) Torpid liver, with chronic gastritis; marked lesion at 4th and 5th dorsal; slight lesion at the 9th dorsal cured.

For HEPATIC ABSCESS the prognosis must be guarded and unfavorable. While limited quantities of pus may be effectually and safely absorbed through increased circulation, any large quantity could probably not be thus disposed of. Some cases have been cured by osteopathic treatment, and there are some chances of curing the ordinary case presented for treatment. The fact that the disease has and can be cured warrants thorough trial.

The TREATMENT must be to absorb the pus and heal the ulcer through increased circulation of the blood. Removal of lesion is naturally the important step in this process, as it is obstructing proper circulation and innervation. The usual lesions in liver diseases must be expected. Full directions have been given for treatment of circulation to the liver. Great care must be taken in local treatment over the liver because of danger of rupturing the abscess. *Pain*, if present, is quieted as before. Attention must be given to the gastro-intestinal disorders; constipation and diarrhoea. As abscess is frequently secondary to some other disease, treatment must be made accordingly in such cases. A bronchial cough, frequently present, may be guarded against by stimulation of the vaso-motors to the lungs.

HYHERTROPHY OF THE LIVER is frequently presented for treatment, and as a rule good results are gotten. Many cases are cured. Many cases cannot, from their nature. be cured. Complete restoration of size and function often results from the treatment. In many other cases, while the size cannot be reduced to normal limits, function is restored. The general prognosis is favorable. In true hypertrophy due to increase of connective tissue the new tissue can probably not be absorbed, but the further increase of it may be checked and the function usually restored.

In true hypertrophy due to increase in size or number of the parenchymatous cells, the treatment may reduce their size or number, and normal size and function of the liver is restored. As the chief causes of true hypertrophy are active and passive congestion (lesion to the vaso-motors), good results follow corrected circulation.

In false hypertrophy due to cancer or abscess, little is expected in the way of reduction. When due to fatty infiltration, the renewed circulation removes the accumulated fatty particles and restores normal size and function. The treatment in these cases consists in the removal of lesion and correction and stimulation of circulation. When secondary, the primary disease is treated.

In fatty degeneration of the liver good results may be expected from the treatment. Recorded facts are lacking, as they are also in regard to amyloid degeneration, cancer, and acute yellow atrophy, of the liver.

SPLENITIS.

DEFINITION: Acute or chronic proliferative inflammation of the spleen. Suppuration may occur.

CASE: Lady, fifty years of age, suffering from chronic inflammation of the spleen. Spleen was much enlarged, and she was unable to wear corsets. Lesion was found in the form of a misplaced rib pressing upon the spleen. Its replacement caused the pain to disappear, and the waist measured two inches less the next morning. The case was cured in one month.

LESIONS occur in downward and forward luxations of the 6th to 12th left ribs. (A. T. Still). Diaphragmmatic lesion thus caused may interfere with position, circulation, or innervation of the organ. Direct pressure of a misplaced rib may irritate the organ, or the rib may, by interference with spinal innervation, cause the trouble.

ANATOMICAL RELATIONS: Stimulation of the peripheral end of the splanchnics causes sudden and large diminution of the volume of the spleen. It is probable that this diminution is due to contraction of its trabeculae and capsule, which are plentifully supplied with involuntary muscle fibres. "The organ is richly supplied with nerve-fibres which, when stimulated directly or reflexly, cause the organ to diminish in volume" (American Text Book of Physiology). According to Schafer, these fibres are contained in the splanchnics, which carry also inhibitory fibres whose stimulation causes dilatation of the spleen.

In view of these facts it seems that treatment over the splanchnic area of the spine and locally over the spleen may produce changes in its volume (through thus directly or indirectly stimulating these nerve-connections) which is most useful in correcting circulation through it. In addition to this, the same work would affect the vaso-motor mechanism of the organ. The splenic plexus, ramifying upon the splenic artery and upon its branches throughout the spleen, is composed of sympathetic fibres from the solar plexus and of branches from the right pneumogastric. Local or spinal treatment affects these. It is readily apparent, in view of the whole mechanism described above, that spinal and rib lesion may seriously affect the organ by disturbance of these nerve-connections, producing inflammatory or congestive conditions.

Anders states that splenitis is probably never primary, but in the case cited above it seems that the disease must have originated primarily in the spleen by action of the disturbance caused by the displaced rib.

TREATMENT: As splenitis and congestion are frequently secondary to some other disease (malaria, typhoid, etc), such disease must be treated primarily. Removal of lesion, as in the above case, may be the only treatment necessary. Stimulation or inhibition of the splanchnics at the spine, and of the capsule and local plexuses by work directly upon the organ, is made. Care must be taken in the latter process to avoid danger of rupture of the organ.

Inhibitive work upon the splanchnics, the solar plexus, and the abdomen will dilate the abdominal vessels and draw the blood to them, away from the spleen.

SPLENIC HYPERAEMIA, active or passive, is readily reduced. Chronic cases may yield at once or may require a patient course of treatment. Contraction of the tissues about the splenic vein has been known to cause great enlargement of the organ by passive congestion. Upon removal of the obstruction the organ quickly returned to its normal limits. The *lesions* and *treatment* are the same as indicated for splenitis.

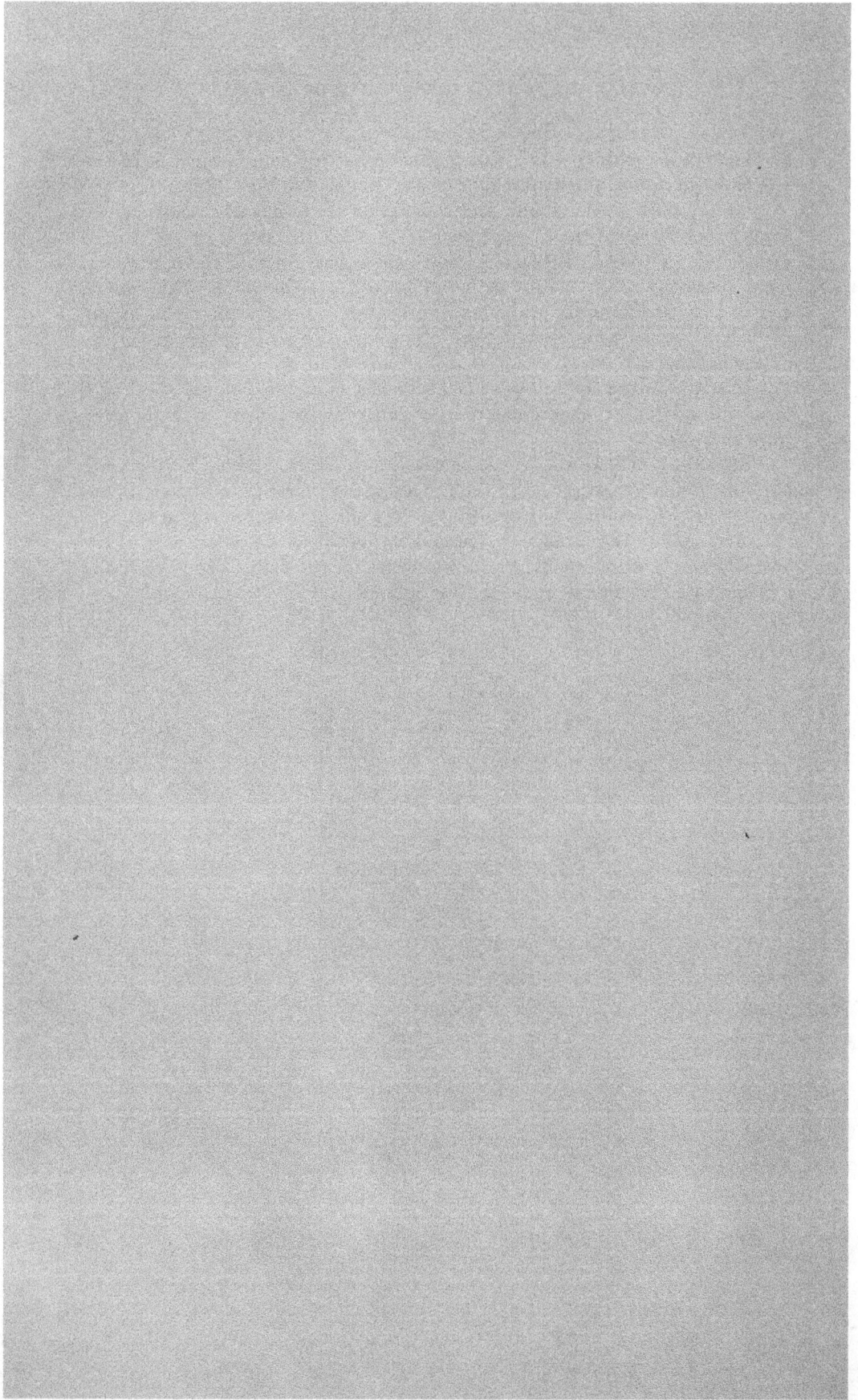

DISEASES OF THE URINARY SYSTEM.

CASES: (1) Lithuria in ′a young girl after typho-malaria. Lesion, a faulty condition of the lower dorsal and lumbar regions. Such quantities of uric acid "sand" appeared as to be easily seen by the naked eye. Dr. A. T. Still found a "hot spot" at the 4th lumbar which was slipped. Also found the 10th right rib off its articulation at its head, interfering with the function of the adrenal bodies. In less than two hours after his treatment normal urine was passed. The previous passage, one half-hour before the treatment, had been cloudy, dark, and contained a heavy precipitate.

(2) Abscess of the kidney and catarrh of the bladder, of three years' standing, in a man. He was obliged to urinate every five or ten minutes, always with great pain. The urine was about one-half sediment and blood, and only about one-half the normal amount. After six weeks' treatment the case was almost well, no pain upon urination; retains urine one hour; practically no sediment; normal amount of urine.

(3) Bright's disease in a mantwenty-nine years of age; diagnosis confirmed by several physicians; great dropsical swelling of feet, limbs and body up to the 12th dorsal vertebra. After five weeks' treatment he was able to go to work at an occupation that kept him constantly upon his feet. After the fourth treatment there had been rapid improvement; in six weeks the urine was almost normal, and the dropsy had disappeared.

(4) Retention of urine from enlarged prostate, and uric acid poisoning, in a man of seventy-three years of age. He was about to be operated upon for "abdominal tumor." The Osteopath used a catheter at once, and drew about a gallon of decomposing urine. The next morning about one quart of urine was drawn, containing much blood and stringy mucous. In three months' treatment the prostate was reduced, and the urination was about normal.

(5) Uremic poisoning (kidney and bladder disease), in which the patient was in a critical condition; had not slept for two days on account of severe pain. In fifteen minutes the pain was relieved by the treatment. Spinal lesion was found at the centers for bladder and kidneys. Great improvement attended one month's treatment.

(6) Chronic Bright's disease after lagrippe. The patient was in a very bad condition, being confined to his room. After five treatments he was able to go out, and was much improved in one month.

(7) Renal calculi, in which operation had been advised. The patient was kept in bed by the great pain of the colic. After two treatments the patient was able to go to the office for treatment, and after a third treatment had no further trouble.

(8) Enuresis. The 5th lumbar vertebra was lateral. The case was entirely cured in six weeks by the removal of this lesion.

(9) Chronic Nephritis (probably) diagnosed as floating kidney. The patient, a lady of fifty-five, was in a very bad general condition; heavy sediment in the urine; painful micturition. Lesions: Upper cervical lateral; posterior curvature from 5th dorsal to 5th lumbar; marked lesion at 10th, 11th and 12th dorsal, and 2d lumbar. The 11th and 12th ribs were subluxated, giving the appearance of tumor, diagnosed as floating kidney. The case began to improve upon the first treatment, and was practically cured in two months.

(10) Kidney disease due to double scoliosis, 6th to 10th dorsal left; 1st to 5th lumbar posterior. Treatment of the curvature improved the kidneys.

(11) Enuresis in a boy of seventeen, of seven years' standing. Occipital pains present. Tissues about 2d cervical tense; about 3d and 4th cervical sore; 7th and 8th dorsal vertebrae anterior and sore. The boy had been thrown from a horse at ten years of age, and the trouble had persisted ever since.

(12) Enuresis in a boy of five, had been present all his life. For four years he had been constantly under medical care. He had no warning of the passage of urine, even in the day time. After eleven treatments but two involuntary passages occurred in eight months. After a recurrence due to an attack of the mumps, two weeks' treatment cured the case. The treatment was given over the sacral and lumbar regions.

(13) Enuresis in a boy of nine. He had been so troubled for eight years during sleep. The usual methods of treatment had been without avail. Great tenderness and a slight lesion occurred at the 2d lumbar, removal of which cured the case.

(14) Enuresis in a boy of twelve who had always had poor health. For eight years nocturnal urination had been constantly present. In the day time the urine passed involuntarily. Lesions were found in the cervical region; pronounced posterior position of the lower dorsal spine; lesions from the 2d to 5th lumbar. Steady improvement took place under treatment, and the case was cured in three months.

(15) Enuresis in a girl of eight cured in five weeks' treatment.

(16) Frequent micturition, varicocele and weak eyes being present. The lesions were at the 3d cervical, lateral spinal curvature, and lesion at the 2d and 4th lumbar.

(17) Acute Nephritis in a man of forty. Lesion was found irritating the renal splanchnics. The treatment was at the 11th and 12th dorsal, and raising of the 11th and 12th ribs.

(18) Acute Bright's Disease, so diagnosed by two physicians. Large quantities of albumen appeared in the urine. The 12th dorsal vertebra was found anterior. One treatment relieved the pain and the patient slept. Good progress was reported.

(19) Acute Bright's Disease. Spinal lesion was found. After seven

weeks' treatment no further symptoms remained. For five weeks a physician examined the urine daily finding no further evidence of the trouble at the end of that time. He said he had never seen a case do so well.

(20) Bright's Disease and Paraplegia; lesion was found as a separation between the 11th and 12th dorsal. There was a history of the patient's having jumped from moving trains for years.

(21) Uremic Poisoning cured by thorough stimulation of the kidneys.

(22) Uremic Poisoning; the case was sleepless, vomiting, and near convulsions. Treatment relieved the case at once.

(23) Enuresis in a boy of five. The lumbar region was very weak, and had a posterior tendency. Treatment here relieved the case.

(24) Renal Calculi. Severe attacks of colic had caused great pain and sleeplessness for three days. Medical treatment for two days was without avail. In the evening of the third day osteopathic treatment was given and the relief was immediate; The patient was out of bed the next morning, and was cured in a few treatments.

(25) Inflammation of the urinary meatus. Constipation was present. There had been congestion of the kidneys one year before. The vertebrae from the 2d to the 5th dorsal were approximated and to the right; those from the 8th dorsal to 3d lumbar were separated. The right innominate was displaced upward and backward, shortening the limb.

(26) Suppression of urine, the patient having not urinated in fifteen hours, was relieved at once by treatment at the renal splanchnics and upper lumbar.

(27) Renal Calculus. Lesion was found at the 11th dorsal. Inhibiting treatment upon the renal splanchnics lessened pain. The calculus was worked along the course of the ureter into the bladder and passed later.

LESIONS: The *centers* of importance osteopathically in urinary diseases are generally stated as follows: 6th dorsal for kidneys; 12th dorsal for renal splanchnics; 2d lumbar for micturition; 3d and 4th sacral for neck and bladder; medulla (sup. cervical, atlas) renal center; 2d to 5th lumbar (Am. Text Bk. Physiol) urino-genital (or genito-spinal) center for bladder; peritoneal sympathetic centers, each side of the umbilicus for the renal plexus; the umbilicus as a landmark for the renal vessels and their sympathetic supply (two inches above.)

The *lesions* usually found in renal diseases are as follows: (1) At the atlas or upper cervical, affecting the superior cervical ganglion and the renal center in the medulla. (2) At the 10th, 11th and 12th dorsal, and the 1st lumbar, the main lesions affecting the kidneys directly. (3) From the 2d lumbar to the 4th sacral for disease in the bladder and urethra. (4) In the female patient it may occur that uterine polapsus, wrinkling the anterior vaginal walls, may twist and obstruct the urethra. (4) In the male patient and enlargement of the prostate gland, especially of its middle lobe, is with considerable frequency found to be the cause, easily overlooked, of stricture of the urethra.

A careful analysis of the lesions in the twenty-seven cases presented above brings out facts representative of this class of cases (urinary diseases.) These facts well illustrate what is usually found in such cases. The lesions are mostly spinal, few being rib lesions; but three of the twenty-seven mention rib lesion. As a matter of fact, spinal lesions are the important causes of urinary troubles. The vast nerve-supply of the kidneys and bladder is delicately balanced. Most of the lesions in renal diseases being spinal, the conclusion is that spinal derangement of this nerve-supply is the most potent and frequent cause of such disease. The kidneys are, at bottom, generally deranged by lesions affecting the nerve-supply, including vaso-motor, i. e. blood-supply, also.

Of these lesions, practically all are low down in the spine, including also the sacral region. Excepting cervical lesion, but one of the above cases mentioned lesion above the 5th dorsal. (This occurred at the 2d dorsal, and was unimportant because of other, lower lesions.) But five showed lesion above the 10th dorsal, and while lesions of some importance occur about the 7th and 8th dorsal, the important lesions all occur lower down.

Eleven of the twenty-seven showed lesion about the 10th, 11th, and 12th dorsal; twenty showed lesion below and including the 10th dorsal; ten showed lesion below the 12th dorsal, i. e., in the lumbar and sacral regions. These latter occur chiefly in bladder and urethral diseases. This is seen in the fact that of the seven cases of enuresis reported, six presented lumbar and sacral lesions. The fact that twenty showed lesion below the 10th dorsal, eleven of them being about the 10th, 11th and 12th dorsal, must be re-marked in considering distinctively kidney diseases. In the cases of Bright's Disease mentioned, all in which the lesion was described showed lesion in the lower dorsal and lumbar regions, practically all of these concentrating about the 10th to 12th dorsal. In nine of these cases the micturition center at the 2d lumbar was affected, participating in both kidney and bladder af-fections. Its anatomical relations make it most important in the latter class, and experience shows that it is more likely to affect bladder than kidneys.

Neck lesion is not important. Only three of the cases showed them, but they occurred at the 2d to 4th vertebrae, where they could all affect the superior cervical ganglion, and through it the medulla. This location of the lesion is mainly important as a secondary or adjuvant lesion in renal diseases.

Without exception, the lesions in these cases fall within areas in which they may affect the sympathetic innervation of the urinary apparatus. It is noticeable, therefore, that only through this nerve-supply could they become the causes of renal disease, even though they should be mainly upon the blood-supply. The vaso-motor function in relation to disease thus has its importance emphasized.

ANATOMICAL RELATIONS: Sensory nerves are distributed through the sympathetic, from the spinal nerves, as follows: To the kidneys from the 10th, 11th and 12th dorsal; to the upper part of the ureter, from the 10th dorsal; at the lower end of the ureter supply from the 1st lumbar tends to appear; to the mucous membrane and neck of the bladder, from the (1st) 2d, 3d and 4th sacral; for sensation of over-distention and ineffectual contraction, from the 11th and 12th dorsal and 1st lumbar (Quain.) This sensory distribution is made use of in relieving spinal pain in kidney and bladder-disease. Disturbed sensations in these parts is usually found associated with lesion in the spinal areas named, generally in connection with more serious trouble.

Vaso-motor fibres for the renal vessel are found in the splanchnics, and somewhat below, occuring from the 6th dorsal to the 2d lumbar nerve. As shown by the American Text Book of Physiology, stimulation of the central endings, not only of the splanchnics, but also of the sciatic, causes constriction of the renal vessels. Thus work upon the spine over the origin of the great sciatic nerve, at the 4th and 5th lumbar, and 1st, 2d and 3d sacral, is useful in controlling the circulation of the kidneys. Actual cases of kidney diseases show spinal lesion as high as the 5th or 6th dorsal, and as low as the 3d or 4th sacral. The continual action of lesion in these situations upon the vaso-motors of the kidneys has most important pathological results through modification of the renal blood-supply. As a rule these lesions are concentrated about the 10th dorsal to 2d lumbar. The main vaso-motor supply, originating as above described, passes from the aortico-renal ganglion, solar and aortic plexuses to the renal plexus. Important branches come from the renal splanchnics, sometimes also from the lesser splanchnic and from the first lumbar ganglion. The branches of this plexus lies upon the renal vessels, and accompany them in their ramifications in the kidneys. Osteopathic work upon this important vaso-motor supply of the kidneys, via the splanchnic area of the spine (by removal of lesion) and the renal plexus, which is reached by abdominal work at the level of the umbilicus, gains marked results upon the circulation, and through it upon the whole metabolism of the kidneys.

The blood-vessels and the muscular coat of the bladder are supplied by the vesical plexus. It consists of numerous nerves from the lower end of the pelvic plexus to the side and lower part of the bladder. The supply to the fundus of the bladder is from the hypogastric plexus. The American Text Book points out that stimulation of the 2nd, 3rd and 4th sacral nerves causes reflex contraction of the bladder. The chief motor fibres of the bladder, probably supplying the longitudinal muscle fibres, pass to the bladder from the sacral nerves. At the same time some of the motor fibres passing to the bladder in the vesical plexus rise in the lumbar nerves and reach their destination via the aortic plexus, inferior mesenteric ganglion and hypogastric and pelvic plexuses. They supply the circular muscle fibres of the bladder and its sphincter.

These facts explain why lower spinal lesion is so often found by the Osteopath to be the cause of motor derangement of the bladder. A good illustration of this is seen in the lack of motor control in enuresis, due as a rule to low lesions. Reference to the case reports above will show that six of the seven cases of enuresis presented lumbar and sacral lesion,

These anatomical facts underlie osteopathic theory of renal diseases. They form a foundation of truth for osteopathic procedure. Lesion to these various important nerve-supplies at their origin along the spine must produce renal disturbance in kind, and this disturbance can be righted only by correction of the anatomical derangement responsible for them.

ACUTE NEPHRITIS.   (Acute Bright's Disease.)

DEFINITION: An acute inflammation of the kidneys, mild or severe, attended by structural changes in the organ..

The LESIONS and ANATOMICAL RELATIONS have been discussed. Lesions occur preferably from the 10th dorsal to the upper lumbar, but may be either higher or lower. Cervical lesions, as low as the 3rd or 4th vertebra, may occur.

The PROGNOSIS is, on the whole, good, still bearing in mind the necessity of guarded prognosis in all renal diseases as above indicated. Considering the seriousness of the disease, it is a matter of remark how many cases of Acute Bright's disease have been apparently entirely cured. Good results are quickly evident under the treatment. The ordinary course of a few days to six weeks is generally shortened.

According to Anders the restoration of the destroyed epithelium and of the glomerular function may occur. The chances of accomplishing the result by the natural method of restored and corrected circulation as brought about by osteopothic treatment would seem of the best. The same author states that in cases due to exposure to cold and wet, irrespective of alcoholic indulgence, it may be presumed with reason that there is some inherent or acquired weakness or a susceptibility of the kidneys rendering them the weak links in the visceral or systemic chain. It is the osteopathic idea that these cases, as a rule, present lesions of the spine of such a nature as to interfere with the vital forces distributed to the kidneys. This, we reason, is the "inherent or acquired weakness or susceptibility of the kidneys that renders their weak links in the visceral chain," and that is the real cause why they fall victims to the various causes ascribed as the active agents in producing the disease. This explains why the poison of acute infectious diseases, as in scarlet fever, producing nephritis in certain cases, has been

able to unbalance the already weakned urinary mechanism. The same explanation holds good for all the ordinary active causes of the disease. It
seems to be the sufficient reason why one person (presumably with spinal
lesion) suffers from the disease while similar circumstances have failed to
cause it in another.

TREATMENT: The general treatment for nephritis, acute and chronic,
have been given with that for congestion of the kidneys, q. v., as stated at
that place. Its object, as stated, is primarily to gain vaso-motor control,
and thus allay inflamation, relieve vascular tension, and, through restored
and corrected circulation, to clear away the debris from the tubules, absorb
the exudates, check degenerative on new growths, and rebuild as far as possible the destroyed or compromised renal epithelium,

Repeated and careful analysis of the urine must be made in all cases of
nephritis for signs of the processes in the kidneys as directed in standard
medical texts.

In *Acute Nephritis*, aside from the main treatment already discussed,
the practitioner must direct his work to the alleviatian of many of the manifestations of the disease. The general treatment will allay many of the
symptoms at once; others may call for special attention. Uremic symptoms,
such as nausea, vomiting, headache, and pain in the back are treated as before directed. For the latter, relaxation of the spinal muscles and inhibition of the sensory nerves (10th to 12th dorsal.) Convulsions are quieted by
inhibitive spinal treatment and by inhibition of the centers or local nerve-
supply for the affected part. The dropsy is relieved by the stimulation of
the general circulation brought about by the general treatment. It is aided
by local treatment of the venous flow from the part affected, e. g., treatment
of the long and short saphenous veins, relaxation of the tissues about the
saphenous opening, and raising the intestines from the femoral veins, in
edema of the lower extremities. Suppression, if it occur, yields at once,
generally, to thorough stimulation of the kidney. The lungs must be stimulated against the occurrence of bronchitis or pneumonia. Perspiration may
be excited by thorough stimulation of the spinal system, heart, and lungs.
It is a necessary measure for the relief of the system from the accumulated
poisons. As a rule, it is readily accomplished by this treatment. Failing
of this, recourse should be had to the hot baths, applications, packs, and the
use of vapor, as described in medical texts,

The *hygiene and diet* of nephritis patients is a most important matter.
These should be carefully looked after according to directions laid down in
standard works.

The patient with acute nephritis should be treated once or twice daily.
More treatment, or less, may be given as the practitioner's judgment dictates.

In CHRONIC EXUDATIVE NEPHRITIS AND CHRONIC NON-EXUDATIVE NE-
PHRITIS the practitioner must be constantly upon his guard. A fair number
of cases of chronic nephritis have been cured or greatly benefited. In the

fomer, the *prognosis*, while guarded, is fair. The patient may be cured, or be helped to enjoy a prolonged and comfortable life. In these cases the practitioner may be thrown off his guard by the fact that the disease may have arisen insidiously without having presented marked symptoms.

In the non-exudative form the prognosis must be unfavorable, owing to the very serious pathological changes that have taken place in the organ. Perhaps much can be done for the comfort of the patient. The slow progress of the case renders thorough treatment useful. The patient may be helped to a long and comfortable life.

Concerning *lesions* and *treatment*, little need be added to what has already been said. Special manifestations of either form may call for special treatment. One must sustain the entire system, and be continually upon his guard against a sudden bad turn in the case, or intercurrent maladies or complications. The retinitis may call for some treatment of the eye locally and through the cervical sympathetic and blood-supply.

Concerning hygiene and diet, the same remark applies as for acute nephritis.

Chronic cases should be treated daily or three times per week, according to the needs of the individual.

CONGESTION OF THE KIDNEYS.

In both acute or arterial hyperemia and chronic or venous hyperemia a good PROGNOSIS can, generally speaking, be expected. This must, however, be *guarded* in all cases, especially in the chronic venous congestion secondary to heart and lung diseases. As both of these conditions of congestion of the kidney are secondary to other diseases, and as each may precede inflammation (acute or chronic) of the kidney, much care must be taken in prognosis and treatment. When the condition is secondary the prognosis must depend upon that for the primary disease. Yet, even though a favorable prognosis is limited by such circumstances, good results are generally gotten upon the kidneys. They are very responsive to treatment; it is usually readily effective in producing good effects. While keeping in mind the difficulties presented by renal cases as a class, we can yet expect improvement under the treatment. Yet, the prognosis for cure is always to be guarded.

The LESIONS for kidney diseases have been discussed above. In cases of congestion specific lesion is expected in the vaso-motor area, 6th dorsal to 2nd lumbar. In cases secondary to other disease the lesion is that producing such disease, though auxiliary lesion to the kidney is often present and has weakened the organ preliminarily to its being thus affected. Though cold and exposure, the toxic products of various acute diseases, and other causes may produce congestion directly, it is still necessary in most cases to account for such agents especially attacking the kidneys, to account for the disease settling upon them. There can be no doubt that in very many cases it is the presence of spinal lesion which determines the disease to the kidneys. This hypothesis not only accounts for the frequency with which spinal lesions are found in such cases, but also explains why one person may become the victim of kidney disease while another under a similar set of circumstances escapes. These general remarks apply with equal force to the subject of nephritis next considered.

The TREATMENT has for its object the correction of the vaso-motor disturbance evident as congestion of the kidneys. It gains vaso-motor control both directly, by treatment to the kidneys, and indirectly, if necessary, by the treatment of the disease to which the congestion is secondary. In the latter case the main treatment must be directed to the primary disease. The spinal lesion to the kidneys must always be removed.

Treatment to gain vaso-motor control is made directly upon the vaso-motor innervation of the kidneys. This consists (in addition to the removal of the lesion obstructing them) of spinal stimulation from the 6th dorsal to the 2nd lumbar, for the vaso-motor fibres to the kidneys originating in this spinal area. This includes the whole splanchnic area. As stimulation over the central ends of the splanchnics and of the great sciatic is known to cause renal constriction, it is well to carry this spinal stimulation down over the origin of the sciatic nerve, including the 4th and 5th lumbar and the upper three sacral.

This treatment for the circulation is aided by direct work over the region of the kidney. Deep pressure, with a spreading motion, applied at the umbilicus and about two inches above it, stimulates the peritoneal nerve-centers said to exist at each side of the umbilicus, it also reaches the renal and supra-renal plexuses and aortico-renal ganglion, lying upon the aorta and renal vessels, the plexus ramifying the kidney upon the blood-vessels. This treatment further affects the renal vessels mechanically, and relieves it of tension in the surrounding tissues.

The spinal treatment should be applied especially to the region of the lesser and renal splanchnic. In these various ways the kidney circulation is equalized and the inflammation or congestion is reduced.

To aid in calling the blood from the kidneys and in equalizing the general body circulation, general deep inhibitive work is made over the abdomen to call the blood to its vessels; a general spinal and neck treatment, particularly directed to stimulation of heart and lungs and to the inhibition of the superior cervical ganglion, tones the general circulation and relieves blood-tension (through the superior cervical).

A valuable spinal treatment for stimulation of the kidneys is performed with the patient lying on his back. The practitioner's hands are slipped palm up beneath the back, one on each side, in the region of the innervation of the kidneys. Now as the fingers are bent at the metacarpo-phalangeal knuckles, making a fulcrum of the latter upon the table, the cushions of the fingers are pressed deeply into the spinal tissues, the weight of the patient is raised by the fingers thus applied, and the tissues are drawn laterally away from the spine. Quick repetetion of this movement a number of times thoroughly manipulates the tissues and stimulates the nerve-connections of the kidneys.

The bowels and skin should be kept free and active by treatment as before described.

The treatment thus described applies not only to congestion of the kidneys, but to nephritis, next to be discussed.

In both forms of congestion of the kidneys the case must be carefully looked after to obviate the danger of its passing into inflammation, acute hyperemia tending to acute nephritis, the passive congestion tending to become chronic nephritis.

The patient should be kept quiet, resting in bed, and upon a liquid diet, in active hyperemia. In venous congestion a light diet must be followed. The patient should drink plenty of pure water. Hot baths and hot applications over the kidneys, may, if necessary, be used with advantage. In the acute form the patient should be seen daily; more than one treatment per diem may be necessary. In the venous form daily treatment should be given.

RENAL CALCULI.

DEFINITION: Fine or coarse concretions in the substance of the kidney or in the renal pelvis resulting from precipitation of the solid constituents of the urine. It is due to spinal lesion which disturbs the normal secretory activities of the kidney and leads to the deposition of certain substances.

The LESIONS AND ANATOMICAL RELATIONS have been discussed under the general consideration of renal diseases. Lesions from the 10th dorsal to the 1st lumbar, including those of the lower two ribs, are the most frequent in these cases. No pathognomonic lesion has been located for this condition. From the nature of the case, any lesion interfering with the proper innervation and circulation of the kidney might so interfere with normal secretions as to render them disproportionate or excessive as to certain constituents. Whether the stone be of uric acid or urates, of calcuim oxalate, phosphates, or some other substance, it is clear that some cause is operating which prevents the natural proportions of the renal constituents from being maintained. While, as Anders states, the causes are not well known, the osteopathic view is that the real cause is found in spinal lesion which deranges the vital forces underlying kidney activity. It is as reasonable that spinal lesion should unbalance the delicate sympathetic nerve-mechanism controlling these organs, leading to disproportionate or excessive secretion of the urinary constituents and the precipitation of the stone, as that spinal lesion should in a similar way disturb intestinal secretion and lead to diarahoea.

The PROGNOSIS is good, both for the removal of the stone and for the prevention of its further formation. Immediate relief is usually given in the case of renal colic, and the case is entirely cured under the treatment. The treatment of these cases is uniformly successful.

The TREATMENT has as its object the removal the stone and the correction of the metabolism of the kidney to prevent stones being formed again. The stone may be removed in one of two ways: Correction of the activities of the organ will lead to disintegration of the stone. Renal secretions dissolve kidney stones. (A. T. Still.) Stones too large to pass, formed by the precipitation of insoluble substances, necessitate operation. This corrective work embraces the removal of lesion, and general stimulation of controlling nerves and circulation. This is accomplished by both spinal and local abdominal treatment as before described in the treatment of the kidney. Under this restorative process normal urine is secreted and the stone is dissolved.

This same procedure would prevent the formation of more calculi. It would be efficient in all cases, and should be administered to cases passing renal sand or gravel without pain as a prophylactic against worse conditions, and to cure the case. It corrects those conditions favoring precipitation; lessens the ascidity of the urine, dispels the uric acid, increases the salines, etc.

The stone may also be removed by manipulation of it along the ureter and into the bladder. The practitioner is generally called to these cases during an attack of renal colic. Under these conditions the first step is to allay the usually extreme pain. First, spinal inhibition is to be made. As the sensory innervation is through the sympathetic, from the 10th dorsal for the upper part of the ureter, while at the lower end the 1st lumbar probably supplies the structure, strong inhibition (as in diarrhoea) must be made. As the pain spreads, and is very likely to extend down the spine to the testacle or inner side of the thigh, it is well to carry the inhibitation from the middle dorsal down over the sacrum. After this treatment obdominal work is better borne. This is a very deep, firm, but not rough, treatment over the course of the ureters. It is slow, inhibitive and relaxative, thus helping to quiet the pain and relaxing the ureter for the passage of the stone. This relaxation may be aided by inhibition of the inferior mesenteric, spermatic, and pelvic (lower hypogastric) plexuses. This treatment aids the ureter to pass the stone by mechanically working along. It should be begun at a point about two inches above and two inches externally from the umbilicus and progress diagonally downward and inward to the promontory of the sacrum and as far below it as possible This treatment reaches the ureter by deep pressure of the overlying tissues down upon the ureter. It must be very deep, but slow and with the careful avoidance of any violence. Usually the stone is readily passed under the treatment, but some cases require nearly continuous treatment for a considerable time, three-quarters of an hour or more. If possible, treatment should not be stopped until the stone is passed. Treatment afterwards over the sore parts may be necessary. The patient's system should be stimulated against syncope or collapse by treatment of the heart, lungs, and cervical region.

The patient should be directed to avoid red meats and those articles of drink and diet favoring uric acid. He should lead a temperate life, taking moderate exercise. The drinking of lemonade, soda-water, and plenty of pure water is a valuable aid and in keeping the kidneys flushed and free.

PYELITIS, if present, must be treated (aside from the removal of the stone from the pelvis) as the inflammatory conditions of the kidney before discussed.

MOVABLE KIDNEY (Nephroptosis, Dislocated Kidney,) may be successfully treated by osteopathic means if it has not that extreme degree of mobility known as "floating kidney." Movable kidney is the term designating the condition in which the upper end of the organ may be pushed down to the level of the umbilicus. The lesions, so far as this condition may be traced to them, are of the sort producing enteroptosis, q. v. There is usually present a slight curvature ofthe dorso-lumbirspine (McConnell). A bid spinal condition, or a definite single lesion, compromises blood and nerve-supply of the organ and its related tissues, weakens the tissues and vessels supporting it in place, and allows of a prolapsus of the organ directly or by allowing other causes to operate. Thus it occurs as a part of enteroptosis, or from falls, heavy lifting, straining at stool, etc. Spinal lesions causing relaxed abdominal walls, also repeated pregnancies producing the same result, favor mobility of the kidney. Lesions and diseases leading to extreme emaciation and consequent wasting of the fatty tissues of the capsule of the kidney may cause this condition, as may also tight lacing.

.TREATMENT: From the nature of these causes it may be seen that one's chances of curing a moderate degree of movable kidney are good, the causes being removable. Much the same treatment would be given as for enteroptosis. The removal of spinal lesion, spinal treatment to restore tone to the support-ing tissues, local treatment at the kidney to mechanically replace it and to re-move the tenderness and swelling in it due to twisting of the renal vessels, and abdominal treatment to restore tone in the surrounding and supporting tissues would all be useful. In cases suffering from extreme emaciation attention should be given to the general health and to incrersing the nutrition of the body. Abdominal supporters and pads should be gradually laid aside, the abdominal muscles being toned to act in their stead. The neurasthenia and general nervous symptoms, indigestion, palpitation, irritable bladder, etc., call for general treatment of the nervous system coupled with special treatment for any particular troublesome manifestation.

The patient should have plenty of rest lying down, and should avoid over-exertion, overeating, straining at stool, etc.

CYSTITIS.

DEFINITION: An acute or chronic inflammation of the mucous membrane of the bladder.

LESIONS AND ANATOMICAL RELATIONS: Lumbar and sacral lesions pre-dominate in bladder troubles. The urino-genital center occurs in the spine from the 2nd to 5th lumbar, while the sensory nerve-supply to the mucous membrane and neck, of the bladder, is derived from the (1st) 2nd, 3rd and 4th sacral. The vescical plexus is derived from the lower end of the pelvic plexus and supplies vaso-motor fibres to the blood-vessels of the bladder. Through the pelvic plexus it is in connection with both lumbar sympathetic and sacral nerves, hence may be subject to the effect of lumbar or sacral lesion, acting to derange the blood-supply of the bladder. Such lesion weakens this circulation and renders the bladder liable to the action of various causes to produce the cystitis. In this way cold or exposure could cause the condition. Through lesion to the motor nerves of the bladder (see Enuresis) a paresis of the bladder walls may be caused, leading to cystitis. An enlarged prostate may cause pressure upon the bladder and retention of urine, leading to the disease. Traumatism, such as the careless use of catheter or sound, irritation of fecal matter or, of a stone in the bladder, or from a pregnant uterus, may be a suf-ficient cause. This is also true of septic causes of cystitis; the introduction of an unclean catheter, the poisonous products of febrile diseases, of gonorrhoea, etc., becoming direct causes of the condition. Yet in many of such cases the weakness of parts due to spinal lesion precedes and predisposes to the trouble. Also lesion is often the direct cause of the condition leading to cystitis, as in inflammation of the surrounding organs; vaginitis, urethritis, etc.

The TREATMENT is to restore normal circulation. It is upon that part of the spine pointed out above as related directly to the vaso-motor innervation of the bladder. Lesion in these areas must be removed. Such treatment is often followed by great relief at once. Local abdominal treatment over the course of the internal iliac venis aids in reducing the inflammation. The abdominal treatment must be carefully applied. It may be made over the hypogastric plexus to aid in controlling the circulation. It should be inhibitive. Inhibitive and relaxing treatment aids in quieting the pain and vesical irritability. It also calls the blood to the abdominal vessels, away from the bladder. An enlarged prostate must be reduced, (Chap. IX. D.) and mechanical irritants must be removed if possible.

For the pain and irritation of the bladder, strong inhibition should be made from the 1st lumbar down, especially over the 2nd, 3rd and 4th sacral nerves. For the vesical and rectal tenesmus, stimulation of the lumbar, and especially of the sacral region should be made after the pain is allayed.

The patient should remain lying down, as it is said that then the intravesical pressure is but one-third as great as in the erect position. The diet should be simple, avoiding highly seasoned foods and alcohol. In the early stages a milk diet is recommended. The patient should drink freely of water for internal irrigation of the bladder. Treatment should be given to keep active the cutaneous circulation (2nd dorsal, 5th lumbar, superior cervical). This is aided by general spinal treatment, by friction of the skin, and by bathing. The bowels must be kept open and the kidneys free. The usual treatments should be given for this purpose. Hot sitz baths and hot applications may be employed to relieve the pain in the intervals between treatments, if necessary.

The patient should be treated once or twice daily.

In the *chronic case* the prognosis is fair, but guarded. Treatment should proceed along the lines laid down above. In this form, and in septic cystitis, washing out the bladder is a valuable aid to the treatment. For the chronic case boiled water, sterile normal salt solution (40-60 gr. to a pint), or a weak solution of mercuric chlorid (1: 50,000 or 100,000) are recommended. For septic cases, a Saturated solution of boric acid may be used.

ENURESIS, (Incontinence of Urine).

DEFINITION: Inability to retain the urine. A neurosis due to sacral or lumbar lesion which so affects the motor nerve mechanism of the bladder as to result in lack of control.

LESIONS AND ANATOMICAL RELATIONS: The lesions usually occur in the lower lumbar and sacral regions. They have been discussed in the beginning of the chapter on renal diseases (see ante). Frequently some single lesion, as of the 2nd or 5th lumbar, is found, the removal of which cures the case at once. A common lesion is weakness and posterior position of the whole lumbar spine. Quite often lower dorsal lesion is found.

As the vescical plexus supplies the muscular coats of the bladder, and as it is in connection, through the pelvic plexuses, with both the lumbar and sacral nerves, lesions of these portions of the spine may readily affect the motor activities of the bladder. This becomes more evident in the light of the fact that the motor fibres of the circular muscles and sphincter of the bladder are derived from the lumbar portion of the sympathetic, by way of the aortic plexus, the inferior mesenteric ganglion, the hypogastric and pelvic plexuses. On the other hand, the sacral nerves furnish the chief motor supply to the longitudinal muscle fibres of the bladder. (Quain.) The American Text Book of Physiology states that stimulation of the sacral nerves (1st, 2nd, 3rd and 4th) causes a reflex contraction of the bladder. It is evident that lumbar and spinal lesion may directly affect this nerve-supply. The lesion involving the sphincteric center of the bladder; the paralytic incontinence; the imperfect vescical innervation and paresis of the walls from over distention; the spasmodic incontinence due to over action of the compressor muscle of the bladder, may all arise from spinal lesion as described occuring at certain or various points in the lumbar and sacral regions. This lesion may cause a stoppage of nerve-supply, resulting in a paralytic condition, or an irritation of the bladder. The anatomical relation between lesion and disease is clear in this case.

The PROGNOSIS is good. Very many cases have been successfully treated. Generally quick results are attained. In some cases a few treatments cause immediate lessening of the trouble.

TREATMENT: The relation of lesion to disease is so close in this disease that the first step is to remove the lesion. This may be all the treatment necessary. A thorough stimulation of the lumbar and sacral region affects the nerve-connections explained above and tones the motor mechanism of the bladder. Spasmodic conditions call for thorough inhibition of these regions. Corrective spinal work restores normal conditions and allows Nature to attend to the result. Abdominal treatment over the hypogastric plexus and over the internal iliac vessels aids the case. When the condition is due to a postrating disease the treatment must be directed as well to the upbuilding of the system. A prolapsed uterus must be replaced, and other irritating causes removed. Among the latter may be intestional worms, an elongated prepuce, etc. Circumcision is advisable in the latter case. In neurotic children treatment must be given to the general nervous system.

Note:—A case of kidney trouble is reported in which insufficiency of urine was overcome solely by stimulation of the superior cervical ganglion. A renal center exists in the medulla. The treatment trebeled the amount of the urine.

No other treatment was given.   Probably the general systemic vaso-constriction set up by stimulation of the general vaso-motor center in the medulla, through the treatment of the superior cervical ganglion, supplied the increased blood-pressure and arterial tension in the kidneys necessary, under the circumstances, to the activity of the organ.

DISEASES OF THE HEART AND CIRCULATORY SYSTEM.

As in considering the disease of the urinary system, a number of cases are here noted for their value in showing various facts in regard to the practice upon cases of this class.   They show either important lesion, the removal of which cured the disease; quickness of results gained by osteopathic treatment in serious or long standing cases, unrelieved by other methods of treatment; and something of the variety and range of the practice in these cases.   These reports, as far as they go, are typical of the practice.   They are not, however, presented as model case reports, nor as representing the whole field of practice in diseases of this class.

CASES: (1) Impeded heart-action, resulting from a fall causing spinal injury and nervous shock.   The marked lesion was found at the atlas.

(2) Fatty degeneration of the heart.   The patient was too weak to walk; the action of the heart was very weak; arrhythmia was present; great dropsy of the lower limbs prevailed.   The patient could sleep only by kneeling over a couch with the chest supported by pillows.   This position relieved irritation from the lesion.   Lesion was marked; there was great contracture of the muscles from the atlas to the 6th dorsal, especially marked in the upper dorsal region.   The patient was very round-shouldered.   These causes caused a drawing together of the sternal ends of the ribs, and lessened the cavity of the chest, allowing of less room for the heart's action.   For two weeks the patient was treated daily, and could then lie down to sleep. After one month he could walk a quarter of a mile to the office for treatment and return unaided.   At the end of a three month course of treatment he returned home to work, and was well two years later.

(3) A case of extreme palpitation was relieved in fifteen minutes.

(4) Great palpitation of the heart, due to marked spinal curvature in the upper dorsal and cervical regions, came upon the patient frequently.   Such an attack was usually treated medically with digitalis and kept the patient in bed for several days.   Osteopathic treatment always relieved the patient of such an attack in a few minutes and the patient could go about her usual duties.   It was a common occurence in this case to slow the heart-beat as much as twenty beats per minute, this effect not being transient, but lasting for several days.

(5) Arrhythmia and a general bad condition of the health; lesion of the

4th left rib; slight lateral lesion of the fifth lumbar vertebra. The latter was probably responsible for uterine trouble present, which may have influenced the heart. After two months' treatment the heart-beat was almost normal.

(6) Palpitation; a smothering sensation had occurred for many years when the patient lay down. This was accompanied by pain in the heart. The case so improved in three weeks under treatment that the patient could with impunity drink coffee and smoke tobacco, whereas these articles had been quite interdicted to him by his previous condition.

(7) A case variously diagnosed as valvular lesion, hypertrophy, angina, pectoris, etc., was cured in one month by osteopathic methods.

(8) Marked arrhythmia, with nervousness and insomnia, was so bene-fitted in four treatments that the heart action became normal. Without further treatment its normal action still continued two months later.

(9) Arrhythmia, in which the patient was very weak. The left 5th rib was down upon the 6th and slightly inward. The cervical and upper thoracic spinal muscles were very much contracted. The treatment was directed to raising the rib and relaxing the contractured muscles, and resulted in regulat-ing the heart-beat in six weeks.

(10) A case of chronic endocarditis, given up by medical practice, was cured in six weeks under osteopathic treatment.

(11) Bad palpitation, of several years' standing, was cured in three months.

(12) Palpitation and a complication of diseases; lesion found at the atlas and in the upper dorsal spine. No palpitation occurred after the third treat-ment.

(13) A case of valvular weakness reported cured in three months.

(14) Enlargement of the heart, mitral and aortic incompetence, and re-gurgitation showed lesion in forward displacement of the atlas, lesion of the left clavicle and upper two or three left ribs. Three treatments produced much improvement, one months treatment corrected the arrhythmia, and constant improvement went on under treatment.

(15) A case of palpitation of the heart, with goitre, uterine disease, etc., presented contracture of the spinal muscles. The clavicles were both down and backward at the sternal end; there was lesion of the 1st right rib and of the 2d left rib; also a general dropping of the ribs which narrowed the chest cavity. Lesion affected the 1st and 2d lumbar, and the pelvis was tilted. In six months all lesions were corrected, and the case showed marked improve-ment.

(16) Palpitation of one years' standing, attending a physical or mental exertion. Sub luxation of the fifth rib was discovered. It was removed in one treatment, and the patient suffered no further trouble.

(17) Angina pectoris after lagrippe; spinal muscles contractured; the 3d to 5th ribs displaced downward. The case was cured in one month.

(18) Angina pectoris showing lesion of the 2d to 5th left ribs. The left

arm could not be raised above the head without extreme pain. Under treatment the pains became gradually less severe, until they had practically ceased at the end of two months.

(19) Pericarditis cured by correction of rib lesions.

(20) Angina pectoris, caused by downward displacement of the left clavicle, and cured by its correction.

(21) Functional weakness; sinking spells occurred upon any exertion, as in climbing stairs. The left thorax was found depressed; the left clavicle was displaced downward at its sternal end, while it was up and forward at its acromial end. All the ribs were crowded together. Relief followed the first treatment, and the case was cured in five weeks.

(22) Cardiac dilatation. In one treatment the pulse was reduced from 140 to 110, and at the end of one month it was 80. Fainting spells, frequent before, did not occur after the first treatment.

(23) Varicose veins and milk leg of fifteen years standing. The tissues surrounding Hunter's canal and the saphenous opening were tense, and the lumbar vertebrae were anterior. An operation had been advised, but the case had been practically cured under osteopathic treatment at the time of the report.

(24) Varicose veins of eight years' standing. Three varicose ulcers were discharging when treatment began. Innominate lesion was discovered. The case was cured in five weeks.

(25) Varicose veins, for which operation had been made without success. The patient was compelled to sit with the limb elevated, and had been thus for five months. The physicians found they could do nothing more, and recommended continued elevation. One month of osteopathic treatment cured the case.

(26) Weakness of the heart of three years' standing. The patient was unable to climb stairs, and had to be assisted to the office for the first treatment. The usual treatment, raising the ribs, gave immediate relief. The patient came alone for the second treatment, and was cured in two weeks.

(27) Varicose veins of two years' standing. Severe and continuous pain in the limb prevented sleep. The muscles over the sacrum and the lower lumbar vertebrae were rigid. In one month of treatment the case showed great improvement.

(28) Disturbed circulation, in which the superficial capillaries of one side of the body were flushed, reddening the skin, while the other half of the body was pale. The line of demarkation between the halves of the body was very prominent. This trouble had come upon the patient as the direct result of a hard bicycle ride. Lesion was found at the fifth lumbar, and its correction cured the case.

(29) Disturbed circulation. The patient had accidentally received a hard blow upon the head, and intense pain developed upon one side of the head. She was unable to turn her head without turning the whole body. If she lay

upon the injured side great pain followed. This condition was of five years' standing. Examination showed a strong contraction of the deep muscles of the neck, which set up irritation of the local sympathetic, affecting the vaso-constrictor fibres of the side of the head in question, causing over-contraction of the vessels, setting up the pain. Treatment was directed entirely to the contractured muscles and in five weeks' time overcame the trouble entirely.

LESIONS: In seeking the lesion and in giving the treatment in cardiac diseases, certain *centers*, prominently connected with the normal activities and pathological manifestations of the heart, must be specially examined for lesion. These centers, given below, do not always relate to specific anatomical or phys-iological centers of the texts, but in some cases refer to bony points become prominent in osteopathic work as locations of lesion or of places where treat-ment produces special results. These are: the first rib (heart flutter); cor-pora striata; 1st, 2d, 3d, 4th, 5th dorsal vertebrae; 2d to 4th dorsal (valves of the heart); 3d and 4th cervical (rhythm of the heart); superior cervical gang-lion (a sympathetic center); upper four or five dorsal nerves, especially the 2d and 3d (accelerator center); medulla (general circulatory.)

General vaso-motor centers which, with the special vaso-motor innerva-tion of a given viscus; suffer from lesion in circulatory disturbances; superior cervical ganglion; 2d dorsal, 5th lumbar, for general superficial capillary circu-lation.

The *lesions* usually present in cardiac disease are: (1) of the atlas and axis; (2) the cervical region generally, both muscular and bony lesion. Les-ions of the atlas, axis and cervical region affect the superior cervical gang-lion and the other sympathetic supply of the heart. (3) Lesions of the clav-icle are found, as are those, (4) of the 1st rib, (5) of the 2d rib, (6) of the upper six ribs, especially on the left side, (7) of the upper five dorsal verte-brae, (8) as a change in the general shape of the thorax, (9) of the fifth left rib in particular, (10) of the diaphragm. i. e., of the lower six ribs, any or all of them, and of certain portions of the spine. (p. 96.)

Lesions were reported in twenty of the above twenty-nine ctses. This number of case reports is too meagre to be used as the basis of conclusive proof as to lesions in the disease, yet an analysis of the cases presents facts typical of those pertaining to general practice in this line. From this stand-point they are instructive.

Five of these twenty cases reporting lesion were not cardiac disease. In thirteen of the fifteen cardiac cases reporting lesion, rib lesion was present. These lesions are of prime importance in such diseases. They seem to be rel-atively more frequent than other sorts, perhaps for the reason that they affect the heart often mechanically, through alteration of the chest cavity, as well as by interference with its nerve connections. A s to kind, the rib lesion is as import-ant as any other lesion, while as to frequency it is of greater importance. Eight of the thirteen rib lesions were of the 4th and 5th ribs, either or both, and usu-ally of the left side. As a matter of fact lesions of these two are the most important of the rib lesions. They may affect both nerve-connections and mechanical relations of the heart. The fact that the apex beat (falling at the fifth interspace) may be interfered with, easily deranging the whole delicate rhythm of the organ, may account in part for the frequency with which such lesion causes cardiac disease. In six of the thirteen the 1st and 2d rib presented lesion, usually on the left side. While these lesions are not so generally the cause of heart disease, they are frequent and important lesions in these cases. Their main effect is through disturbance of the nerve connections. The first rib may derange circulation through the sub-clavian vessels, as may the clavicle. In four of the fifteen cases lesion of the clavicle occurred. While not frequent, these lesions may be the cause of serious trouble.

Spinal lesions, including both muscular and bony, are of the greatest importance when it is considered that rib lesion contributes to them by disturbance of the spinal nerve-connections. They occur in seven of the above fifteen cases. They act by producing derangement of the important nerve-connections in the upper dorsal region. From this point of view bony and muscular lesions in the cervical region become significant, while not so frequently the sole cause of heart disease, they yet often occur and derange the important sympathetic nerve connections of the heart and this region. Lesions of the atlas, axis, or of any of the first three or four cervical vertebrae, also of the rectus capitis anticus major muscle, may affect the superior cervical ganglion as well as other cervical sympathetics. In six of the fifteen cases cervical lesion occurred, three of the six being dislocation of the athas.

It may be noted that practically all of the above lesions affect the heart, in whole or in part, through its nerve-connections. This seems to be the most important avenue over which abnormal influences travel from lesion to heart. By working directly upon nerve distribution to the heart, irrespective of lesion, important changes are readily made in its activities. Physiologically this organ is markedly affected by nervous influences. It seems that a viscus whose nervous equilibrium is so readily disturbed or influenced, should be peculiarly susceptible to the influence of lesions to its regulative mechanism. Such lesions as osteopathy considers, affecting this mechanism directly as it does, must be the true cause of many pathological states. Their removal is therefore a rational means of cure.

The diaphragmatic lesion is of some importance in heart diseases, as mentioned above. In four of the fifteen cases such lesion was present as may have affected the diaphragm.

In the cases of varicose veins reported the importance of lumbar, sacral and innominate lesion becomes apparent, also of the stoppage of venous return. The two cases of vascular disturbance showed lesion of the cervical region and of the 5th lumbar vertebra, it being noticable that each came at a place at which it could effect the center for superficial circulation. (Superior cervical and 5th lumbar.)

In seventeen of the twenty cases benefit or cure was made in a short time, considering the case. In periods varying from one or a few treatments to three months results were attained in long standing or serious cases that well demonstrated the superiority of osteopathic therapeutics. In one case the pulse was reduced from 140 to 110 at the first treatment, and was kept down and constantly improved thereafter. In case 4 it is pointed out that the pulse could be slowed as much as twenty beats per minute. Considering the fact that a cardiac medicine that reduces the heart beat one per minute is a successful one, it is readily seen that osteopathic control of the heart is most successful.

The ANATOMICAL RELATIONS between the lesion and the heart-disease are made clear by the following facts : In view of them it seems that the science of Osteopathy, by its methods of diagnosis, arrives at the real cause of the disease. This is true also with reference to diseases in general.

The pneumogastric nerves and the sympathetics are the cardiac nerves. The pneumogastric is the heart inhibitor, and its center has been definitely located in the medulla. It is a well-known osteopathic fact that lesion in the superior cervical region, acting through the superior cervical ganglion, may disturb the centers contained in the medulla. In such case the heart may be affected by disturbance of the center of cardiac inhibition.

Special details of the action of the vagus in inhibiting the heart have been observed. Strong stimulation of the nerve lengthens both systole and diastole, i. e. slows the beat. It also lessens the force of contraction, and causes the heart to beat not only more slowly, but more weakly. At the same time this stimulation results in the heart handling less blood, as the output and the input of the ventricle are both diminished. The ventricular tonus is diminished, and the heart dilates furher by vagus stimulation, while at the same time the walls of the ventricle have been found to be softer.

Osteopathic lesion to the vagi is a demonstrated fact. In view of the above functions of these nerves, it becomes at once apparent that lesion to them might cause serious disturbance. An irritative lesion, keeping up stimulation of the nerve, would permanently slow the beat, lessen cardiac force, retard circulation, and possibly lead to dilated and flaccid heart. On the other hand, should the lesion be of a nature to cut off or to inhibit to a degree the vagal impulse normally retarding the heart within limits, the accelerator sympathetics would be left free to run the heart too fast. In either case the removal of the lesion to the pneumogastric would be of prime importance in curing the condition. Aside from removal of lesion, osteopathic treatment of the vagi has been demonstrated to influence heart action. The after effect of vagus stimulation Gaskell notes to be increased force of cardiac contraction. This is an indication that upon removal of lesion Nature would make special effort to repair the former deficiency of function. As it is known that section of the vagus is followed by atrophy of the cardiac muscle, it would be possible that serious lesion might approximate such a result.

The vagus supplies the heart by its upper and lower cervical and thoracic cardiac branches, which join with the sympathetic and go to the cardiac plexus. It also has connection with the superior cervical ganglion. As this nerve is known to be amenable to osteopathic treatment, at many points, likewise susceptible of lesion at various places, as at the atlas, axis, and upper dorsal via its sympathetic connections, along the sterno-mastoid muscle and at the clavicle, its importance in relation to the cause and cure of heart disease is apparent.

The cardiac depressor nerve, whose presence has been demonstrated in man, as well as in various other mammals, retards heart action in a manner different from that of the vagus. Its stimulative impulses come from the heart and act upon its sympathetic connections with the splanchnics to produce a reflex vaso-dilatation in the abdominal vessels. They dilate and receive a large amount of blood from the general system, the general blood pressure is lessened, arterial tension falls, and the heart is thus quieted.

An important avenue to the heart is through the cervical sympathetic ganglia, each of which sends a cardiac branch to the cardiac plexus. Between these branches, the branches of the vagus, and the thoracic sympathetic, there are numerous points of communication. Each ganglion is so situated and so connected with the spinal nerves that it is susceptible to lesion. The upper ganglion lies in front of the second and third cervical vertebrae and communicates with the upper four cervical nerves. It may suffer from lesion of the upper three vertebrae. Its branches of communication with the third and 4th cervical nerves often pierce the rectus capitis anticus major muscle, on the sheath of which the ganglion lies. Contracture of this muscle may act as lesion to them. The middle ganglion lies in front of 6th and 7th cervical vertebrae and connects with the 5th and 6th cervical nerves. The lower ganglion lies in front of the 1st costo-vertebral articulation, and connects with the 7th and 8th cervical nerves. They are susceptible to lesion respectively of the 5th and 6th cervical vertebrae and of the 7th cervical vertebrae and the first rib. All three are liable to muscular lesion. Hence the importance of neck lesion in cardiac disease.

The accelerator or augmentor nerves of the heart are sympathetic. They are antagonistic to the vagi. That they are likely to suffer from spinal lesion is at once apparent from their anatomical relations. They are derived from the upper four or five dorsal nerves, especially from the 2nd and 3rd. They join the sympathetic at the middle and lower cervical, perhaps also first thoracic, ganglia. (Quain) The most important treatments for cardiac stimulation or inhibition are made in the upper dorsal region, at the origins of these nerves, by stimulation or inhibition of them. Important heart lesions occur in the upper dorsal region (spine or rib) and probably affect the heart through these conections. The connection of these glanglia with the middle and inferior cervical ganglia lends the latter added importance in these matters.

When these accelerators are stimulated they increase the frequency of the heart-beat from 7 to 70 per cent, but a long stimulation produces no greater acceleration than a short one. This marked increase in the pulse is quickly apparent under osteopathic stimulation of the accelerators. Further results of stimulating them are an increased force of the ventricular beat, the ventricles are more completely filled by the auricles and their volume is increased. The strength and volume of the auricular contractions are also increased. Hence our treatment both quickens and invigorates the heat muscle.

Lesions of the lower cervical, upper dorsal, or upper thoracic (rib) region might be of such a nature as to maintain continual stimulation of the accelerators, lead to permanently quickened and strengthened heart-beat, and produce such an affect as hypertrophy of the heart. Or the lesion might cut off or lessen the accelerator impulse, leading to abnormally slow heart-beat, lack of strength of heart action, etc. Hence the importance of correcting lesion in these regions.

Jacobson (in Hilton's "Rest and Pain") points out that the cardiac plexus, through the aortic plexus, is connected with the 4th, 5th, and 6th spinal nerves. This fact may in part explain the importance of lesion of the 4th and 5th ribs in heart disease. The 1st, 2nd and 3rd spinal nerves, through the sympathetic, supply sensory fibers to the heart. (Quain) The above facts explain why secondary lesion as contractured muscles may occur along the upper dorsal spine as far as the 6th in cardiac disease.

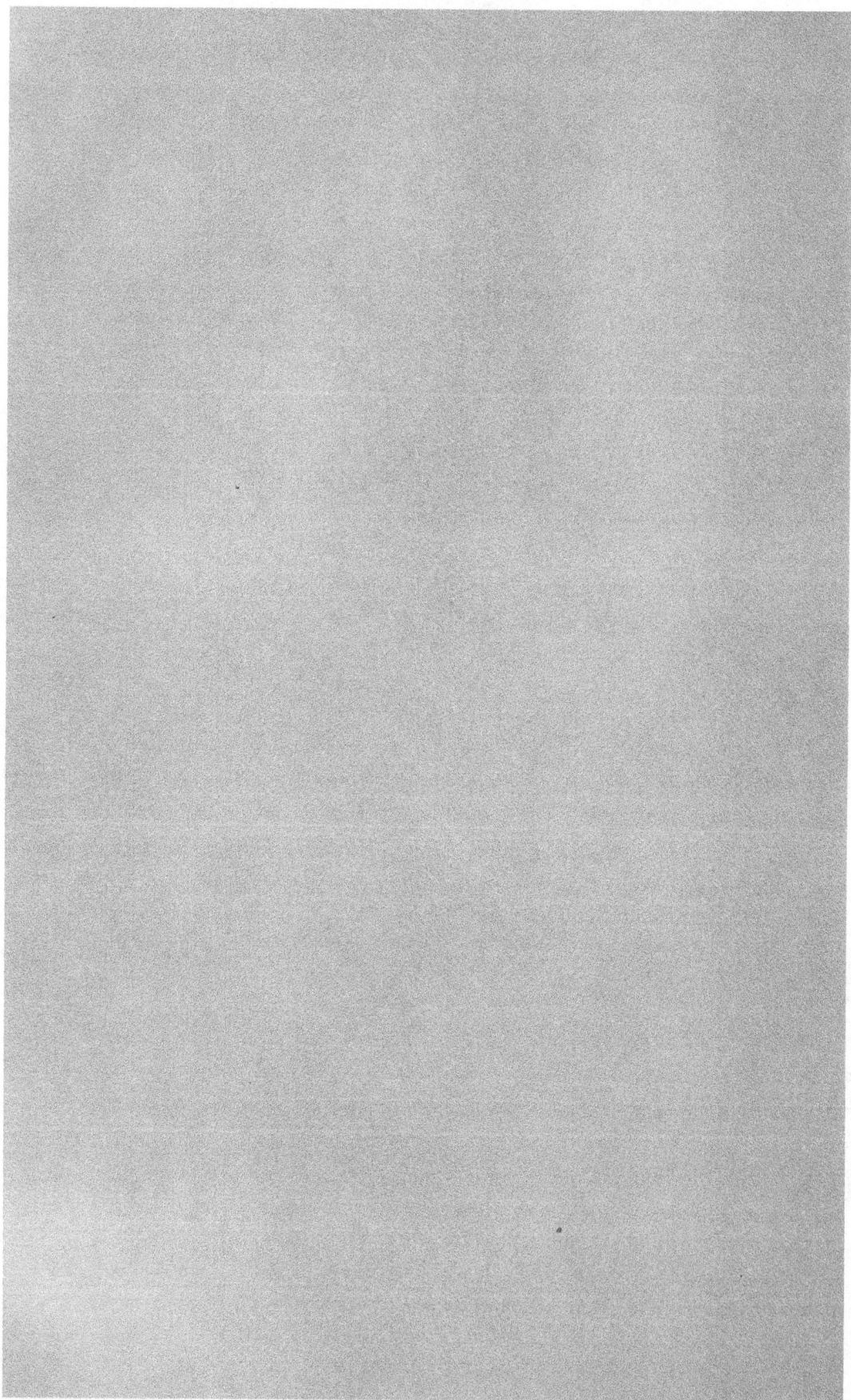

ANATOMICAL RELATIONS. Continued.

The cardiac plexus is made up of the cardiac branches of the vagus and from the cervical ganglia, whose functions and relations to cardiac disease were pointed out above. This plexus suffers from lesion of those nerves, and is the medium through which such lesion acts upon the heart. The right and left coronary plexuses derived from the cardiac, supply the coronary arteries. Lesion to them, through the cardiac, would influence nutrition and circulation in the heart substance.

The intercostal nerves may become important paths of transmission of the effects of lesion to the heart. It is well known that rib lesions are among the most frequent causes of heart-disease. Possibly much of their influence is by irritation to the intercostal nerves. These nerves are the anterior primary branches of the spinal nerves, and the ramus communicans from each thoracic sympathetic ganglion passes directly to the intercostal nerve corresponding. As shown above, the heart is in connection with the upper six dorsal nerves through its sympathetic supply. The upper four or five give origin to the accelerators. The 1st, 2nd, and 3rd contribute sensory branches to the heart. The 4th, 5th, and 6th connect with the cardiac plexus through the aortic. Hence, on account of this direct connection between heart and the anterior primary divisions of the upper six dorsal nerves the immediate effect of lesion in this portion of the thorax might be upon the heart. Hence the importance of luxated ribs, sore and contractured intercostal muscles, a narrowed chest and changed shape of the thorax. These facts emphasize the importance of the maintainence of free thoracic play in the maintainence of the health of the thoracic viscera.

A general changed shape of the thorax may have its bearing upon the etiology of cardiac trouble in other ways. The total intercostal circulation represents a considerable portion of the general circulation. If this whole circulation be obstructed, as may occur in those conditions in which a general alteration in the shape of the thorax has produced narrowing of the intercostal spaces, the heart must be put to greater exertion to force the blood through this area of obstructed vessels. Furthermore, such a condition of narrowed thorax is just the one pointed out as the cause of lesion to the diaphragm which obstructs the flow of blood through the aorta and still further embarrases the heart. Take these obstructions to intercostal and aortic circulation in conjunction with rib lesions to intercostal nerves, a frequent occurance, and it could hardly result otherwise than that cardiac derangement must follow.

The phrenic nerve innervates both heart and diaphragm. Lesion to it may affect this organ, or treatment of it may aid in cardiac cases. It is joined by branches from the middle or lower cervical sympathetic ganglia and from the thoracic sympathetic, both of which are connected with the heart innervation. It perforates the diaphragm and joins the abdominal sympathetic. It supplies the right pericardium, the right auricle, and the inferior vena cava. Perhaps it, a motor nerve, coordinates the activities of of heart and diaphragm, so closely related in function. Its inhibition is our common method of relaxing the diaphragm in hiccough.

Its inhibition would be important in securing a lax or quiet diaphragm, so desirable in the treatment of certain forms of cardiac diseases, the more so as it may likely be suffering from the irritation of the disease affecting the heart or its coverings.

Clavicular lesion may affect the subclavian vessels, dam back the flow of blood through the artery, or by preventing the return flow through the vein cause the periodic loss of a heart-beat through insufficient filling of the organ.

The intimate relations between the cardiac nerves and the general nervous system is seen in the fact that stimulation of the sciatic increases the force and frequency of the heart-beat, while stimulation of the abdominal sympathetics inhibits heart-action. These facts are of value in treatment for the general circulation.

———

PERICARDITIS.

Under osteopethic treatment the *prognosis* for cure is good in the dry or plastic form and in that with serous effusion. In the purulent form, and in chronic adhesive pericarditis the prognosis must be unfavorable, though much might be done to benefit the patient's condition.

The LESIONS affect the blood-supply by derangement of the spinal sympathetics. Irritative rib lesions, bringing pressure directly upon the heart, cause the disease by mechanical irritation of the pericardium. This is especially likely to occur in lesion to the fourth and fifth left ribs, they occuring at the site of apex beat where the greater range of motion is more likely to be interfered with by narrowing of the thoracic cavity or by inward displacement of these ribs. Lesions to the subclavian vein at the first rib or clavicle, and to the anterior intercostal vessels, preventing venous drainage of the pericardium, may predispose to the condition. A narrowed thoracic cavity and a deranged diaphragm may, by pressure or traction upon the pericardium, allow special causes to set up irritation and inflammation in the structure. These various lesions may lay the foundation for the disease, some special active acause producing it directly. Thus spinal and other lesion to the cardiac nerves weakens the tissues and lays them liable to the effect of such diseases as rheumatism, gout, scarlatina, influenza, etc., secondarily to which pericarditis occurs. In such cases also attention must be given to the lesion accountable for the primary disease.

In the TREATMENT the patient must be kept at rest in the recumbens position to aid in slowing the beat of the heart. This object is directly accomplished by stimulation of the vagi and inhibition of the accelerators. The former is treated by manipulation along its course behind the sterno-mastoid mnscle. Inhibition of the accelerators is applied along the spine from the 6th cervical to the 5th dorsal. With the patient lying upon his back the left arm is raised and held well above and behind the head, while steady pressure is applied along the upper dorsal region as far down as the fifth vertebra.

The lesion must be removed. The ribs may be carefully raised to free the venous circulation through the internal mammary veins, which drain the anterior intercostal veins. This aids in allaying the inflammation, as does all the inhibitive abdominal treatment by drawing the blood to the abdomen. The latter operation is assisted by inhibition along the splanchnics at the spine. Calling the blood to the abdomen not only aids in allaying the inflammation, but may very likely slow the heart by decreasing arterial tension. As this reflex dilatation of the abdominal veins is a result the same as that produced by the heart depressor nerve in functioning to quiet the heart, it is supposable that treatment given to dilate these vessels produces a result similar to that resulting from depressor nerve action.

As all the ribs are carefully raised to expand the thorax and give freedom to the heart, the various intercostal muscles should be gently manifested and relaxed. On account of the close connection pointed out above between the intercostal nerves and the sympathetics connected with the heart, it is probable that reflex sensations are transmitted from the diseased cardiac apparatus to the intercostal nerves, leading to a contractured condition of the intercostal muscles generally.

The phrenic nerves should be inhibited to relax the diaphragm, (and pericardium (?) which it supplies.) This treatment is the more important in pericarditis, as the diaphragm is probably irritated by the inflammation in the pericardium directly contiguous to it. Irritation would mean contracture. This relaxation of the diaphragm would aid in quieting the heart and in relieving the whole local condition. The desirability of securing a lax state of diaphragm and pericardium in the treatment of pericarditis is suggested by Hilton.

The pain about the heart is lessened by the whole treatment. Direct treatment may be made for it by inhibition of the 1st, 2nd, and 3rd dorsal nerves (sensory to the heart), and the 4th, 5th, and 6sh dorsal nerves, which apparently convey sensory impressions from the heart.

The dyspnea is relieved by the allaying of the inflammation, quieting the heart, and raising of all the ribs. Effusion is prevented or resorbed by keeping up free circulation, especially after the acute stage for the latter object. If necessary, the ice-bag may be applied to the precordial region to allay the inflammation. Its use may become necessary in the intervals between treatment.   The diet should be of milk and broths during the acute stage. Later it should be light.

Treatment should be given daily. More than one treatment *per diem* may be necessary, especially attention to various phases.

PALPITATION.

DEFINITION: A paroxysmal rapidity of heart-action, perceptible to the patient, and usually accompanied by increased force, disturbed rhythm, precordial distress, anxiety, and dyspnea. This condition is caused by special lesion, usually a bony one, that interferes with the nerve-mechanism or with the heart mechanically. This, and the so-called neuroses of the heart, are, from the osteopathic standpoint, neuroses mainly because of their being caused by disturbed nerve-mechanism of the organ. This is no more nor less true in such diseases than in the general diseases of the heart.

LESIONS AND ANATOMICAL RELATIONS have been discussed in a general way above. An examination of the several cases of palpitation reported at the beginning of the chapter shows a wide range of lesion, namely from the atlas to the last rib, when considering as a lesion producing this condition these changes in the shape of the thorax and those lesions of the lower six ribs responsible for lesion of the diaphragm embarrasing the heart. These lesions may act by disturbing the nerve-connections of the heart, by occluding certain vascular areas or single vessels, or by direct mechanical pressure upon the heart. Lesions of the clavicle and first rib are frequent, and they by damming back the blood in the sub-clavian artery, may cause periods of labored beat of the heart to force it through. Or by lessening venous flow from the sub-clavian vein such lesion may cause a paroxysm of rapid beating of the heart in the endeavor to fill itself. Cervical and upper dorsal lesions, curvatures of the upper spine, lesions of the upper five ribs, and general contracture of the spinal muscles could all act as irritants upon the accelerator sympathetics noted as rising from the upper four or five dorsal nerves and passing to the middle and lower cervical sympathetic ganglia. Stimulation of these accelerators thus caused could produce the rapid beating of the heart found in palpitation. This class of lesion is most frequent in these cases.

Atlas lesion may affect the heart through the superior cervical ganglion and its upper cardiac branch. But through this ganglion such lesion is able to affect the inhibitory center in the medulla, or it may affect the vagus itself by way of its sympathetic connections with the ganglion mentioned. The result is over-activity of the inhibitor function of the vagus and the rapid beat thus allowed as the result of unapposed activity of the accelerator. This style of lesion is not a frequent cause of palpitation.

It may be argued that as bony lesions are by nature continuous, the paroxysmal rapidity of the heart in palpitation could not be thus caused, that the effect of this continuous lesion must itself be continuous as opposed to paroxysmal. Such is not the case, however. The lesion may not be so excessive in degree as to keep up continual irritation. Its irritation may become active only in certain motions or postures of the affected parts. It may be the neuropathic basis weakening the nerve tissues and leaving the heart liable to the effects of special emotions, stimulants, etc. The lesion might even *per se* be of a nature to cause continuous irritation and yet its effects not be continually apparent as rapid heart-beat on account of the natural variation in the activity of the accelerator centers and in the condition of the nervous system.

Luxation of the fifth left rib mechanically irritates the heart and causes palpitation. Occuring as it does at the site of the apex-beat, it is just as likely a cause of palpitation as is the pressure from a stomach dilated with gas. Displacement of this rib and of the 4th is a common cause of palpitation. Rib lesions in general are quite apt to be found in cases in which palpilation is brought on by slight muscular exertion. The movable rib, being luxated, is readily thrown into an exaggerated condition of lesion upon muscular effort. Cases are continually met in which some special form of muscular activity, perhaps necessitated by the patient's occupation, has first caused the displacement and has then bcome the repeatedly-acting cause of the various attacks of palpitation which have followed.

A frequent and serious cause of heart disease in general, as well as of palpitation in particular, is found in a general downward luxation of the ribs resulting in a narrowed thorax. Such a condition becomes a three-fold lesion. Looked at as the cause of palpitation it acts: (1) By partially occluding the calibre of the arteries in the total intercostal area, aggregating a considerable vascular total. (2) By causing lesion to the diaphragm of a nature allowing it to constrict the aorta. As a result of all this arterial obstruction the heart labors (palpitation) to force the blood along its accustomed channels. (3) By irritation to the intercostal nerves in the narrowed intercostal spaces. The upper six of these nerves, as above explained, are in direct sympathetic connection with the heart and convey to it the irritation engendered in the intercostal spaces, causing it to palpitate.

It will be noted that chronic heart sufferers are very often the possessors of flat chests and narrowed thoraxes.

Dyspepsia, flatulence and diseased abdominal organs often reflexly set up palpitation. It may be that both effects are the results of a common lesion, i. e., one to the splanchnic nerves (abdominally or spinally). It has been explained that the depressor nerve of the heart acts reflexly through the splanchnics to produce vaso-dilatation in the great abdominal vascular area, "bleeding the patient into his own veins," and cause a fall of blood-pressure with a quieting of the heart. On the other hand, splanchnic lesion may set up intense vaso-constriction in this area, oppose the circulation of the blood in this way, and cause the labored beat or palpitation of the heart to force the blood through.

The common cause assigned for palpitation, such as a strong emotion, the use of tea, coffee, tobacco, and alcohol; reflex disturbances from the ovaries, uterus, and other pelvic organs, etc., seem to be but incidental. There must be some cause determining the effects of these agents upon the heart. Otherwise it is hard to explain why these things effect one patient's heart and not that of another. The real cause weakening the heart and allowing these incidental causes to disturb it lies in the anatomical weak point affecting the organ or its connections. A multitude of cases cured by replacement of a displaced rib, or the like, leads to the conclusion that these so-called causes had little to do with the real cause; cf case 6 above, in which three week's treatment cured palpitation of many year's standing, and rendered the patient immune to the effects of coffee and tobacco, which before he could not use.

In cases where the palpitation is purely secondary, as in anemia, from the changed state of the blood, and in acute infections diseases, from the irritation of toxic substances circulating in the blood, the lesions belong to the primary disease.

The PROGNOSIS is good. The most marked and long standing cases have yielded readily to treatment. The case is generally relieved at once and soon cured.

The TREATMENT at the time of attack must look at once to quieting the the nerve irritation that is causing the trouble. (1) Often the immediate removal of the lesion is practicable and is the sole treatment necessary.

(2) Inhibition of the accelerators in the manner described in detail in the previous pages is the most efficient method of at once relieving the palpitation. Considerable pressure may be applied to the accelerator area of the spine, the left arm meanwhile being strongly held above the head (see Pericarditis). Steady pressure at each point along these nerves for several minutes is necessary. During this treatment one hand is slipped beneath the patient, the arm may be held down above the head against the table by the pressure of the practitioner's trunk against it, while with his free hand relaxes the intercostal tissues all about the precordial region. This is to release contractions in the intercostal muscles set up by the irritation carried from the cardiac plexus to the upper intercostal nerves, with which it is closely connected.

(3) Stimulation of the pneumogastric nerves in the neck aids in inhibit the heart action (IV, Chap. IV).

(4) Stimulation of the abdominal sympathetics, by a quick treatment, will aid in inhibiting the heart beat. A better method, however, is to dilate the vast abdominal vascular system by the deep, inhibitive abdominal treatment. This drains the blood into the abdomen, decreases general arterial

tension, and quiets the heart. It is the exact process by which the depressor nerve quiets the heart, and may possibly cause it to function, Strong inhibition of the spinal splanchnics aids this process.

(5) All the ribs should be carefully elevated to allow free play to respiration and heart. The dyspnea is a reflex from the disturbed heart. It is relieved by this treatment, and by the relieving of the heart.

(6) Other sources of irritation, as anemia, pelvic disease, etc., call for special treatment.

(7) Upon the attack the patient should be laid upon his back at once, and the clothing about the chest and neck should be loosened. Treatment (2) should be at once applied. In case of necessity during the practitioner's absence an ice-bag applied to the precordial region is a good domestic remedy. The patient may swallow bits of ice or drink plentifully of cold water. Hot and somewhat stimulating drinks are recommended.

If the attacks are frequent or persistent the treatment must be often given. In treatment to prevent the recurrence of attacks a course of treatment may be carried out along the lines laid down. Special attention would naturally be given the lesion. Heart action and circulation would be built np, etc.

TACHYCARDIA, BRACHYCARDIAANDARRHYTHMIA.

The first is a rapid beating of the heart in paroxysms of variable duration, unaccompanied by any marked subjective sensations. The second is an abnormal slowness of the heart, temporary or permanent. The third is irregular beating of the heart, the irregularity being manifest in volume and force only, in time only, or in both in various combinations, presenting various peculiarities.

The lesion and its mode of causing disease described for palpitation are essentially the same for these three manifestations of disturbance to the cardiac mechanism. The treatment, also, would proceed along the same general lines there laid down, being varied to suit the requirements of the disease and of the individual case. As a matter of fact the lesions found as the actual causes of these different diseases are practically the same in kind. affect the same areas, nerve connections, and vascular relations, but differ in degree, in concentration upon a particular region, e. g., chiefly upon the accelerators in the upper dorsal region to produce tachycardia, and therefore in the particular manifestation or results of their presence.

It is natural that these lesions producing palpitation should be greater in degree and more continuous and severe in action, thus producing tachycardia; that upper dorsal lesion should so excessively affect the accelerators as to permanently inhibit their activity to a degree great enough to cause brachycardia, or that the periodic or irregular manifestations of such lesion should produce arrhythmia. The latter is generally a feature of ordinary palpitation. In the same way arterial, venous, or other nerve lesion might become the cause of either disease. In other words, a purely osteopathic classification of diseases would regard these conditions as essentially the same, both as to lesion and as to general manner of treatment.

The fact that tachycardia is looked upon as being a manifestation of paralysis of the pneumogastric or stimulation of the sympathetic is significant from the osteopathic view point.

The *prognosis* for these conditions is ordinarily good. The results attained are very satisfactory and cases are often readily cured. The fact that they are frequently symptomatic of other disease, or secondary thereto, makes the prognosis and treatment depend upon the primary condition. When, as is often the case, they are found to depend upon specific removable lesion the prognosis is good. It is not good when organic heart disease is present.

The *treatment* for these conditions must be primarily the removal of lesion or irritating cause, or the treatment of the primary disease to which either may be secondary or symptomatic. That for tachycardia and arrhythmia is practically that for palpitation. The treatment for brachycardia is mainly stimulation of the accelerators. In the treatment of brachycardia or the tachycardia following acute infectious disease, e. g., typhoid fever, the excretory organs must be stimulated to free the system of poison, and the centers controlling the activities of the heart must be built up, as they have been invaded by the poison of the disease. In brachycardia the heart and lungs must be kept stimulated against the occurrence of syncope or physical prostration. Treatment in the intervals may be directed to up-building the general health, mechanical correction of the body, etc.

ANGINA PECTORIS.

DEFINITION: Paroxysms of violent pain in the pecordial region, extending to the neck, back and arms, and accompanied by a sense of impending death. It is said to be largely symptomatic.

The *lesions* presented in the above cases were mainly to the left ribs over the heart. One case showed lesion to the left clavicle, affecting the subclavian circulation. Another case is reported with the lesion as a spreading of the sixth and seventh left ribs anteriorly. Lesions to the ribs over the heart are very common in this disease. The upper dorsal spine is often affected. The nature of the pain of angina pectoris is not well understood. Upper dorsal lesion may irritate the sensory nerves of the heart. (1st, 2d, and 3d dorsal.) The irritation of the lesion upon the heart may result in a neurosis of the sensory branches of the vagi. Other lesion to the vagi through their sympathetic connections may cause it. Some writers advance the theory that an aortitis is present and causes it. A deranged nerve-mechanism as the result of spinal, rib and other lesion, seems sufficient, from an osteopathic point of view, to cause this disturbance. The fact that it is usually associated with some form of organic heart lesion, arterio-sclerosis, etc., is not contrary to the idea that bony lesion is at bottom the cause of the whole bad condition.

The *prognosis* must be guarded because of the frequent presence of organic heart disease in cases manifesting angina pectoris. The prognosis for relief is good, and cases are often entirely cured.

The *treatment* consists mainly in relieving the pain. This may be best accomplished by raising the left lower ribs in the region of the heart, especially in case of lesion here, by adopting the motion described for inhibition of the accelerators, bringing pressure over the upper three spinal nerves (cardiac sensory) at the same time, and also relaxing the tissues of the pecordial region, with additional inhibition of the pneumogastric nerves.

Spinal inhibition may be carried down along the spine as low as the 6th dorsal nerve. Inhibition should be made upon the local nerves of the parts to which the pain has radiated, as to the brachial plexus, the cervical and spinal nerves, etc.

A general course of treatment, should be giqen to strengthen the patient's general health, to correct heart-action, and to remove all lesions. In this way much may be done to prevent the recurrence of the attacks. The patient should lead a quiet life free from physical, mental and emotional extremes. In case of emergency the use of the ice bag, or of hot applications over the heart may be useful.

ENDOCARDITIS AND MYOCARDITIS.

These are inflammations of the endocardium and of the heart muscle, attended by various pathological and degenerative changes in the part attacked. The extent to which the pathological changes go in most of these cases renders a cure hopeless. All forms of these diseases are apt to produce serious valvular lesions. Aside from simple acute endocarditis, death is immanent in most of these cases, yet much may be done in individual cases to alleviate conditions and to prolong life.

THE LESIONS AND ANATOMICAL RELATIONS as pointed out at the opening of the chapter apply here. It is seldom that myocarditis or any of the several forms of endocarditis seems to occur idiopathically. How far the actual causes of these diseases may be shown, from the accumulation of osteopathic data, to be specific osteopathic lesions to the heart remains to the future to decide. The accepted cause of these conditions generally is the irritation of the organ by the poisonous products of disease. Acute articular rheumatism is made accountable for 40 per cent of simple acute endocarditis. Rheumatism, malaria, scarlet fever, pulmonary tuberculosis, syphilis, gout, lead poisoning, etc., are looked upon as the primary diseases in which poisonous products are generated and cause endocarditis or myocarditis as a secondary condition. Various other causes are assigned.

While poison in the system is admitted by the Osteopath to be sufficient cause of disease, it seems likely that specific lesion to the cardiac apparatus has much to do in weakening the heart and laying it liable to the invasion of these diseases. Circulation to the substance of the heart is under control of the coronary plexuses, derived from the cardiac plexus. Lesion to the latter through its spinal connections may affect the former and disturb the nutrition of the organ. The same result may be produced by lesion to the pneumogastries, said to contain vaso-motor fibers to the heart and to have charge of trophic condition. It is obvious that the usual cardiac lesions may predispose the heart to these diseases. The direct irritation of the left ribs upon the heart, when they are displaced, may directly cause pericarditis and myocarditis. As medical etiology lays most of these cases to the action of bacteria, it is reasonable to conclude that some direct lesion to the heart deteriorates the vitality of its tissues and allows them to gain a foothold.

This conclusion is strengthened by the fact that endocarditis sometimes follows chronic wasting diseases, such as diabetes and gleet. The fact that chronic endocarditis may be due to mechanicel influences, may be caused by heavy muscular effort, straining, etc., and the further fact that myocarditis is ascribed by Anders to injuries of the antero-lateral thoracic region emphasizes the idea that mechanical lesions regarded as important by the Osteopath may directly cause these conditions.

The PROGNOSIS for simple acute endocarditis is good. It depends some upon the primary disease. The prognosis for chronic and ulcerative endocarditis and for myocarditis is grave. If specific lesion is found and may be removed, perhaps much may be done for the case—generally speaking, much may be done in all of these cases to limit the disease and to prolong life. Chronic endocarditis has been cured.

The TREATMENT is practically that described for pericarditis, q. v. Knowledge of the nerve and blood-supply and of lesions gives one the key to the situation. The lesion and all cause of irritation must be removed, and the patient, in the acute stages, is kept in bed to keep the heart quiet. Inhibition of the accelerators and stimulation of the vagi is done as directed. The ribs are raised to give the best freedom, and the abdominal treatment may be applied to draw the blood away from the heart and aid in keeping it quiet.

Strict attention must be given the primary disease. In those generating toxins in the system the bowels, kidneys and liver are stimulated to excrete the poisons. In the chronic forms the heart and its connected nerves may be carefully stimulated to increase its tone and nutrition. The vegetation in acute endocarditis may be absorbed.

Prophylactic treatment in rheumatism aud in those diseases leading to these conditions consists in keeping the heart well stimulated, and in maintaining free action of kidneys and bowels to excrete the poison.

VALVULAR DISEASES.

The *prognosis* in cases of this kind is not generally favorable. As a rule, valvular disease is incurable. Yet some cases may be cured, and a fair number have been cured by osteopathic treatment. In cases not curable much may be done to better the patient's condition. Cases caused by simple dilatation or diminished contractile power may be cured. Also when occuring in simple acute endocarditis the prognosis for cure is good.

LESIONS: In many cases of valvular lesion, in the left heart especially, the lesions present would be as described for endocarditis, to which disease these may be secondary, In tricuspid insufficiency due to obstructed pulmonary circuit lesion to the lung, as described in the chapter on lung diseases, may cause the valvular trouble.

In aortic stenosis from increased tension in the aorta the condition may be due to lesion to the diaphragm as explained impeding circulation through the aorta. The same result may follow extensive arterial obstruction, as of all the intercostals, the sub-clavians, the abdominals, etc., as explained under *Anatomical Relations* at the opening of this chapter. Aortic valvular lesions due to heavy muscular strains, etc., may be due to the presence of some one of the various lesions described as affecting the heart, which forms a predisposing cause. Lesions to the vagus and to the sympathetic supply of the heart may lead to lack of tone and diminished contractile power (See gen. anatomical relations) which sometimes causes valvular disease, General lesions to the cardiac mechanism, as of upper vertebrae, ribs, diaphragm, vagi and sympathetics, doubtless weaken the heart and act as predisposing causes to the valvular lesion which so frequently follows other disease.

The TREATMENT in ordinary cases would be to sustain the heart and to maintain compensation. It should look to the removal of any lesion, or of any obstruction to the blood-current, especially in tricuspid insufficiency caused by obstructed pulmonary circulation, and in aortic stenosis due to increased tension in the aorta. Diaphrammatic lesion or important arterial obstruction may be present. In the obstructed pulmonary circulation the lungs should be kept stimulated and any lesion to the lung should be removed. In cases in athletes or due to heavy muscular strains one should suspect the presence of definite spinal or rib lesion due to such activities.

The primary disease which may be causing the trouble calls for treatment according to its kind. In diminished contractile power or dilatation of the left ventricle causing mitral insufficiency the accelerators, should be stimulated, as this increases cardiac tonus and strength of beat, and contracts the heart. In such cases lesion should be suspected to the vagus, as lesion to this nerve may diminish ventricular tonus, dilate the heart, and weaken its walls.

In all such cases the patient should lead a quiet life, free from excitement or great exertion. He should be much out of doors, and live upon a light nutritious diet. He should avoid straining at stool, exposure, the use of alcohol, tobacco, etc. Bathing is recommended with exception of Turkish baths.

HYPERTROPHY OF THE HEART.

In these conditions the *prognosis* is fair. Much may be done to maintain the patient in a state of comfortable health, preventing dilatation. Cases may sometimes be cured by osteopathic theropeutics. The prognosis depends upon that for the condtion producing the hypertrophy. In such forms of valvular diseases as are curable it may be cured. In cases due to exophthalmic goitre it may be curable.

Such LESIONS as before described in cardiac disease may affect the nerve connections, etc., of the cardiac mechanism, and cause or predispose to the condition. A common cause is obstruction to the circulation through the small arteries. In the light of such fact, lesions before pointed out causing obstructed pulmonary circulation, obstructed aorta, intercostals, subclavians, abdominals, etc., are important. As the heart hypertrophies in valvular disease frequently, lesions would have to be sought according to primary conditions.

Lesion to the sympathetics, as in exophthalmic goitre, causing hypertrophy are important. Lesion to vagi and accelerators, resulting in overactivity of the heart may cause hypertrophy. When such simple causes as the use of alcohol, coffee, tobacco, etc., and lead poisoning, etc., are alleged, one is bound to suspect one of the ordinary lesions present as the real cause allowing the heart to be affected by such agents.

The TREATMENT looks to be removal lesion, obstruction to the blood flow, etc. It is directed to the primary disease when the hypertrophy, as is the rule, is a secondary condition. The circulation through the lungs should be kept free. The patient should remain quiet. Attention should be given the sympathetics to slow the beat as much as possible.

The patient should lead a quiet life, free from excitement. His diet should be chosen with care, and he should particularly avoid overeating, alcohol, coffee, etc.

DILATATION OF THE HEART.

DEFINITION: There may be simple dilatation of a cavity, causing increase in its size and thinning of its walls. The dilatation may be accompanied with hypertrophy, in which there is both increase in the size of the cavity and in the thickness of the muscular wall.

As to CAUSES, the lesions as discussed would be sufficient. No specific lesion has been pointed out for this condition. Lesions to the cardiac mechanism weaken the heart and thus are especially apt to predispose to dilatation. Under such conditions over-exertion and great physical strain would be more likely to cause dilatation of the right ventricle. As the vagus nerve has been shown to have a trophic influence upon the heart walls, also upon their dilatation, lack of tone, and a softened condition of them, lesion to it would have an important part in the production of dilatation. Obstructed circulation, and any cause producing increased intra- cardiac pressure may result in dilatation. This is seen in mitral diseases. Osteopathic lesion causing obstruction or the aorta by the diaphragm, obstruction to the intercostals, abdominals, pulmonary circulation, etc., as before discussed, may become the direct cause of dilatation of the heart.

The PROGNOSIS is not good. It depends upon that for the primary condition often, as in valvular diseases where the prognosis is bad. When due to specific removable lesion the prognosis may become favorable.

The TREATMENT consists in righting of mechancal relations and removal of lesion. Obstruction to the circulation must be relieved, and heart and lungs must be kept well stimulated to empty the chambers of the heart of the clotted blood that is retained in them. Stimulation of the accelerators aids the process by steadying and strengthening the heart beat, contracting it and adding tone.

When secondary to acute infectious disease, valvular disease, etc., the primary condition must be treated. The dropsy and dyspepsia present depend upon the bad circulation and are treated in the usual ways. Stimulation of the lungs and raising the ribs relieve the dyspnea. Stimulation to the kidneys increases the flow of urine, which has been lessened, and aids in overcoming the dropsy.

In the acute form the patient should rest in bed. In the chronic form he should avoid fatigue. General directions for the care of the patient are as before given.

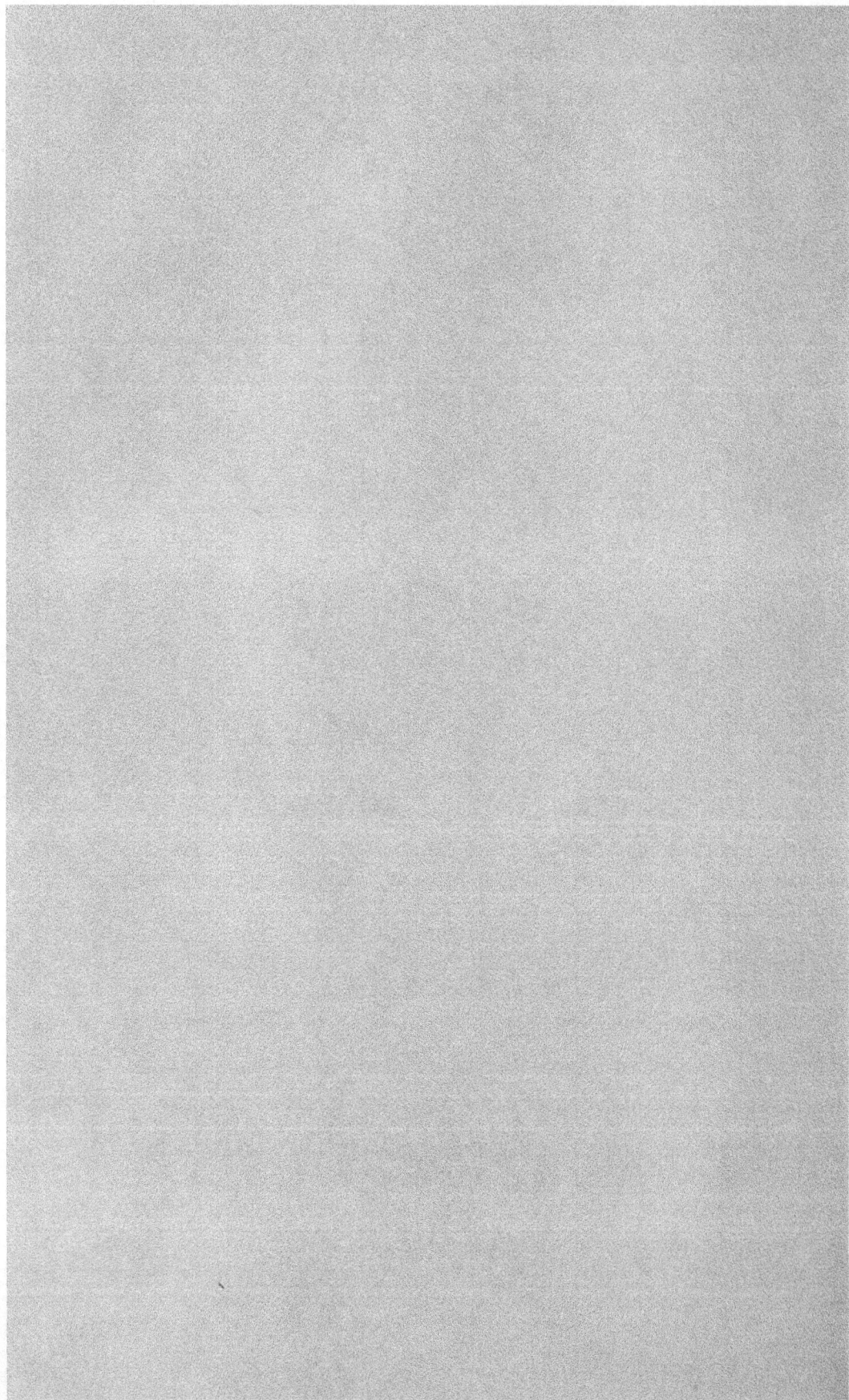

DISEASES OF THE NERVOUS SYSTEM.

CHOREA. (St. Vitus Dance.)

DEFINITION: A disease of the nervous system characterized by involuntary contraction of muscle groups, accompanied by weakness, and often by slight mental derangement, due to spinal lesions interfering with motor function of brain or cord.

CASES: (1) A case in a young girl, of three or four months standing; very severe; had lost all control of hands and feet, and of speech; could lake only liquid food. It was thought she could not live. Lesions were found at the atlas and 4th dorsal vertebrae. The case was cured.

(2) In a boy of nine, chorea followed vaccination. Lesion was found at the atlas and at the 2d to 4th dorsal vertebrae. Case cured in five weeks.

(3) A case in a child of eleven, of nine months standing. Very severe; no sleep for six nights; power of articulation was lost. Six weeks of treatment showed great improvement.

(4) A girl of ten; marked lesion of the atlas, and of the 3d and 4th cervical vertebrae; the 2d to 6th dorsal vertebrae were irregular and lateral; 5th lumbar posterior; cured in four manths.

(5) Case of two years' standing in a boy of twelve; right hand useless and carried in a sling; lesion at 1st to 3d dorsal. Under treatment he became able to write well in one month. The case was cured.

(6) A case of two years' standing in a girl of thirteen. She had grown continually worse under usual treatment. The atlas was found displaced to the left, and upon its being replaced at the second treatment the jerking of the muscles began to grow less at once. The case was cured in one month, and the child, previously undersized, grew rapidly thereafter.

(7) The patient was a girl of thirteen; confined to the bed; arms and limbs drawn and useless; she could not sleep or speak intelligently. Bony lesions were found in the cervical and lower dorsal regions, and all the spinal muscles were contractured. The case, of three months' standing, was cured in one month.

LESIONS AND ANATOMICAL RELATIONS: The lesions in these cases are found in the majority of cases in the upper dorsal and cervical regions. Six of the above seven cases described lesion and are illustrative of the facts generally observed in such cases. All showed lesion in the cervical or upper dorsal region, one or both. Neck lesion is important in these cases.

Five of the above showed cervical lesion, four of the five being atlas lesions. The fact that atlas lesions alone may cause the disease is illustrated by case (6) The fact that the upper dorsal lesion alone may cause it is illustrated by case (5). But frequently, as in three of those reported, combined lesion of the cervical and upper dorsal regions occur. The upper dorsal lesion is perhaps the most important one.   Four of the above six showed lesion somewhere in the upper six dorsal vertebrae.   The spinal area from the atlas to the 6th dorsal may be regarded as the important locality for lesions producing chorea.   They may occur lower or affect the ribs as well as vertebrae.

These lesions high up in the spine may involve the cord and brain, in a similar manner but lesser degree, as in paralytic affections of the whole body.   The frequent occurrence of high lesion explains the usual general effect of the disease upon the whole body, including the upper and lower limbs and suggests the idea that the cord, brain, or both are involved by the lesion.

The authors state that the pathology of this condition is obscure, no constant lesions being found.   Probably, as McConnell observes, this is due to the fact that spinal lesion may often involve simply nerve-fibers.   Some writers hold the disease to be a functional brain disturbance affecting the centers controlling the motor apparatus.   From this point of view cervical and atlas lesion have an important bearing, as they may influence brain centers by interference with blood-supply to the brain through direct impingement upon the vertebral arteries and by disturbance of the cervical sympathetics.   Upper dorsal lesion may aid this effect by sympathetic disturbance.   From this view either atlas, other cervical, or upper dorsal lesion alone could cause the disease.

It is worthy of note that the upper dorsal lesion (1st to 6th) falls upon a portion of the cord richer, perhaps, than any other in sympathetic centers.   The cilio-spinal center, vaso-motors to face and mouth, pupillo-dilator fibers, motor fibers to involuntary muscles of the orbit, vaso-motors to the lungs, accelerators to the heart, etc., all occur within this spinal area.   This disturbance to the sympathetic may have much to do in unbalancing the nervous system in such cases.   This lesion could also effect spinal fibers by impingement or the nutrition of the cord through sympathetic disturbance of its blood-supply.

On the whole the likely pathology in this disease is that there is cord lesion or brain lesion due to mechanical irritation or to cut off nutrition.   These various lesions weaken the portions of the nerve-system involved, and lay it liable to the action of such reflex causes as irritation due to parasites, eye-strain, nasal disease, sexual disorders, etc., or to such causes as over-study, shock, worry, strain, etc.

The PROGNOSIS is good.   It is rare that the treatment fails to cure or greatly relieve the case.   Cure in a short time is the rule, even in serious and long-standing cases.

The TREATMENT consists mainly in removal of lesion as the real cause.   In some cases this is the sole treatment necessary.   Ordinarily it is necessary to carry the patient through a course of treatment.   All causes of irritation or nerve-strain should be removed. Such are intestinal worms, causes of worry, etc., as noted above. An important measure in these cases is the treatment upon the neck and spine for the general nervous system. The neck treatment reaches the sympathetic system, the medulla, the circulation to the brain, and influences the whole nervous system. It consists of the removal of lesion, relaxation of tissues, inhibition or stimulation of the cervical nerves and centers, etc. The spinal treatment is upon the same plan. It should be carried down along the spine. These treatments quickly relieve nervous tension and quiet the nervous system. They correct the circulation to the brain and central nervous system, increasing their nutrition, and stopping the muscular twitching characteristic of these conditions. An important treatment is the removal of contracture of the muscles all along the spine, common in these cases. Attention must be given to the patient's general health. The heart is often very fast and should be slowed in the way already described. The kidneys should be stimulated and general metabolism in the body looked to, to increase the too light specific gravity of the urine. The bowels must be kept regular.

A thorough general treatment should be given to the muscular system, especially to those muscle groups involved in the disease. This includes flexion and circumduction of limbs and arms, etc.

In some cases inhibition of the cervical sympathetic will cause the muscular twitching to cease at once. It has been accomplisned by pressure between the 3d and 4th cervical vertebrae.

In the hygienic treatment of the case all causes of nerve-strain, overwork mentally, excessive physical exertion, etc., must be removed. Muscular exertion may lead to heart involvement. especially as cervical and upper dorsal lesion favor such conditions, The diet should be light and nutritious. Fruits and vegetables may be taken, but meats and highly seasoned foods should be avoided. Sponging of the back, chest and neck with cold water is useful.

The various CHOREIFORM AFFECTIONS, such as the spasmodic ties, habit chorea, laryngeal tic, choreic wry-neck, facial tic, jumping disease, etc., also rhythmic or hysteric chorea, fibrillary chorea, athetosis, and varions other forms, are met in the same way.

Huntingdon's chorea; a hereditary disease with progressive dementia, is a very grave disease. There is no record of its ever having been treated osteopathically.

EPILEPSY.

DEFINITION: A disease in which there is loss of consciousness, with or without convulsions. From the osteopathic point of view it is caused by lesions interfering with the nutrition of cord or brain, or irritating the motor nerve strands running to the peripheral motor structures, or exciting connected nerves.

CASES: (1) A case showing lesions at 7th and 11th dorsal vertebrae. Under the treatment the attacks were much decreased in frequency, not having appeared for a considerable period.

(2) A case of more than one year's standing in a girl of thirteen; three to twelve attacks daily; lesions in upper cervical spine, posterior curvature from 6th dorsal to lower lumbar, marked lesions occuring at the 6th dorsal and at the 5th lumbar; all spinal muscles very rigid. Improvement began at once upon treatment, and the case was cured in three months.

(3) A case of fifteen years' standing in a man of thirty. No attacks occured after the first treatment, and the case was cured in four months. No recurrence of attacks nineteen months later.

(4) A case of twelve years' standing in a boy of twelve cured by the treatment.

(5) Daily attacks in a boy of eighteen, apparently due to a nervous stomach disease. The latter was cured in three months, and no further attack had occured six months afterward.

(6) A case of fourteen years' duration in a lady of eighty was cured in two treatments. No attack occured after the first treatment. The report was made two and a half years after the cure, no further attack having occured.

(7) In a boy of twelve, monthly spells of two days' duration occured, during which he would have from three to five spasms. The 3rd cervical vertebra was found turned far to the right. Under a three months' course of treatment he had not had the last two monthly spells.

(8) A case of petit mal in a young man of thirty. Lesions at the atlas, which was to the right and turned with the right transverse process backward, and at the axis, displaced to the left. Case still under treatment.

LESIONS AND ANATOMICAL RELATIONS: It seems that lesion along the neck and spine anywhere may cause epilepsy—Dr. A. T. Still is credited with the statement that there is usually lesion between the 2nd and 3rd cervical vertebrae. Lesions in the above cases occured at the atlas, cervical region, and from the middle dorsal down to the last lumbar. McConnell states that lesions occur often in the splanchnic area and to the ribs, especially in the spinal region between the 4th and 8th dorsal vertebrae, also that the prominent lesions occur in the neck from the 3rd to 7th vertebra. He notes a case caused by displacement of the right 5th rib. An attack could be caused by irritation of this lesion, or be relieved at once by replacing the rib.

The neck lesion seems, on the whole, to be the most important. Neck and spinal lesion may act by obstructing the blood-supply to brain or cord. They may affect the cord directly by mechanical irritation, or may affect brain, cord, or nervous-system generally through the sympathetics. In this way they may bring about these morbid conditions of cord, brain and and meninges said to cause the disease. While the pathology of epilepsy is unknown, it yet appears that osteopa thic lesion may account from any of the various conditions assigned as causes. Such lesions, disturbing the sympathetic system, may act as does peripheral irritation from dentition, worms, cicatrices, adherent prepuce, etc. Various of these lesions may directly irritate peripheral nerve structures. As traumatism is assigned as a cause, osteopathic lesion as cause or effect of traumatic conditions may be the real cause.

According to Gray the best accepted modern theory of the cause of epilepsy is that it is due to direct or indirect excitation of the cortex or of *the nerve-strands leading from the cortex to the peripheral ctructures*; that there is a *peculiar molecular condition of the motor tract which runs from the motor convolutions to the peripheral motor structures and muscles*. He states that we are ignorant of the nature of this molecular condition; that muscles can be convulsed only by direct excitation of the muscle itself, or of the motor tract leading from the muscle up to the motor convolutions; but that same varieties of epilepsy are evidenly due to an *excitation that extende into this motor tract from some part of the nervous system beyond it*. It would seem clear that osteopathic lesion may irritate these motor tracts somewhere in their course, as by direct pressure of luxated spinal vertebrae, etc., or that in a multitude of ways it may produce excitation in some other part of the nervous system from which it extends to the motor tract. As nerve irritation by lesion is the important point in osteopathic etiology generally, being well supported by numerous instances in which its removal has cured the disease, it is a reasonable conclusion that the various bony lesions found in epilepsy are causing it by excitation of the sort mentioned. This point is likewise supported by the fact that removal of such lesion has often cured epilepsy.

The PROGNOSIS is fair in the ordinary case, a fair number of the cases coming under osteopathic treatment being cured entirely. A large percentage not cured are benefitted. There seems to be but little difference in the prognosis in favor of petit mal. In Jacksonian Epilepsy the prognosis is not good.

TREATMENT: At the time of attacks but little can be done for the patient. If the patient can be reached at the aura the attack may be prevented by pushing the patient's head strongly back against a hand applying deep pressure in the sub-occipital fossae. This treatment seems to arouse reflex stimulation or to equalize blood-flow to the brain by affect upon the superior cervical ganglion and medulla.

Anders states that constriction of the limb in which the aura occurs, forcibly moving the patient's head, placing snuff to the patient's nose, applying ice to his spine, etc,, will sometimes prevent the attack. McConnell calls attention to the fact that in cases where the exciting factor seems to be in the intestine and there is reversed peristalsis of the intestines, causing a reversion of the nerve current in the vagi, thorough rapid abdominal treatment will normalize peristalsis and aid in preventing an impending attack. Stimulation of the solar plexus may lesson the attack by calling the blood to the intestines and thus reducing pressure in the cranium.

At the time of the attack the patient must be prevented from having serious falls, if possible. The clothing about the neck should be loosened so that it may not restrict circulation. Some object should be slipped between the teeth to prevent the patient's biting his tongue. Small objects that may fall into the wind-pipe should not be used for this purpose.

A general course of treatment is depended upon to prevent recurrence of attacks and to cure the case. This consists in the removal of lesion, whatever it be, and of all causes of reflex irritation mentioned above. It is especially important to remove lesion acting to irritate the motor fibers of the central nervous system, in view of the fact pointed out above that such excitation is probably the most efficient cause of epilepsy. Treatment should be given to correct blood-flow to and from the brain, including such treatments as opening the mouth against resistance, treatments above the course of the carotids, elevation of the clavicles, treatment of the cervical sympathetics, etc. Attention should be given to upbuilding the general health, and to keeping bowels and stomach in good condition. All causes of worry or nerve-strain should be avoided and the patient should lead an out-door life. The food should be light and easily digested, consisting of some meat, fruit, vegetables, cereals, etc. Cold sponge baths are recommended.

MIGRAINE, (Hemicrania, Sick Headache) and OTHER FORMS OF HEADACHE (Cephalalgia).

DEFINITION : Migraine is "a neurosis characterized by severe attacks of headache, often paroxysmal and more or less periodic, with or without nausea and vomiting." It is of obscure pathology; there seems to be nothing to connect it with stomach lesion, and from an osteopathic point of view it is generally found to be due to cervical bony lesions.

Headache is the general term used to describe pain in the head. It may be either symptomatic or idiopathic, the latter being generally chronic and due to specific bony lesion, usually in the cervical vertebrae. A large class of the latter come under osteopathic treatment, generally in very bad condition after having suffered far beyond the power of drugs to cure. These may almost be considered as suffering from a hitherto undescribed form of headache, depending upon specific lesion, often the result of accident, and usually immediately relieved and cured upon removal of the lesion. The form embraces many of the kinds of heahache generally described under one or other of the usual classifications.

CASES : (1) Extremely severe frontal headache in a man of thirty-two, since boyhood. He had taken every known remedy without avail. Lesions were found in muscular contractions on the right side of the neck; the dorsal spine was anterior in its upper half ; the 11th dorsal vertebra was luxated to the left ; the 2d and 5th lumbar vertebrae were prominent ; the sacrum was tilted forward and the left innominate was slipped, lengthening the limb. The lesions were corrected and the case cured.

(2) Nervous headache of years' standing in a lady was cured in three months.

(3) Chronic headache of twenty years' standing cured in six weeks.

(4) Acute headache, very severe ; pulse 128, temperature 103 3-5° ; relieved in one treatment and soon cured.

(5) Migraine in a man of thirty, since his sixteenth year, when he fell from a wagon. Lesion existed at the 3d cervical vertebra and at the atlas. The case was relieved at once and cured.

(6) In a boy of twelve a very severe headache was caused by a fall on his head from a bar in the gymnasium. The atlas was found displaced laterally, and the case was cured in two treatments.

(7) In a chronic case of occipital headache persisting for years, no ordinary remedy would affect the condition. The atlas was found slipped and the muscles about it very much contracted and tender. Relief was given at one treatment, and the case was practically cured in one month.

(8) Migraine, with constipation, stomach disease, temporary blindness, etc., was cured in nine months.

(9) A man of forty-five, troubled for many years by occipital headache, mostly upon the left side. Lesion was found at the atlas, impinging upon a cervical nerve. Cure was accomplished in two months.

(10) In a lady of thirty there was constant occipito-frontal headache. The eyes were weak and painful; the glasses had been changed six times in one year. The muscles of neck and shoulder were found much contracted, the atlas was luxated to the right and painful upon pressure. But one severe headache occurred during one month's treatment, and the eyes were much improved. In two months the glasses were laid aside and the headache was cured.

(11) Headache, with blind spells, in a woman of forty-one; the 1st and 2d cervical vertebrae were approximated and sore; the muscles of the upper cervical region very tense; headache constant; 1st to 8th dorsal vertebrae were flattened anteriorly; 11th dorsal to 3d lumbar posterior. The patient had suffered a sunstroke, and had had two or three attacks monthly since.

(12) Congestive headache in a man of thirty-seven, of twelve years' standing. Violent attacks occurred daily, and every known remedy had been used in vain. The sole lesion was a depressed clavical interfering

with the venous flow from the head.   Two treatments restored the bone to place ann cured the case.

(13) Catamenial headache (migraine) occurred each month, lasting two or three days. It was of six years' standing. A cure was made in two month's treatment, no headache occurring after the first treatment.

(14) Chronic headache of four years' standing, caused by a fall upon the back of the head, which rendered the neck partly stiff.   There was contracture of the tissues over the spinous process of the axis, which was displaced to the right.   After four treatments the pain had disappeared.

LESIONS :   Migraine, with other forms shows the usual lesions.   Lesions found to produce it are of the atlas : 1st, 2nd and 3d cervical; upper dorsal; 8th and 10th dorsal; 7th and 8th ribs.

When headache is symptomatic purely, lesion depends upon the primary diseae, but specific lesion is often present and determines the effect in the head.

Nine of the above fifteen cases report lesion.   Eight of the nine were cervical lesions; one was clavicular; six of the eight cervical were of the atlas. Atlas, axis, cervical, and, to some extent, spinal lesions are the important ones producing headache. They result in chronic, idiopathic headaches. Often these may develop into insanity.

Lesions act by disturbing sympathetic relations, reflexly causing the headaches, just as may be the case in reflex headache from uterine prolapsus. They all act by stoppage of blood-flow. This may occur in several ways. The vertebral arteries may be occluded by pressure from the displaced cervical vertebra; the clavicle may hinder venous flow in the external and internal jugulars, the sympathetic irritation may set up vaso-motor reflexes prevent proper circulation. A lesion may cause headache by direct pressure of the luxated vertebra upon a nerve-fibre. A very common place for this to occur is at the atlas which impinges branches of the of the suboccipital nerve sent to supply the occipito-atlantal articulation. The same thing is apt to occur at any of the upper three cervical vertebrae, the corresponding nerves sending branches to supply sensation to the scalp. Contraction of tissues over branches of the fifth nerve, or at their foramia of exit may cause headache. Reflex or direct irritation of the fifth nerve may cause it.

The kinds of pain in headache aid in diagnosing the variety. Dana notes the fact that a pulsating or throbbing pain occurs in headache due to vaso-motor disturbance, as in migraine, a dull, heavy pain in toxic or dyspeptic forms; a constrictive, squeezing, or pressing pain in neurotic or neurasthenic cases; a hot, burning, or sore pain in rheumatic or anemic headache; a sharp, boring pain in hysteric, epileptic, or neurotic forms.

The pain is usually found to be localized in or referred to the peripheral ends of the fifth nerve, they supplying the antero-lateral parts of the scalp and the dura mater with sensation. Hence treatment is directed to the branches of the fifth nerve upon the face and scalp. The chief local treatment in occipital headache is made to the upper four cervical nerves, as their branches are here involved.

The PROGNOSIS is good in all forms of headache, even in migraine. The most long standing and severe cases yield readily to treatment, even when all other remedies have failed.

The TREATMENT described will apply to any of the numerous kinds of headache described, though special postions of the treatment laid down may apply to any given case as sufficient for it. The treatment must be adapted to the case, each one needing a special study of its features to enable one to discover the cause and apply the proper treatment. The treatment successful in one case may not apply to another.

The lesion must be removed, and this often constitutes the sole treatment necessary. All causes of irritation must be removed, such as eye strain, sympathetic disturbance, uterine or stomach disease, etc. Ordinarily the first step is the relaxation of contractured muscles in the neck and upper dorsal region. This relives irritation to nerv es, frees circulation and prepares for the replacing of a displaced vertebra. Attention should be given to freeing all points of venous flow from the head. Treatment may be made in the course of the veins across the forehead to the outer canthus of the eye and down toward the angle of the jaw, along the jugular veins, raising the clavicle and relaxing all the tissues.

Inhibition along the back and sides of the neck in the region of the upper four vertebrae, and in the sub-occipital fossae quiets the upper four cervical nerves and aids in restoring equality of circulation through affect upon the superior cervical ganglion.

Often pressure made as follows is efficient: in the mid-line of the neck, just below the occiput; below the ears, upon and below the transverse processes of the atlas; along the upper dorsal region at the upper three or four vertebrae. These treatments quiet cerebro-spinal nerves and correct vasomotion.

Treatment should be made upon the face over the points of the fifth nerve (Chap. V. B). Relax tissues over the nerves and at the foramina. Manipulation to relax the tissues all along the course of the longitudinal, sinus, from nasion to occipital protuberance, and thence laterally toward the mastoid processes, over the course of the lateral sinuses, aids in freeing the circulation in them. As this treatment is carried over the vertex the terminals of the various sensory nerves of the scalp are affected and quieted.

Deep pressure over the solar plexus and inhibitive abdominal treatment aid in relieving the headache some times by quieting the reflexes and calling the blood away from the head.

Exciting causes should be avoided. It is well in such cases as need it to give attention to regulating the condition of stomach and bowels. Cold applied to the forehead and temples, and heat applied to the base of the skull and the extremities aid in relief.

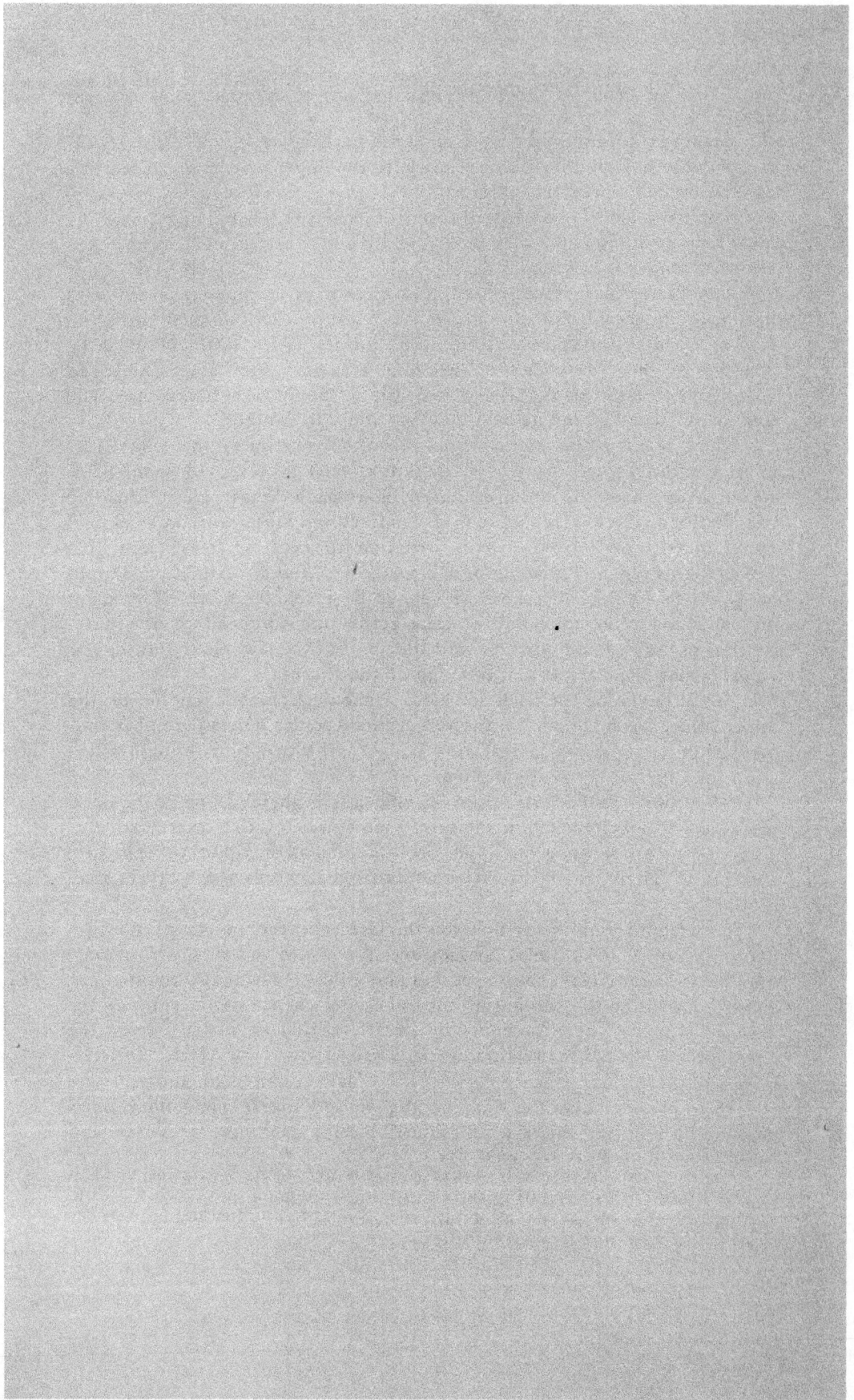

LOCOMOTOR ATAXIA AND SPASTIC PARAPLEGIA.

DEFINITION: Locomotor Ataxia, or Tabes Dorsalis, is a disease characterized by sclerosis of the posterior columns of the cord, loss of co-ordination in the muscles of the limbs, absence of the patellar reflex, lightning pains in the limbs, and the Argyll-Robertson pupil, which reacts to accomodation but not to light.

CASES: (1) In a woman of thirty-two, lesions were found at the atlas and upper lumbar region. Under treatment she regained control of bladder and bowels, became able to walk well, and the progress of the disease had apparently been terminated.

(2) In a man of twenty-nine, the lesion was a complex curvature of the spine. It was lateral to the right from the 5th dorsal to 2nd lumbar, and posterior in the lower lumbar region, being so marked that the left lower ribs came within the iliac fossa, while the right ones descended over the hip. The whole thorax was misshaped. The right limb was atrophied to one-half its original size. After eight months' treatment the patient could walk thirty-five blocks without a cane; his general health was good, and the disease was showing rapid improvement.

(3) A case in a young man of twenty, in which there was marked scoliosis of the dorsal spine, involving the thorax, some improvement in the locomotor ataxia was gained under treatment.

(4) A case in a man of thirty-five showed spinal lesion in the dorsal spine between the shoulders, the vertebrae being irregular and posterior. Under continued treatment his walking was much improved, visceral crises were prevented, the control of bladder and rectum were regained, and the pains in the lower limbs were done away.

(5) A case which could not rise from his chair nor walk, could do both after three weeks' treatment.

(6) A case of eleven years' standing in a man. In several weeks treatment the pain was stopped and the case showed marked improvement.

(7) A case presented spinal lesion in the form of a too great anterior sweep of the lumbar region of the spine.

SPASTIC PARAPLEGIA (Spastic Spinal Paralysis) is a cord disease with loss of muscular power, exaggerated patellar reflexes, a peculiar gait, and precipitate micturition, It is a primary lateral sclerosis of the cord.

CASE: A middle-aged man, after injury to the spine in a mine accident, was affected with complete motor and sensory paraplegia. Operation for supposed fracture of the 7th dorsal vertebra removed pressure and restored sensation for the greater part. Spastic paraplegia developed. The lesions were found to be a posterior 7th dorsal vertebra; 8th, 9th and 10th posterior and toward the left. Considerable improvement was made under treatment.

Lesions in both of these diseases are found at various places along the spine. In spastic paraplegia they are generally in the lower dorsal, lumbar and sacral regions.

In locomotor ataxia spinal curvature is often found as the cause. Derangement of the thoracic vertebrae in the region between the shoulders often causes it. Atlas, cervical and lumbar lesions are often found.

The PROGNOSIS in neither disease is promising as to cure. Most cases are benefited, some to a marked extent. Locomotor ataxia is more frequently met with and on the whole more successfully treated. The progress of the disease is often checked; the lightning pains and visceral crises are prevented or checked; control of bladder and rectum are established; the power of walking, even after complete loss in some cases, is restored. These cases are generally benefited, but sometimes do not yield to treatment. In cases of spastic paraplegia the sum-total of results is not so great. The walking is often improved, and precipitate micturition is bettered.

The sclerotic changes in the cord in these diseases renders them incurable even after removal of specific lesion, yet the sclerotic process is often checked by the removal of lesion and the attendant treatment.

A few cases of both diseases, in early stages and resulting from injury, are reported cured.

The TREATMENT of locomotor ataxia consists in the removal of lesion and general spinal treatment. The removal of lesion alone is insufficient. The thorough spinal treatment must be made to influence spinal nerve connections, the central distribution of the sympathetics, and the blood-circulation about and to the spine. This treatment should be given especially from the middle dorsal down, as the degenerative changes in cord and changes begin in the lower part. If the ataxic condition has not yet appeared in the arms, and cerebral symptoms have not developed the indication is especially for treatment to the lower spine. Treatment to the upper spinal and cervical regions should be given, however, at any stage, to limit or prevent the spread of the pathological cord changes in these regions.

The nerve-supply to the limbs, upper and lower, as well as the limbs themselves, should be treated. Care must be taken in this matter, as the tendency of the long bones to fracture is marked in locomotor ataxia. The arthropathies, if present, call for special treatment to the joint involved, and its nerve and blood-supply. As the knee-joints are most frequently attacked, the treatment to the lower limbs will serve to lessen the danger of their occurance. The spinal treatment should include springing the spine, and various other methods of separating the vertebrae from each other, increasing circulation about them and keeping up their nutritive integrity, as the articular surfaces and interarticular fibro-cartilages are liable respectively to absorption and atrophy.

Abdominal treatment should be maintained to prevent visceral crises, most common about the stomach. Treatment should be upon the abdominal nerve-plexuses and blood-circulation. The stomach and bowels may thus be kept in good condition. Lumbar and sacral treatment, together with treatment to the internal iliac blood-vessels from the abdominal aspect, aid in restoring the spincters of bladder and rectum to good conditions. In case of necessity a catheter should be used to empty the bladder. To relieve the lightning pains in the limbs strong inhibition should be made upon the anterior crural nerve in Scarpa's triangle; upon the great sciatic at the back of the thigh between the tuberosity and the great trochanter, slightly nearer the latter; and upon the lumbar and sacral portions of the spine.

The treatment of spastic paraplegia proceeds upon the same lines as the general treatment for locomotor ataxia, including removal of lesion, thorough general spinal treatment, and treatment of the lower limbs. The spasticity in the latter sometimes hinders treatment, but may be overcome by inhibition of the anterior crural and sciatic as above.

Other forms, such as Secondary Spastic Paralysis, in which the symptoms are not so well marked; Congenital Spastic Paraplegia, usually due to injury at birth; Ataxic Paraplegia, combining spastic and ataxic features retaining the reflexes; and the Combined System Scleroses, etc., are approached in the same manner for discovery of lesions and treatment.

PARALYSIS AGITANS.

(Parkinson's Disease. Shaking Palsy,)

DEFINITION:—A chronic disease, in which there is tremor, peculiar character of speech and gait, and progressive loss of muscular power.

The LESIONS found in this disease usually occur in the cervical and upper dorsal regions, and among the upper ribs. These lesions, being present, doubtless determine the victim of the disease.

It occurs in those whose central nervous system is thus weakened and laid liable to the action of such secondary causes as exhausting illness, mental strain, worry, traumatism, etc. The latter may directly result in such lesions. The fact that the pathology of the disease is obscure, it being by many regarded as a functional disturbance, and the further fact that the causes are not well known, lends color to the 'theory that such lesions as are recognized by Osteopathy, being always such as are not sought for by the regular practitioner, are the real causes of the condition. They occur high in the spine, at a point where, acting upon the central nervous system, they could produce the effect in the whole body, as noted in the tremor of both upper and lower limbs, as well as of the head sometimes.

The PROGNOSIS:—There is a reasonable expectation of limiting the progress of the disease and bettering the patient's general condition. The fact that there is no pathological change in the cord, and that the disease is probably functional, leaves ground for hope that very much benefit, perhaps cure, can be attained under osteopathic treatment. A number of cases have been cured.

The practitioner must bear in mind that it is a feature of the disease for the patient to sometimes be better, and he must not too strongly encourage the patient when such a period occurs, without reason to expect the permanence of such gain.

The TREATMENT consists in removal of lesion; the thorough relaxation of all spinal and cervical muscles, particularly apt to be set and hardened about the neck and shoulders; and a most thorough general spinal treatment. Particular attention should be paid to the condition of the nerve-plexuses supplying the upper and lower limbs- These, and the circulation to the limbs, should be strongly stimulated. The general health is usually good, but it is not amiss to keep bowels, kidneys and liver well stimulated.

Light exercise and baths are good for the case.

OCCUPATION NEUROSES.

DEFINITION:—A neurosis due to constant use of certain groups of muscles in occupations which necessitate delicate movements, resulting in cramp, spasm, paralysis, tremor or neuralgia, and due to specific lesion to the nerves supplying the affected groups of muscles.

The very numerous varieties of this disease, various forms of musician's cramp, telegrapher's, seamstress', driver's, milker's, cigar-makers, etc., are all manifestations, more or less severe, of obstruction to the nerves supplying the parts involved. These obstructions generally act upon the nerve-supply of the upper limbs, but in a few varieties, as in ballet-dancers and tailors, those of the lower limbs may be involved.

CASES:—Numerous cases of telegrapher's, writer's and piansit's paralysis are known and recalled in this connection, although the data as to lesions, etc., are not now available. These cases were generally cured. The following cases are typical.

(1) A marked case of telegrapher's paralysis, of three years' standing. For two years the hands had been almost useless, and the patient could not distinguish by touch between an ink-stand and a pencil, sensation and motion were both much impaired. The lesions were found in the 1st, 2d, and 3d right ribs being close together; the clavicle down upon the right first rib and the cervical origin of the brachial plexus covered with much contracured muscles. After one month's treatment the patient could write his name. In six weeks he could distinguish between coins by touch, and in three months the case was cured.

(2)   A case of telegrapher's paralysis of three months' standing. The patient had stopped work to go to a hospital, but took osteopathic treatment instead.   In three days he was able to return to work, and was cured in five weeks.

(3)   Pianist's paralysis, showing lesions in the upper dorsal spine.

(4)   Pianist's paralysis showing lesions in the cervical and upper dorsal regions of the spine, depression of both clavicles, and contracture of muscles in the posterior cervical, upper dorsal, and shoulder regions.

The LESIONS in these cases are doubtless often directly due to the occupation.   Case (1) above is a good illustration of the result of an occupation requiring the elevation of the right shoulder, resulted in drawing together the upper three ribs, and in approximating the clavicle and first rib in such a manner as to bring pressure upon the brachial plexus.   A faulty posture, involving bad position of the shoulder, neck and upper spine, is quite as likely to result in bony lesions in these parts as is faulty posture to result in spinal curvature.

In a certain number of cases the lesions are likely present in the spine and other parts, and determine an early breakdown in the anatomical parts concerned in the occupation, from over-use.   Over use of an arm, as in writing, no doubt plays its part in wearing out the nerve-mechanism, but the fact that many young people suffering from an occupation neurosis are found to have these lesions while many other persons labor assiduously for years at the same occupations without disability, indicates that the lesions behind the excessive use is the real cause of the trouble.   Use of the arm is really excessive only in proportion as the parts do not recuperate after use.   The lesion to nerve-supply prevents proper recuperation and the arm wears out because of the presence of lesion.

In pianists spinal disease is often found to be due to sitting for hours at the instrument.   It may as reasonably cause spinal lesions of a nature to result in the neurosis of the arms.   That central, i. e. spinal, lesion is present is indicated by the fact that in penmen who learn to write with the left hand after an attack of paralysis in the right the disease usually soon makes its appearance in that member also.   In pianists the trouble is generally bilateral from spinal lesion.

Lesions may occur high in the cervical region, but such is not likely to be the case.   Lesions from the origin of the brachial plexus to the sixth dorsal vertebra are met with.   Most commonly the lesion lies between the 5th cervical and fourth dorsal, favoring a position still lower in the cervical and about the upper three or four dorsal.   Lesion of the clavicle and upper two ribs, especially upon the right side, are very common.   It is readily seen from the nature of the causes producing lesion that the ribs below the upper two may be involved.   Ribs and vertebrae as low as the 5th or 6th may be luxated and cause the trouble.   Vaso-motor, secretory and trophic affections occur in the affected member.   Vaso-motors to the arms are found as low as the first thoracic ganglion, or lower. The connection of the inter-costal nerves with the sympathetic system may explain why rib lesions this low may cause the trouble. The first and second intercostal nerves are con-nected with the brachial plexus. They are often impinged by the corres-ponding ribs in these troubles. McConnell calls attention to the fact that slight luxations of shoulder and elbow-joints may cause this disease. In such case the affect would probably be through lesion to the articular branches supplied from the brachial plexus.

While Dana states that this condition is "a neurosis having no appre-ciable anatomical basis," it seems from the results gotten by the removal of lesion that Osteopathy discovers the real anatomical cause of disease.

The PROGNOSIS is good. Even the worst cases are cured. Cure is the rule, though some cases may be intractable.

TREATMENT:—The removal of lesion as the direct cause, as in displace-ment of the clavicle onto the brachial plexus, is often the only treatment necessary. The nerve and blood-supply of the affected part should be kept free by treatment upon them and by relaxation of all contractured muscles and hardened tissues. The arms should be stretched and treated as de-scribed in Chap. X. The brachial plexus may be stimulated on the inner side of the arm just below the axilla, and in the neck behind the clavicle. Treatment should be carried up along the plexus to the spine. The elbow and shoulder joints should be sprung and adjusted if necessary. (Chap. X.)

It may be necessary to have the patient rest from his occupation dur-ing the treatment, particularly at first for a few weeks. This matter depends upon conditions. Some cases have been cured while the customary work is continued. In some cases it is well to give a general treatment to the nervous system, as nervous symptoms may appear. Vertigo and insomnia are sometimes present, doubtless due to the upper spinal lesions affecting the blood-circulation to the brain.

Local work should be carried over the brachial artery, and over the fore-arm and hand. This increases local circulation and does away with the local congestion and secretory disturbance found in the affected mem-bers. It may be useful for the patient to develop the arms by systematic gymnastics. The various mechanical appliances used to lessen the work upon the affected muscle groups and to call into play other and larger groups, may be useful if the patient finds it necessary to continue his occu-pation. Sleeves that interfere with free motion of the hand in writing, cuffs that bind the wrist, constricting bands that may be used as sleeve support-ers, and any agency limiting motion and circulation must be avoided.

The pain frequently present in arms and shoulders may be quieted by inhibition of the plexus and its spinal origin, but generally yields to the general process of relaxing muscles, etc.

NEURASTHENIA.

(NERVOUS PROSTRATION.)

DEFINITION: "A functional disease of the nervous system, character-ized by mental and bodily weakness." It is not a psychosis. There is functional exhaustion and irritablity of the nerve centers.

CASES: (1) Well marked neurasthenia in a child of five, a neurotic. It had never walked, and had never slept in the daytime. In one month it became able to walk under the treatment.

(2) In a lady a case of three years' standing, with attendant consti-pation, was cured in two months.

(3) In a woman of thirty-two, neurasthenia developed after confine-ment and sickness. Symptoms of the disease were all very well marked. Lesions were found in a displacement of the third cervical vertebra to the right, general depression of the ribs, separation of the 11th and 12th dorsal vertebrae, a posterior luxation of the fifth lumbar vertebra, and contracture of the lumbar muscles. The neurasthenia was apparently reflex from uter-ine disease. Two weeks' daily treatment re-established menstruation, which had been suppressed for some time. Under one month's treatment all the symptoms had disappeared.

(4) A case of neurasthenia in a lady of sixty, following overwork and runaway accident. The whole spine and body was hyperesthetic, the spinal tissues, from occiput to sacrum, were exceedingly tense. Treatment was beneficial from the first. One year's treatment produced great improve-ment.

(5) In a lady of fifty, with uterine disease, lesions were found in a posterior luxation of the atlas and depression of all the ribs, narrowing the thorax. The patient was benefitted.

(6) Neurasthenia in a lady of thirty-five, complicated with constipa-tion, ovarian disease, and many other symptoms, was almost cured in one month's treatment.

(7) In neurasthenia of eight year's standing, due to cigarette smoking, six weeks' treatment cured the cigarette habit and materially bettered the general condition.

(8) Neurasthenia and exophthalmic goitre of one month's standing. The goitre was cured in two week's treatment. In one month's treatment the neurasthenia was cured and the patient had gained twenty pounds.

(9) Traumatic neurasthenia developed after the patient was thrown from a buggy. Lesion was found in a slip at the fourth lumbar and marked lateral luxation of the tenth dorsal vertebra. The spinal lesion was cor-rected in three weeks, but no improvement occurred in the patient's gener-al condition until ten weeks' treatment had been taken. After two weeks' further treatment the case was well.

(10) In a man of thirty neurasthenia of three year's standing was cured in two months.

(11) In a young lady a case of several month's standing was cured in four months.

The LESIONS found in neurasthenia are general spinal lesions. Different cases present different lesions, and no typical lesion may be described for all cases. Yet perhaps a majority of these cases show a depression of all of the ribs, narrowing the thorax and often causing enteropsis. Floating kidney and enteroptosis are well known as causes of neurasthenia. There is no doubt that many cases of neurasthenia apparently thus caused are really due to bad spinal condition and flattening of the thorax through depresssion of all the ribs. These extensive lesions effect the cerebro spinal system directly, also the sympathetic system, thus causing the neurasthenia and the enteroptosis, (p. 98.)

Often the lesion in these cases is such as produce disease in some organ, secondary to which neurasthenia is developed. This is well illustrated in these lower spinal lesions producing uterine disease, from which neurasthenia is reflexly caused. Thus a variety of lesions may be found in neurasthenia, different cases presenting different lesions. Each case demands an individual study. For the production of neurasthenia there is necessary merely a lesion producing an irritation upon the nerve system, reflexly or directly, allowing a leakage of nerve-force, and determining the victim of neurasthenia from overwork, worry, uterine disease, naso-pharyngeal disease, the use of coffee, alcohol, etc.

The different varieties of neurrasthenia may be caused by the predominance of lesion, e. g., the cerebral type by upper dorsal and cervical lesions, the gastric by splanchnic lesions, the lithemic by lower dorsal and upper lumbar lesions, etc. Iefluenza, a common cause of this disease, is a malady particularly noted by osteopathy as producing serious spinal lesions, mostly in the shape of contractured muscles and tenseness of the other tissues, but sometimes actual bony lesions by drawing parts out of place through contracture of attached tissues. Lesions thus produced may cause neurasthenia. Neurasthenia is common as the result of traumatism, such as caused by railway accidents, bony lesions thus being produced as irritants to nerves.

The PROGNOSIS for cure is good. Those cases that have not yielded to any of the usual modes of treatment often readily yield to osteopathic treatment. The best of results may be expected in the worst cases. Cases are often quickly cured f gotten in the early stages. The average case demands a somewhat long course of treatment, varying from a few months to a year or more.

The TREATMENT must be adapted to the case in hand after a special study of its peculiarities and requirements. The removal of every source of reflex irritation is necessary, but these sources must be studied out in each individual case. The lesions present should be removed, but the case is not always at once benefitted thereby, as a course of treatment is generally necessary to recuperate the exhausted nerve-centers. Consequently a most systematic and thorough course of treatment be devoted to this end. The various spinal treatments as described, for relaxation of all spinal tissues, springing the vertebrae apart for freedom of circulation and stimulation of the spinal nerve-system and the circulation thereto, is given to increase nutrition of the nervous system and upbuild the exhausted centers. This spinal treatment affects the sympathetic system markedly. Cervical treatment is also important in this connection. Good results are usually at once apparent in relief of nerve-tension, reduction of irritability, and correction of function.

Special manifestations of the condition, as headache, insomnia, vertigo, etc., call for cervical treatment particularly. Bowels, kidneys, liver, etc., must be carefully looked after to relieve the constipation, lithemia, anorexia and other such symptoms usually present. A thorough general treatment of the whole body is not amiss in these cases.

The patient must be kept free from excitement and from all causes of drain upon nervous vitality. The diet should be light and nutritious. The use of cold sponge or shower baths may be helpful. Advising the patient to take gentle exercise, baths, etc,, will aid him to preserve a cheerful state of mind. Some cases may be treated daily with advantage, in the beginning of the treatment. Later, the treatments may be decreased in number to three or two per week.

HYSTERIA.

This is a condition frequently met and treated osteopathically. One needs to be continually upon guard against its simulation of other conditions, being equally careful not to overlook other diseases because of a hurried diagnosis of hysteria. Being a functional disease of the nervous system, and a psychosis, it is frequently found to depend upon some spinal bony lesion acting as the cause disturbing the nervous equilibrium. The *lesion* varies. One cannot expect a certain kind of lesion in these cases, but generally finds some actual derangement which is at bottom, responsible for the altered nerve-conditions making it possible for a neurotic disposition, infectious fevers, poisons of various kinds, emotional disturbances, mental or physical strain, and other causes to result in hysterical attacks.

Correction of lesion removes the primary cause of irritation to the nervous system, perhaps cures a certain disease to which the hysteria is secondary, and is an important step in the radical cure of the condition.

The *Prognosis* for cure is good. The treatment relieves nervous tension and quiets the overwrought system at once.

In the *Treatment* considerable tact must be used. The primary treatment embraces the removal of all lesions and causes of irritation. A course of treatment for the general nervous system must be carried through. The general treatment as described for upbuilding the nervous system in neurasthenia would be applicable here.

During an hysterical attack the practitioner must use great firmness, but not violence, with the patient. He must gain mental and moral control, and while applying a general relaxing and inhibitive spinal and cervical treatment to relieve nerve-tension and to quiet the nervous system, by a strong show of authority compel the patient to cease various motions, unbend a clinched hand, stop incoherent talking, etc. Sometimes a dash of cold water upon the face or abdomen, or pressure over the ovaries will end the attack. All sympathetic friends must be dismissed from the room, and moral suasion, with isolation of the patient, be tried. The practitioner must gain the patient's confidence. Hysterical joints, hysterical pains, contractures, eye-symptoms, paralyses, etc., call for no special treatment; all disappear upon regulation of the mental condition and upbuilding of the general nervous system.

Many chronic cases, as in bed-ridden hysterics, must be carried through a course of education in performing simple motions and acts which they thought beyond their power. The patient should lead a regular life, and her mind should be kept occupied by some engrossing occupation.

Judicious management of the case, authority over the patient, and a careful general course of treatment for the health of the body and particularly of the nervous system, will be successful in the majority of cases.

INSOMNIA.

DEFINITION. Incomplete, disturbed, or lacking sleep. A condition frequently idiopathic and caused by specific lesions, usually bony. Idiopathic insomnia embraces many forms generally looked upon as symptomatic or secondary. Many really symptomatic or secondary cases are noted, especially in nervous diseases, the primary condition itself being usually found to depend, at bottom, upon bony lesion.

CASES: Very numerous cases are met and treated osteopathically. The following cases illustrate various points in connection with such cases:

(1) Insomnia, nervousness, and a complication of troubles. Sleep could not be induced by the most powerful soporifics. Lesion was found among the cervical and upper dorsal vertebrae. The case was cured in two months' treatment.

(2) Insomnia and general nervousness, pronounced incurable. The patient had had no good nights' sleep in five years, and had become a

nervous wreck.   Lesion was found in the shape of contractured condition of all the cervical muscles.   The case was cured in one month.

(3)   A case of several years' standing, in which the lesion affected the atlas, which was displaced a little to the right, was cured by the correction of the lesion in six treatments.

(4)   A case of insomnia as an accompaniment of neurasthenia, in which the patient had depended upon soporifics for a number of years, slept well after the second or third treatment.   The use of artificial aid to sleep was necessary but at rare intervals thereafter.   The case was practically cured at the time of report.

(5)   A case of insomnia of some years' standing, due to cervical and upper dorsal lesions, cured in six months' treatment.

(6)   A case of three years' standing, in which the heart-beat had become very irregular from the resulting nervousness.   Four treatments corrected the heart-beat, and the case had been practically cured, at the time of report, by two months' treatment.

(7)   A case of paroxysmal sleep, or narcolepsy, presenting lesion in the form of a luxation of the second cervical vertebra toward the right.   The case was not observed under treatment.

(8)   A case of narcolepsy due to cervical lesions successfully treated.

LESIONS AND ANATOMICAL RELATIONS: The lesions, both in insomnia and in the various other disorders of sleep, are generally found in the atlas and cervical and upper dorsal regions.   All such cases, perhaps constituting a majority of all cases of these diseases, should be regarded from the osteopathic point of view as idiopathic insomnia, dependent upon specific lesion interfering with circulation to the brain.   Lesions to the atlas and second cervical vertebra are very common causes, and lesions usually occur within the cervical region or among the upper five dorsal vertebrae.   Lesions to clavicle and to corresponding ribs may be present.   It will be observed that from the occiput to 5th dorsal all these lesions fall within a area particularly rich in sympathetic and vaso-motor centers for the head, as before pointed out.   Atlas and axis lesion acting upon the superior cervical ganglion, medulla, or curvical sympathetic, and other cervical and the upper dorsal lesions acting upon the sympathetic nerves supplying vaso-motor control to the blood vessels of neck and head, disturb circulation to the brain and cause the insomnia.   Direct pressure of the cervical vertebrae upon the vertebral arteries may contribute to or produce, the same result.

It is probable that in many cases of insomnia there is an anemic state of the brain caused by the interference of such lesions with the sympathetics or by direct pressure upon the arteries.   The insomnia in various diseases of the heart and arteries, in general anemia, and in Bright's disease, is said to be due to an anemic condition of the brain.   On the other hand it is doubtless true that there is in many cases a sluggish or impeded cerebral circulation as a result of the disturbance of sympathetic vaso-motors, impeded venous return, etc., caused by these lesions. In neurasthenic insomnia, it is said, there is loss of vaso-motor tone in the cerebral vessels. The use of various mechanical remedies is based upon the idea of calling the blood from the head to the skin or abdominal organs, e. g., a hot foot-bath, eating a light lunch, etc.

In some cases the symptoms indicate the necessity of increasing or decreasing the amount of blood in the cerebral vessels, and these results may be readily attained by the appropriate treatment. But, from the nature of the case, removal of lesion and the restoration of free circulation result in restoring normal quiet to the nerve mechanism and normal flow of the blood in the vessels, characteristic of the normal body which enjoys healthful sleep. Such a result is the most rational object of the treatment.

When insomnia is symptomatic or secondary, lesions must be sought according to the primary condition.

In some cases of disturbed vaso-motor conditions of the brain, lesion is found in the form of much thickened, tensed, and overgrown tissues at the base of the skull, above and about the spine of the axis, extending laterally toward the mastoid process. With this condition there frequently exists an approximation of the second cervical spine to the occiput.

The PROGNOSIS in insomnia is good. No class of cases presents more striking results in the shape of cure of the most long-standing and intractable cases. It is a frequent occurrence that a case of some year's standing is made to sleep naturally after a single or few treatments.

Not all cases thus easily yield to treatment. Often great patience and persistence are necessary to secure good results.

The TREATMENT calls for the removal of lesion primarily, and of any cause of irritation to the nervous system. The treatment as described in detail for headache, q. v., is applicable here. It embraces inhibition of the superior cervical ganglion and of all the cervical vaso-motors, including the middle and inferior cervical ganglion and the upper dorsal centers, deep pressure beneath the ears and beneath the occiput (p. 187.) All the cervical muscles and other tissues should be thoroughly relaxed. A general spinal treatment, in nervous cases, at once relieves nerve-tension and irritation, and materially aids in producing sleep. It is sometimes well to add to this a general body treatment as an aid in equalizing circulation and toning up the nervous system. All points of cervical circulation should be attended to. The treatment begun over forehead and face may be continued down over the neck, opening the mouth against resistance, stimulating the carotid arteries and jugular veins, raising the clavicles, and even the upper few ribs, and thus entirely freeing the circulation to and from the head.

In cases of congestion of the cerebral vessels the inhibitive abdominal treatment should be used to draw the blood away from the head to the abdominal vessels.

In anemic cases one should add treatment to liver, kidneys, stomach, bowels and spleen. The heart and lungs should be stimulated. In insomnia due to auto-intoxication, as in lithemia, uremia, malaria, etc., one should look particularly to the excretions. Various domestic remedies may prove useful in simple cases, such as a warm general bath, a hot foot-bath, a cold douche down the spine, exercise and light massage, sleeping in cold rooms, avoidance of late meals, and the avoidance of mental work several hours before retiring.

The various perversions of sleep, such as dreams and nightmare, sommolentia, or incomplete sleep, sommambulism, morbid drowsiness, narcolepsy, catalepsy and prolonged sleep, would all be approached and treated upon the same lines as laid down for insomnia.

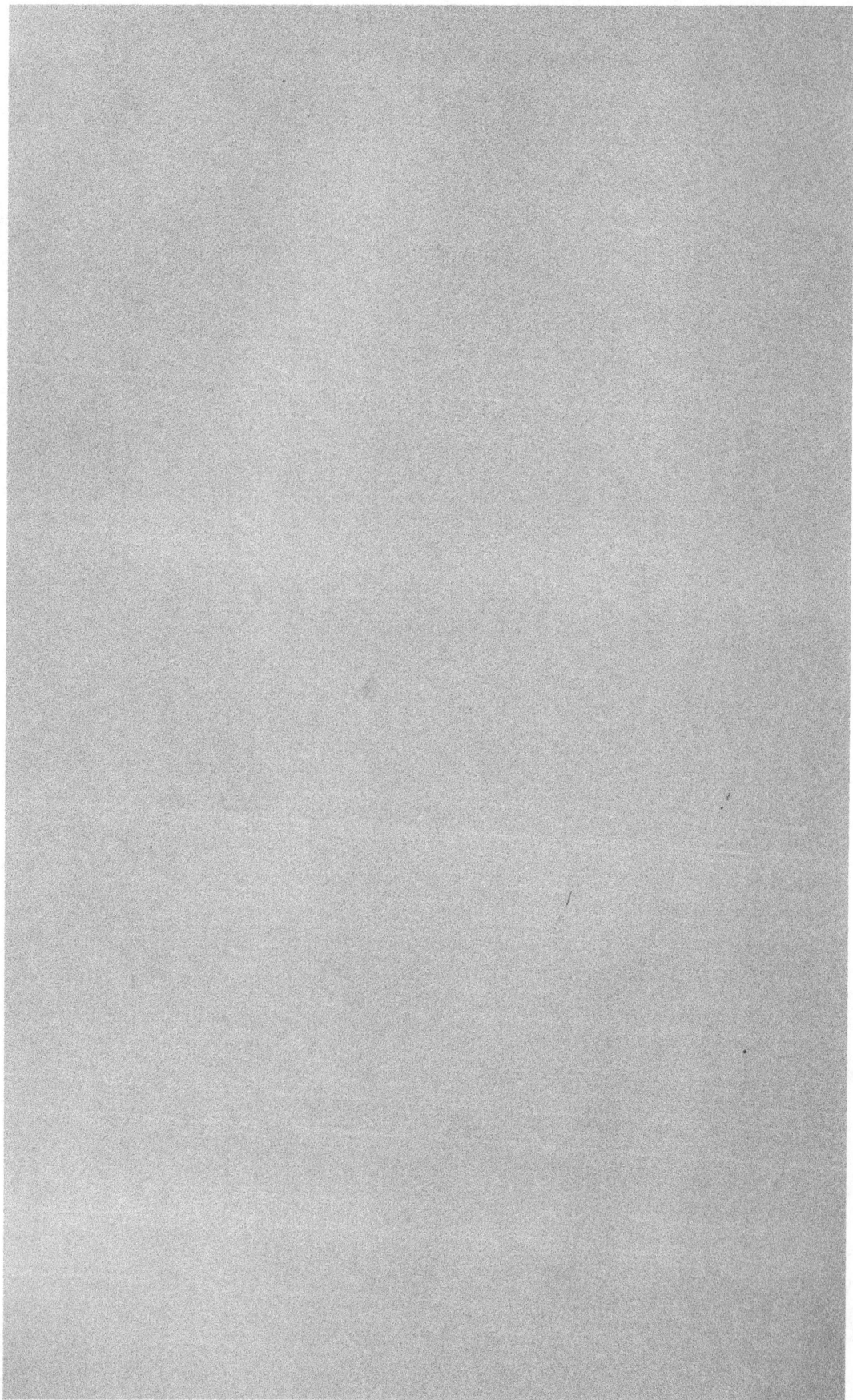

PARALYSIS,

The various forms of paralysis come, with much frequency, under osteopathic treatment. Paralysis of every part of the body, and from various causes, is successfully treated. The following cases are illustrative.

CASES:—(1) Paraplegia in a young lady, caused by fall of eighteen feet. The lower half of the body, and the lower limbs were paralyzed; control of the bladder was lost; within a certain period of five months she had passed twenty-eight calculi about the size of peas, never before the accident having had any urinary trouble. Lesions as follows: Marked posterior and slight lateral curvature of the spine, involving the lower and upper lumbar regions; the coccyx was bent and twisted; the right innominate bone was luxated backward. The condition was of nine and one-half months standing. After the first treatment she was able to sleep without the customary opiate. During the second week's treatment she began to gain control of the bladder; and the bowels acted naturally. The urine became normal at this time. During the course of the treatment an ulcer upon the right foot healed. A course of two month's treatment had almost cured the patient at the time of reporting the case.

(2) Paraplegia in a man, due to an injury in a runaway accident in which he was thrown, striking the lower dorsal and lumbar regions of the spine. After two weeks he gradually began to lose the use of his limbs, and in seven months he was confined to a chair, soon becoming unable to move a muscle of either limb. Lesions were as follows: 9th, 10th and 11th dorsal vertebrae displaced backward sufficiently to simulate the posterior angular projection in Potts' disease; a marked contraction of the muscles of the right side of the spine from the ninth dorsal down; slight swerving of the spine to the same side as the contracture and limited by its extent; great tension and slight lesion at the junction of the fifth lumbar vertebra with the sacrum; a binding together of all the spinal vertebrae by an apparent contracture of the ligaments. After a few treatments motion returned, and the patient was able to go about upon crutches. The case had been almost cured after a course of five weeks' treatment.

(3) Complete paralysis of the body below the waist, and of the lower limbs, caused by spinal curvature. The case was entirely cured, sensation, motion, and function of abdominal and pelvic organs being restored.

(4) Lack of free use of the feet due to a paralytic stroke six years before. A disarticulation among the tarsal bones was discovered, and its removal practically cured the case.

(5) Monoplegia, partial in one lower limb, of a number of years' standing was cured by the treatment.

(6) Paraplegia, partial, was cured by correction of lesion of the sixth dorsal vertebrae.

(7) General paralysis in a case which gradually for six years lost the use of all the voluntary muscles, the eyes were crossed and nearly blind, bowels and bladder were involved. The case was cured by adjusting lesion between the atlas and occiput, the latter being displaced anteriorly upon the former.

(8) Infantile paralysis involving the left lower limb. The case was in a child two years old. A sacro-iliac lesion was found as the cause, and was treated. The child could move the limb slightly after the first treatment, and after the sixth treatment perfect use was restored.

(9) A case of paralysis was found presenting lesions at the occipito-atlantal and lumbo-sacral articulations, and from the sixth to the tenth dorsal vertebrae. There was a history of exposure, alcoholism, sexual excess and great physical strain. Correction of the lesions effected a cure in five months.

(10) A case of paraplegia in a man of fifty-five, due to injury in a railroad wreck. Both innominate bones were found displaced anteriorly, and lesions were found involving the whole lumbar and lower dorsal regions of the spine. The paralysis of the limbs was total. After three treatments the patient could walk with crutches. After two weeks treatment the patient could walk without crutch or cane, being as well as ever, excepting some weakness of the spine.

(11) Paraplegia, involving the bowels, in a lady of fifty-three, and of fifteen years' standing. Sensation was lacking in the limbs, and there was very little motion. In less than one month's treatment sensation and motion were both perfectly restored and the bowels were acting naturally.

(12) Hemiplegia of the left side following two strokes, one fifteen years previously, one four years. The patient was cured in one month.

(13) Paralysis following a stroke. The cervical muscles were found contractured. Their correction was accomplished in five weeks, and none of the paralytic condition remained.

(14) Paralysis affecting the fingers and thumbs of both hands in a boy of fourteen. The only lesion was contracture of the muscles along the lower cervical and upper dorsal regions of the spine. There was also some atrophy of the muscles over the brachial plexus and the axillary artery. Five months' treatment restored the thumbs and first two fingers to nearly normal condition, the condition of the other fingers was much improved, and the hands could be used considerably.

(15) Paralysis and muscular atrophy of both arms in a boy six years of age. The condition followed an attack of malaria. The condition spread to involve both lower limbs. Spinal lesions were found preventing circulation to the cord. The child began at once to improve under the treatment. After the third treatment he could move his fingers. In two weeks he could use his hands well enough to feed himself. In one month he was practically cured.

(16) Disseminated subacute cervical and lumbar myelitis in a boy of seven, following the swallowing of two pins. Severe illness at once followed, and in the fifth week the pins were located by the X-ray on the left side about the level of the third cervical vertebra. They were later ejected, he becoming immediately totally paralyzed. For two weeks it was thought he could not live. After about seven weeks the case came under osteopathic treatment. The tissues of the entire cervical region were badly swollen and intensely painful, and this condition was found along the whole spine. Control of the bowels and bladder was lost, and the muscles of both upper and lower limbs atrophied. After the first treatment the patient slept soundly for the first time in two weeks. After about four months' treatment the case was practically cured.

(17) Monoplegia attacking the right lower limb of a girl of six, paralyzed since the age of ten as the result of spinal meningitis. No bony lesion was found, but the treatment was directed to increasing the circulation to the cord. The case was practically cured in three months' treatment.

(18) Paraplegia in a girl of four, which had been gradually developing for one year, showed improvement after the first treatment and was cured in less than one month.

(19) Paraplegia of eight months' standing. The patient was bedridden. Lesion was found as a posterior condition of all the lumbar vertebrae and a slip of the last lumbar upon the sacrum. The case was cured in three months.

(20) Bell's disease (facial paralysis), due to lesion at the second cervical vertebra, cured in three weeks.

(21) Partial paralysis of the lower limbs of four months' standing, due to lesions at the sacro-iliac articulation and at the 5th dorsal vertebra, cured in two months.

(22) Partial paralysis in a lower limb in a girl of six, since infancy, accompanied by under-developement of the limb, was found to be due to a partial dislocation of the hip, and was cured in two months.

(23) Paralysis, probably Progressive Spinal Muscular Atrophy, in a woman of thirty-five, of fifteen years' standing. The last two years had been spent in bed. Lesions were found at the 7th curvical and 1st dorsal vertebrae, which were anterior. The case was cured in ten months'.

(24) Paralysis of the fingers, affecting the last two, and partly the middle finger of the right hand. The patient was a lady of seventy-nine years of age. A fall upon the hand had occured a short time previously. A slight lateral lesion of the first dorsal vertebra was found and corrected, curing the case in six weeks.

(25) Hemiparesis or *Hemiplegia* in a lady of sixty, of six weeks' standing. The right side was affected. Lesion was found in the 3rd cervical and 5th lumbar vertebrae, the spinal muscles also being much contracted. The patient walked after the third treatment and was cured in six weeks.

(26) Hemiplegia, alternate or crossed, following a stroke a year before, affected the left side of the face and the right arm and lower limb. Case was practically cured in three and one-half months' treatment.

(27) Hemiplegia, partial, of the right side, following lightning-stroke. A displacement of the atlas was found and righted at once, immediately curing the case.

(28) Paralysis and Dysentery. The paralysis affected the lower limbs, and had been of seven years' standing. Lesion was found as great tenderness at the lumbo-sacral joint, a slip forward of the 5th lumbar, luxation of the innominates, and a lateral swerve of the lumbar and lower dorsal region of the spine. A tremor of the head was present, the cervical muscles being very tense. After seven months' treatment the lesion were about overcome and the patient was nearly well.

(29) Paralysis affecting certain muscles of the throat, also affecting the speech. The lesion was found in a contracture holding the hyoid bone out of place. The patient was cured by relaxing the contracture.

(30) Facial paralysis of more than one years' standing, was cured in three weeks' treatment. The lesion was found in a displacement of the second cervical vertebra.

(31) Facial paralysis caused by luxation of the atlas and axis to the left. There was also tension of the tissues at the base of the skull and on the left side of the neck. The case, still under treatment, was improving satisfactorily.

(32) Facial paralysis was seen on the day following its first appearance. The lesion was marked muscular contraction at the angle of the jaw on the affected side Treatment gave immediate relief, and the case had almost been cured in ten treatments.

(33) Progressive paralysis in a case after two falls causing serious illness. Motion in the lower limbs was lost, blindness ensued, and speech became unintelligible. There was formication in the hands and arms, and extreme pain along the spine, occuring in agonizing paroxysms. Lesions were found as a lateral dislocation of the third cervical vertebra, luxation of 7th and 8th right ribs, and a posterior protrusion of the lumbar vertebrae One treatment brought the first sleep possible in three days. Under treatment the spinal pain was relieved. vision was restored, and the patient had been practically cured at the time of the report.

(34) Crutch paralysis in a man of sixty-five, causing loss of use of the left hand. A crutch had been used on the left side. The head of the second left rib was found displaced, and the head of the humerus was slightly dislocated anteriorly. After eleven treatments the patient was well.

(35) Myotonia Congenita (Thomsen's Disease) in a man, of ten years' standing. Lesion of a lumbar vertebra was removed, curing the case.

(36) Hemiplegia in a child twenty months old, of ten months stand-

ing. Lesion was found at the atlas, which was immediately replaced, and rapid improvement followed. In three weeks the child could walk, and recovery was almost perfect.

(37) Brachial Neuritis of five months' standing, causing severe pain in amrs and shoulders, and partial paralysis of the hands. Lesions were found in luxation of the 2nd, 3rd and 4th right ribs, and the 2nd left rib, with irregularities of the lower cervical and upper dorsal vertebrae. One treatment greatly relieved the pain; three treatments enabled the patient to close his hands and snap his fingers; and in three months' treatment the case was entirely cured.

(38) Partial paralysis of one hand, loss of memory, and at times inability to articulate. Lesion was found at the 2nd cervical vertebra. The case was cured by one month's treatment.

LESIONS: Thirty-two of the above cases reported lesion. Twenty-seven of the thirty-two were bony lesions, while five of the lesions were contractures as the sole apparent anatomical derangements. Twenty-one of the bony lesions were vertebral; three were rib lesions; one was a hip lesion; five were of the innominates; one of the coccyx; five of the atlas. In but seven was there serious accident as the obvious circumstance resulting in such injury as to cause the paralysis. Minor accidents were doubtless the causes of many of these lesions. Thirty-five of the thirty-eight cases reported were reported as cured. In twenty-eight of these cases cured, quick results were gotten by the treatment, either in the form of immediate betterment or of cure.

These facts are typical, and illustrate much that is seen in the practice upon this class of cases. They point prominently to importance of anatomical lesion, of the kind most regarded by osteopathy, as the cause of paralytic diseases. The necessity of the removal of such lesion in curing the condition is obvious. These facts clearly indicate the great potency of actual bony lesion, derangement of a bony part, in causing paralysis. They illustrate also what experience shows to be a fact, that displacement of spinal vertebrae occurs as the real cause of a majority of the cases of paralysis. Rib lesions sometimes occur, but do not seem to be important as causes of such disease. The finding of a partial dislocation of a hip as the cause of paralysis in a limb is a fine point of osteopathic diagnosis. These lesions are occasionally found and are of prime importance. They are almost invariably overlooked in the usual line of practice. Their reduction is the sole and immediate remedy of the monoplegia. In a few cases both hips have been found thus luxated causing apparent paraplegia.

Contractured muscles are no doubt generally secondary lesions. But with some frequency they have been found as the sole discoverable cause of paralysis, and their removal has resulted in cure,

Innominate lesion if found to be of the greatest importance in causing paralysis of the lower extremities. The coccyx lesion does not seem to be

important in this connection. The atlas lesion is perhaps the most important single lesion, notwithstanding the fact that it does not with great frequency occur as the sole cause of a paralytic condition. Occuring at a part
of the spine where the bones are small and the contained portion of the
cord large, it is particularly likely to impinge upon the medulla and cause
paralytic effects in the whole body below, upon one side of the body, or in
the head and its parts. As shown above, lesions of the atlas occured in five
of these cases. It was present in two of these cases suffering paralysis of
both upper and lower limbs. In one of these cases, in which also there was
blindness and crossing of the eyes, it was the sole lesion. This circumstance
is well illustrative of the importance of the atlas lesion. In two cases it was
the sole lesion causing hemiplegia. It was present with lesion of the axis
in a case of facial paralysis.

A glance at the summary of the lesions will show the very general
range of these bony lesions. Atlas, axis, cervical, upper dorsal, middle dorsal, lower dorsal, lumbar, innominate, coccyx, hip, rib, and shoulder lesions
were found. It seems that any movable part along the spine, or in relation
with the various nerve-plexuses concerned in the various paralysis, may become misplaced and become a factor in producing a paralytic condition.
Yet there is a great deal of constancy of lesion. It tends as much toward
the specific in this class of cases as in any. Generally in paraplegia, monoplegia or paralysis of the two upper limbs the lesion is local at a place where
it may affect the origin of the nerves concerned in the innervation of the
parts involved. All of the seven cases of paraplegia show this in low lesion
along the spine. All the six cases of monoplegia show it in local lesions to
the origins of the plexuses involved.

It often happens that in cases of paralysis involving the upper and
lower limbs, one or both, there is a high lesion affecting the upper and a
low lesion affecting the lower members. Yet a single lesion high up more
frequently perhaps causes the tronble in upper and lower limbs. Lesions
of the fifth lumbar and of the innominates are frequent in paralysis and in
hemiparaplegias. These are important lesions.

An inspection of the lesions reported in seven of the above paraplegia
cases shows that the lower dorsal and upper lumbar region is a favorite
place for lesions in such cases; that spinal curvatures may cause the condition; that fifth lumbar and innominate lesions are much in evidence.

In case of general paralysis involving upper and lower limbs it is noted
that atlas lesion alone may be the cause; that often there are both upper
and lower lesions, respectively affecting upper and lower limbs; and that
contractured muscles and causes obstructing circulation to the cord may be
sufficient.

The monoplegias show much constancy of lesion to the origin of the
plexuses. The hip-joint, shoulder-joint, and sacro-iliac lesion all attract

attention. The hemiplegias seem more apt to show single high lesion, as of the atlas, but both high and low spinal lesions may be present.

The facial paralysis shows almost specific bony lesions. In three of the four cases the 2nd cervical vertebra is involved. In one of these three the atlas is also at fault. In a fourth case there was merely contracture of muscles occuring over the course of the trunk of the nerve were it crosses the ramus of the jaw. In these cases, bony lesions if present, are expected to occur among the upper three cervical vertebra.

ANATOMICAL RELATIONS: The close relation between the lesion and the disease is shown by several facts. The early development of paralysis after accident giving origin to those lesions found upon examination to exist at important points indicates the correctness of the osteopathic idea that such lesions are the direct causes. The further fact that recovery is dependent upon the removal of such lesions, that it actually is accomplished by their removal, also shows the close relation of lesion to paralytic disease. Finally the Osteopath's experience directs him to expect bony lesion at certain spinal areas, according to nerve-distribution from the spine to affected parts. In all these cases we speak of lesion significant to the Osteopath only.

The various lesions, bony and otherwise, act in several was to cause the paralytic effect that follows their presence In the first place, a misplaced vertebra or bony part, or a contractured muscle, may bring direct pressure upon a nerve, a fibre, or a plexus, cutting off its function and causing paralysis in its area of distribution. This fact is well shown in case 24. Here pressure of the first dorsal vertebra upon the last cervical and first dorsal nerves, one or both, which make up the ulnar nerve, resulted in paralysis in the ulnar distribution in the hand, affecting the little finger, ring-finger, and in part the middle finger. The same conclusion is indicated by the facts in case 29. Contracture of the hyoid muscles drew the bone against the pneumogastric nerve, causing paralysis of the laryngeal muscles, affecting deglutition and speech. The same evidence of direct pressure upon nerves is seen in case 32, where the muscles contracted over the trunk of the facial nerve; in case 34, where the head of the humerus impinged the brachial plexus; in case 8, where the sacro-iliac lesion affected the sacral nerves. In all of these cases quick results following the removal of pressure show that the effect of the lesion must have been directly upon the nerves involved by pressure.

In such cases the result is seen to be directly upon the part supplied by the impinged nerves, it is uncomplicated by results in other parts of the body, and is manifested in a circumscribed area, namely, in the muscle groups supplied by the nerve or nerves in question. In diagnosis a practical point is to expect lesion of a kind exerting direct pressure in cases presenting general features as described above. The lesion is known at once to be located some where in the path or at the origin of the nerves involved,

On the other hand, a certain class of lesions is found causing paralytic disease by lesion to the cord. The effect to the cord may be through direct pressure upon it, or in other ways. An example of such conditions is seen in case 38. Here lesion of the 2nd cervical vertebra caused partial paralysis in one hand, loss of memory, and at times inability to articulate. There was evident involvement of brain and cord, and the lesion was too high to affect the brachial plexus by direct pressure. In such case there is possibility of the lesion affecting the cord either by direct pressure or by interference with the sympathetic or with cord-nutrition. The supposition of direct pressure is supported by the fact that removal of the lesion cured the case in one month. In case 33, formication in the upper, and paralysis in the lower limbs, blindness, unintelligible speech, and paroxysms of spinal pain, clearly indicate involvement of cord and brain. The lesion of the 3rd cervical vertebra was too high to affect the brachial plexus by direct pressure; the lesion to the lumbar vertebra likewise could not have pressed directly upon the nerve-supply to the lower limbs. Yet the paralytic condition in lower limbs, referable to the posterior displacement or protrusion of the lumbar vertebrae, favors the theory of direct pressure upon the cord, since such paralysis of the lower limbs is known to follow actual lesion to the lumbar segments of the spinal cord.

In case 30, the hemiplegia resulted from lesion at the atlas, and was cured by its removal. The fact that the child could walk in three weeks after treatment began, and the highness of the lesion, both favor the idea that there was pressure upon the cord. In case 7, where there was paralysis of the voluntary muscles, crossed eyes, and partial blindness, the lesion was again at the atlas (occipitoa-tlantal) and the same reasoning would apply. So in case 6, paraplegia following lesion of the 6th dorsal vertebra.

It must be noted that in all these cases the results are quite unlike those in the first group considered. The results, instead of being direct upon nerve or plexus, are indirect; they are also complicated with effects in more than one part of the body, and are not circumscribed by being limited to one muscle group. It is an indication in diagnosis to expect such cord lesions in cases showing this style of effects from lesion.

In some cases the lesions no doubt do shut off nutrition to the cord or brain. It is seen in cases where cervical bony lesion results in atrophy of the optic nerve, causing blindness through interference with its nutrition. (case 33; case 7.) In case 15, lesions were described as being present and preventing circulation to the cord. Treatment with the idea of restoring this circulation resulted in quick benefit and cure. In case 17, the lasting effects of the meningitis upon the cord were overcome by building up circulation to it.

Quickness of results in many cases indicates functional derangement from pressure of the lesion, which being removed leads to immediate restoration of function. On the other hand a course of treatment must look to regeneration of nerves and of ganglion cells in many cases where degeneration has taken place in these tissues because of the effect of the lesion.

In hip cases, as in case 22, the underdevelopement accompanying the paralysis is often due to pressure upon blood-vessels as well as upon nerves. The pressure is from the displaced bone and the contractures of tissues.

The PROGNOSIS in paralytic cases is very favorable. A large percentage of the cases is entirely cured. Few cases are neither benefitted nor cured. The apparent greatness of the lesion bears no proportionate relation to the degree of the effect. A small or very limited lesion often causes the most serious paralysis.

Many cases are slow and difficult. Some cannot be cured.

The length of standing of the case should not determine the prognosis. Recent cases may be the most difficult to cure. Many of the most long standing and worst cases are quickly benefitted and cured. The prognosis is good, even after "strokes," and often in cases where there is blood-clot on the brain.

TREATMENT: The bony lesion must be removed. This is often the only necessary treatment. But most cases require a course of treatment to regenerate, through the blood-supply, the nerves and centers effected. This necessitates insuring a good quality of blood, and in many such cases the important first step consists in sufficient treatment to bowels, stomach, liver and kidneys to improve the general health and expel all impurities from the blood.

The general spinal and cervical treatment should be applied to tone the general nervous system and to increase the circulation and nutrition of it. This is accomplished by relaxation of all the spinal tissues, separation of the spinal vertebrae to allow free circulation, and stimulation of the central distribution of the sympathetic having control of circulation to the spine.

In case of blood-clot upon the brain the treatment is to increase cervical circulation to absorb it. This can be accomplished in cases where the clot has not had time to become organized or encysted. After cerebral hemorrhage, treatment should keep this object constantly in mind. But in many old cases of hemiplegia after cerebral apoplexy, where doubtless the clot has become organized, much benefit can be given by the treatment.

Local treatment is made upon the paralyzed limb or part to soften contractures, build up circulation, increase nutrition of the tissues, and to tone the local nerve-mechanism.

Lesions as described in this chapter will be found in most of the various diseases of brain and spinal cord. The same principles and methods of treatment, varied to suit the case, may be applied to them.

For example, in CEREBRAL HEMORRHAGE, OR CEREBRAL APOPLEXY, strong inhibition is made at once upon the sub-occipital regions to dilate the blood-vessels and to aid in reducing the congestion. This object is aided in a most important manner by the general cervical, spinal and abdominal treatment, relaxing all tissues and calling the blood to these parts away from the head. These treatments should be relaxing and inhibitive in nature as before described. The head should be kept raised to aid in drawing the blood from it. In the intervals of treatment the ice-bag may be applied to the head, hot applications to the feet, and counterirritants to the spine. The patient should remain quietly in bed and be fed upon a liquid diet.

After the acute stage the treatment should be carried on to remove the blood-clot from the brain and to overcome the hemiplegia. The former is accomplished by the usual cervical treatments to increase circulation to the brain; the latter by such treatment as described in detail above for cases of paralysis. The clot may, if taken in time, be completely removed, and the patient may be completely cured of all paralysis. During the acute stages the patient should be seen twice or several times daily. Later he may be treated daily or three times a week.

In the various forms of SPINAL MENINGITIS, often met in our practice, good prognosis is the rule. Cases are made to recover entirely, all paralysis or lingering stiffness of the muscles being overcome. The *treatment* in the acute form is the general spinal, cervical, and abdominal, to control the circulation of the cord and call the blood away from it. The rigidity of the muscles is overcome by manipulation and by careful, inhibitive spinal treatment. Bowels and kidneys must be kept active by treatment, to aid in removing toxic products from the system. It may be necessary to use a catheter on account of the paralysis of the sphincter of the bladder. In the intervals of treatment ice-bags may be applied along the spine. A course of treatment should be carried on to insure complete resorption of the inflammatory products from about the cord, and to prevent or overcome any paralytic sequel to the condition.

In MYELITIS the same general plan of treatment should be adopted to gain vaso-motor control and lessen the inflammatory process in the cord. Diagnosis should be made of the portions of the cord affected, and treatment should be applied here particularly to absorb the extravasated blood and do away with the danger of softening or degeneration of the cord following. The patient should be keep quiet, and attention be given to any special manifestation in the case requiring alleviation. Care must be taken in the manipulation to avoid all irritation of the skin on account of the liability to bed-sores. Rigidity and spasm in the affected muscles may be overcome by inhibitive manipulation of them, and by inhibition of the nerves. Guard against renal and pulmonary complications by keeping the lungs and kidneys well stimulated. A course of treatment must follow to guard against or overcome paralysis. The prognosis is good in the acute case. A chronic case may be cured, or much may be done for its benefit.

In meningitis, myelitis, apolexy, etc., various spinal and cervical lesions occur, of the kinds pointed out in the general consideration of the subject of paralysis.

INSANITY.

CASES: (1) Farmer, injured while at work, later became insane. Treatment by the usual methods did not avail and preparations were made to take him to an asylum. He had been insane for some months, when the osteopathic examination was made. Four men were required to hold the patient during the examination, so violent had he become. Lesion was found as a marked displacement of the third cervical vertebra to the right. It was set at once, and the patient immediately fell asleep, sleeping for twelve hours and awaking rational. In a few days the patient was well.

(2) A young lady, violently insane for six years. Lesion was found as a slightly misplaced atlas, which was corrected at one treatment. The symptoms of insanity all disappeared in a few days. There was history of a fall six years previous to the development of the insanity, and it was thought that the luxation of the atlas was caused then.

(3) A young woman of twenty-four, insane and confined in an asylum for eight months. Lesion existed in the form of a double lateral curvature in the lumbo-dorsal region; 5th lumbar vertebra posterior; 4th dorsal markedly posterior; 3rd and 5th dorsal anterior; 7th and 8th right ribs pressing upon the liver; innominates, one forward and the other back, one limb being 1 inch longer than than the other. Treatment directed to the correction of these lesions caused immediate benefit, and the patient was apparently well after two weeks' treatment.

(4) In a lady of twenty, insanity of two months' standing. There was a history of attacks of marked cerebral congestion. At times she became violent. The lesions were great tenderness and tension in the cervical region above the 4th vertebra, but no bony lesion; tenderness at the 5th lumbar vertebra and over the left ovary. Dysmenorrhoea was present. After the first treatment she slept for eleven hours, and awoke sane for the first time in eight months. After three weeks' treatment the patient was well.

(5) A boy acted in an insane manner after a fall upon his head from a window. A cervical vertebra was found luxated, and one treatment sufficed to cure the case.

(6) A lady of thirty-eight, who had been a chronic sufferer from rheumatism, had become insane ten years previously to treatment. At the time of becoming insane the menses had ceased. She had been in an asylum for six months, growing continually worse. She was much excited and suffered hallucinations. The lesions were such as pertained to the rheumatic condition; general muscular contracture, joints somewhat stiffened, tenderness over the kidneys, feeble pulse, and subnormal temperature. One month of treatment showed great improvement; after two months the menses were reestablished and the mind was nearly normal. Recovery was complete.

(7) Insanity in a man followed injury in a runaway accident. Lesion existed as anterior displacement of the atlas and a twist of the second and third vertebrae, one being turned forward and the other backward. There was also contraction and soreness of the posterior cervical muscles. Continued pain existed at the top of the head, there was an eruption upon the face, and a marked abnormal pulsation of the abdominal aorta. Treatment soon cured the case.

The cases are illustrative of osteopathic practice in insanity, numerous cases of which come under treatment. As a rule bony lesions are found. Sometimes lesion exists in the form of merely muscular contracture in the cervical region. The LESIONS are generally in the cervical region. Five of the above seven cases presented such lesion. Atlas lesion is frequent. In some cases are general spinal lesions leading to effects upon the nervous system. Often marked lesion is found in the dorsal region. McConnell notes the occurrence in insanity of middle dorsal, renal splanchnic, and rib lesions. The latter occur among the middle ribs on the right side. Case 3 above shows such lesions.

Lesions act by interfering with cerebral circulation, probably in some cases by pressure upon the cord, and also by affecting the nervous system and setting up reflexes. On the whole but little can be said definitely in regard to the pathology of insanity from the osteopathic point of view. That lesions exist as the cause of such conditions, and that their removal cures, and alone can cure, them, cannot be doubted from the facts. But just how lesion is acting to cause derangement of the mental functions is not known. It is noticable that quick results usually follow treatment, as in the seven cases above. Often the patient falls at once into a deep and lasting sleep. These facts indicate some marked and immediate relief to the brain. It seems as if some great pressure had been taken off the brain, leaving the mind free and Nature unopposed in her work of repair. This is doubtless literally true in those cases of insanity attended by cerebral congestion, in which the impeded circulation is at once restored to normal tension by removal of that which impedes the venous flow from the head. When the lesion is cervical it is altogether likely that its action upon the brain is by deranging the cerebral circulation, either by direct pressure upon the vertebral arteries by a displaced vertebra, by irritation to cervical sympathetics and the vaso-motor center in the medulla, or by a combination of these two. In this way may be set up either hyperemia or anemia of the brain. For example, pressure upon the vertebral arteries and irritation to the vaso-motors causing vaso-constriction might co-operate to cause marked anemia of the brain. On the other hand, impeded venous return and increased arterial tension in this region might result from lesion and cause cerebral hyperemia. Many cases of insanity are met in which there is hyperemia, as in cases 4 and 7.

That hyperemia and anemia are important in relation to insanity is shown by the statement of Kellogg that "insanity from circulatory disorders of the brain arises chiefly in intense hyperemic and anemic forms." That osteopathic lesion profoundly affects cerebral circulation is evidenced by many facts in the treatment of various diseases. The importance of these circulatory disturbances is further indicated by Kellogg's statement that vascular degenerations deprive the brain of its customary blood-supply and also prevent elimination of the waste products of cellular activity. It is evident that the lesion shutting off the arterial supply or preventing free circulation in the brain could act as could vascular degenerations in producing the effects mentioned. Kellogg says it is freely admitted that then is a previous link in the chain of events leading to insanity from such causes as he mentions above. This link the Osteopath supplies by noting these important bony and other lesions, without the removal of which these cases fail to be cured.

It is likely that the atlas lesion, so often found in insanity, acts chiefly by deranging the circulation through its close relations to the superior cervical ganglion and the medulla. It does not seem that this and other cervical bony lesion cause direct pressure upon the cord, as in such case one would expect paralysis in the body below, yet it is not impossible that it may press directly upon the cord, getting its effect upon the brain through ascending tracts.

The general spinal, vertebral and rib lesions mentioned may affect the general nervous system, as is known to be a fact from a study of nervous diseases, (see Paralysis) in this way leading to nervous diseases, reflex and otherwise, which are at the basis of insanity "All the (various influences) acting in the production of general diseases of the nervous system are those fundamentally involved in the causation of insanity," (Kellogg). The splanchnic, right rib, and renal lesions noted by osteopathy as present in insanity cases may cause insanity through derangement of kidneys, liver and gastro-intestinal tract. The fact is noted by writers upon insanity that kidney diseases, notably Bright's disease, and gastro-intestinal conditions, as gastric and intestinal catarrh, are sometimes closely associated with the causation of insanity. Likewise liver disease is well known to be closely connected with insanity, gall-stones and icterus being common in insanity. These visceral diseases, as well as some nervous diseases seem to be related to insanity through the vaso-motor reflexes they arouse. Kellogg says, "vaso-motor disorders essentially constitute the connecting link in the causation of insanity by visceral affections and peripheral nervous diseases. The vaso-motor center in the medulla is under the reflex control not alone of the cerebral cortex, but of the entire peripheral distribution of the sensory nervous system, so that not only emotional stimuli, but peripheral irritations, may affect circulatory changes and variations in the blood-pressure which stand in poximate relation to mental disorder."

It is a well demonstrated fact that osteopathic lesion causes not only the visceral diseases, but likewise marked vaso-motor disorders, etc., apparently so closely related to these brain conditions.

In view of these various facts it seems that the Osteopath has in insanity a broad field for his labors. Nor would he be confined to that class of cases in which the traumatic effects of lesions due to violent accidents and the like are the causes of insanity. But as it is evident that the various lesions, bony and otherwise, that he finds may become fundamental to the causation of insanity through producing visceral, nervous, and vaso-motor disorders, his field in insanity must be as broad as the disease.

The PROGNOSIS is good. The most brilliant and quickest results are often attained. A large percentage of the cases treated are cured. It is needless to say that many cannot be cured.

The TREATMENT looks to the removal of lesion, and of all causes of irritation, reflex, emotional and otherwise. The whole nervous system should be upbuilt by general spinal and cervical treatment. One of the main objects is to correct cerebral circulation. A congested condition is treated as in congestive headache or apoplexy, q. v. The abdominal inhibition may be employed. The general health is looked to, kidneys, liver, stomach, bowels, pelvic viscera, heart and lungs are all regulated in case of affection in them. The patient should lead a quiet, regular life.

Diseases of Women (3nd edition).

Cases: (1) Dysmenorrhoea and irregularity of menstruation with a complication of troubles in a young lady of 25. The lower dorsal and lumbar vertebrae were ant. The case was cured in ten weeks, having gained 22 lbs. (2) Dysmenorrhoea in a married woman of 38. At each period she was confined to her bed, there being menorrhagia, headache, nausea, etc. The condition was of 12 yrs. standing since childbirth. The uterus was prolapsed and retroverted. The right innominate was post. The bone was replaced, the uterus put into correct position, and the case was discharged cured in two months.
3 Dysmenorrhoea of 3 yrs. standing in a

young lady of 21. Lesions were: 5th lumbar to the right, and surrounding tissues much contracted; 9th, 10th, & 11th D. vertebrae luxated and that portion of the spine rigid. Patient's general health was much affected. The case was cured by removal of lesion in two months.

(4) Amenorrhoea with a complication of troubles in a woman of 22 of 13 mos' standing. The greatest gynecologist of Cincinnati said the uterus was atrophied and she would never menstruate again. Lesions were: 7th D. spine to Right and whole spine rather irregular. Pelvis twisted with apparent lengthening of right limb. The case was benefited from the beginning of the treatment and was cured in four months. Menses appeared in six weeks.

(5) Amenorrhea of 7 mos' standing in a case in which the periods had been very irregular often not occurring for three or four months. General health much affected. After two weeks' treatment she was much better and the menses appeared. Under the treatment the patient gained rapidly in weight, the normal period being reëstablished.

(6) Amenorrhea in a young woman of over 8 mos' standing. Lesions were: 2nd L Post. 1, 2 & 3 D lat; 5 L ant. Treatment corrected the lesions and cured the case in 3 mos, the patient having gained 12 lbs.

(7) Amenorrhea of more than 1 yr's standing in a young woman. Lesions: 4th & 5th L ant.

luxation of 8th & 9th D. stricture of the os. Lesions were corrected and os relaxed by spinal work. Menstruation came on normally.

(8.) Menorrhagia and dysmenorrhea. Menstrual flow started upon the least exercise. The curves of the spine were straightened and there were many slight irregularities in it. The coccyx was lateral to the right and ant. The case was first treated during the period and the flow ceased at once, not returning for four mos., after which it was normal.

(9.) Uterine hemorrhage suddenly appearing with abdominal pains. The latter were intense and hemorrhage profuse. One treatment entirely relieved the trouble.

(10) Uterine hemorrhage, frequent and profuse, in a married woman who had previously undergone operation for the removal of uterine fibroid tumors. The uterus was retroverted, the left innominate ant., the 2nd & 3rd L luxated. The hemorrhages ceased after the second treatment.

(11.) Metrorrhagia of 2 yrs. standing. The right innominate slipped upward and its correction entirely cured the trouble.

(12.) Prolapsus of the uterus in a lady of 40 who had suffered with spinal trouble and dysmenorrhea for 26 yrs. The patient had been taking local treatment for uterine displacement and other trouble twice a week, for 2 yrs. After three mos. of osteopathic treatment in which time about five local treatments were given, the prolapsus, leucorrhea etc. were cured. Practically all the treatment was upon spinal lesion, the spine having been found swerved one and one-half inches laterally. It was corrected. June to pg 248.

DISEASES OF THE EYE.

CASES: (1) Impaired vision in a boy of seventeen, who had been wearing glasses over three years. Severe headache and inability to read followed removal of them. Lesion was found as lateral luxation of the atlas and third cervical vertebra. After three weeks' treatment the glasses were removed, and at the end of two months the eyes were completely cured. The report was made six months later, the eyes still being well.

(2) In a case of weak eyes the glasses were laid aside permanently after one month's treatment.

(3) Weak eyes, which for two years, had required the use of spectacles, were cured at the second treatment by adjustment of cervical bony lesion. The glasses were at once laid aside.

(4) A young man of eighteen had, for twelve years, been forced to wear spectacles, in spite of which the eyes continued to grow weaker. He had to give up school work. Under osteopathic treatment he laid aside the glasses after three treatments. No further treatment was required. Five months later the eyes were still well.

(5) A case in which weakness of the eyes and rheumatic pains in the shoulder were caused lesion in the form of closeness of the second and third cervical vertebrae. After one treatment the glasses were laid aside and the pain in the shoulder was gone. The trouble, caused by a fall in a gymnasium, affected but one eye and one side of the body, a nervous twitching of the muscles being present.

(6) A young lady had suffered with weak eyes for two years. The eyes would be very painful if the glasses were laid aside even for five minutes. Lesion was of the 2nd dorsal vertebra, lateral to the left. After five treatments the glasses were discarded.

(7) In a lady of forty, weakness of the eyes, accompanied by great pain in the eyeballs and at the base of the brain. Lesion existed at the atlas and third cervical vertebra. Constipation and uterine prolapsus were present, with characteristic lesions. After one month the eyes were almost well. Photophobia was a feature of the case.

(8) In a cases of weak eyes, with pain in the neck, occipital headache, and a complication, ot troubles lesions were found as anterior luxation of 3rd, 4th, and 5th cervical vertebrae, the 5th being sore. The whole spinal column was stiff and stooped forward.

(9) In a case of weak eyes in a young man of twenty, of two month's standing, the patient was unable to read, the balls were injected and painful, and the lids were inflamed. The atlas and axis were too close.

(10) In a lady of thirty-two, weakness of the eye and chronic hoarseness had existed for twenty-two years. The left cervical muscles were very sore, there was a separation between the atlas and axis, and the 5th cervical vertebra was sore. The right tear duct was closed.

(11) In a case of weakness of the eyes, coupled with indigestion, jaundice and hemorrhoids, the 7th to 11th dorsal vertebrae were posterior; coccyx anterior; an innominate forward.

(12) Extreme weakness of the eyes, together with female disease. A few minutes' use of the eyes caused violent headache. Lesions were at the atlas and in a tilting of an innominate bone. The case was cured by removal of the lesions.

(13) Eye trouble in a boy of thirteen, not benefitted by glasses. Patient was very nervous. The atlas was slipped forward. The lesion was corrected and the case cured in six weeks.

(14) A case of pterygium due to granulated lids of sixteen years' duration. The left pupil was covered by the growth, and the right one was nearly so. The case was cured by the adjustment of cervical lesion.

(15) Pterygium over each eye due to lesion of the atlas. Under treatment gradual correction of the lesion was accompanied by gradual absorption of the growth.

(16) Partial blindness and strabismus, associated with general paralysis, due to a forward slip of the head upon the atlas. The case was cured in two months.

(17) A case of blindness from optic-nerve-atrophy, due to a fall from a swing, resulting in lesion of the atlas and several cervical and upper dorsal vertebrae. The disease was of twenty-three years' standing It was cured by two years' treatment.

(18) Blindness of one eye, and almost total loss of sight in the other of about a years' duration, was cured in two weeks by correction of lesion of the atlas, which was displaced to the right, and of one of the first ribs, which was luxated upwards.

(19) Partial blindness, the patient being unable to read or to recognize a person ten feet away. The trouble was due to starvation of the optic nerve from lesion of the upper cervical vertebrae. In four months the patient had been cured.

(20) Blindness, almost total, in a man of sixty, due to a fall when he was a child. Lesion was found as luxation of a cervical vertebra. The treatment so benefitted the eye that it could see to read coarse print.

(21) A case of cataract reported cured, the patient's oculist verifying the report.

(22) Total blindness in the left eye for more than two years, due to lesion of the atlas. The pupil was much dilated. After one treatment sight was partly restored, and at the end of a month of treatment the case was nearly entirely well.

(23) Total blindness with paralysis of lower limbs, formication of upper limbs, etc. Lesion was found in lateral luxation of the third cervical vertebra, of the 7th and 8th right ribs, and posterior protrusion of the lumar vertebrae. Soon vision was partly restored, but with diplopia. Slight

pressure upon the seventh cervical vertebra would at once restore perfect vision. When pressure was removed diplopia again occured. Under the treatment the sight was entirely restored. Speech had been lacking, but was restored, and the paralysis was cured.

(24) In a young man of twenty, diplopia of two years' duration had followed a severe attack of measles. The 3rd cervical vertebra was displaced anteriorly and the tissues about it were sore. Tenderness existed also at the 5th and 6th cervical vertebrae. The first dorsal was posterior, the 2nd to 6th flattened, the 8th to 12th weak, with a separation between the 12th dorsal and 1st lumbar, and the 1st to 4th lumbar vertebrae were posterior, The case was cured in one month. There had been supposed hemorrhagic retinitis.

(25) A case of strabismus due to lesion of the 2nd dorsal vertebra was cured by correction of the lesion. During the course of treatment, after the eyes had first become straightened pressure upon the second dorsal vertebra would cross them again.

(26) A case of strabismus, unilateral, convergent, due to a fall in a runaway accident. The atlas was displaced to the right; 4th and 5th cervical vertebrae anterior. The case was improving under treatment.

(27) Kerito-conjunctivitis, in the left eye, of four years' standing. There was opacity of the upper two-thirds of the cornea, with marked vascularization, inflammation and granulation of the eyelids, and injection of the sclerotic. The atlas was luxated to the left, the fifth and sixth cervical vertebrae were anterior and to the left, and the upper dorsal vertebrae were posterior. Under the treatment the case was almost cured in less than two months.

(28) In a man of thirty-seven, glaucoma was present, and total blindness of the left eye was predicted by the oculist. The patient was a neurasthenic probably of the cerebral type, pain in the head and eye being extreme. The eye trouble was overcome and the patient's general condition much improved by three months' treatment. No especial lesions were found.

(29) Partial blindness, in which the blindness was limited to a circular portion of each eye. Lesion was found as a luxation of the atlas to the right and backwards. The case is still under treatment.

(30) A case in which the tear-duct was closed. It had been growing worse under the usual form of treatment for two years. The eye was much inflamed. Relief was experienced at the first treatment, after the second the duct was permanently opened, and the inflammation about the eye gradually disappeared. The case was well a year later.

(31) Eye-strain, causing constant headache, due to a luxated atlas. Glasses gave no relief. The headache did not recur after the first treatment, and the eyes were well after seven treatments. The case had been of but two or three months' standing.

(32) Astigmatism in a girl of ten. Lesion was found at the 2nd dor-

sal. Treatment was directed to correction of this lesion and to stimulation of the ocular blood and nerve-supply. The case was soon cured.

(33) In astigmatism for which the patient had worn spectacles for nine years, lesion was found in anterior luxation of the atlas and a twist of the inferior maxillary bone. The glasses were permanently discarded after one treatment, and the case was soon entirely cured.

LESIONS: Of the 33 cases above, 27 report lesion, and in each case bony lesions were present. Contracture was also noted in one case. Of these 27 lesions, 23 were cervical bony lesions and two were muscular contractures. Preponderance of atlas lesion was seen in the cervical region, 16 of the 27 being such. Numerous lesions occured. Among the other cervical vertebrae were lesions as follows: Axis, 3; 3rd cervical, 6; 4th cervical, 2; 5th cervical, 5; 6th cervical, 2.

Upper dorsal lesions were present in 8 cases, 7 being bony lesions. These lesions extended as low as the 6th dorsal vertebra, as follows: 1st dorsal, 2; 2nd dorsal, 5; 3rd dorsal, 2; 4th dorsal, 2; 5th and 6th dorsal each one.

Other bony lesions occuring in these cases, and of importance in eye troubles generally, are luxation of the inferior maxillary bone and of the first rib, sometimes also of the clavicle.

These reports illustrate very well the general lesions found in diseases of the eye. The most important lesions occur among the vertebrae of the cervical and upper dorsal region. Muscular lesions are often found in this region, and are of considerable importance. The whole cervical region is frequently involved, or any one or several of the vertebrae may be luxated. Perhaps the more important lesions are of the atlas, axis, and 3rd cervical vertebra. The 4th and 5th are also important.

There is a form of neck lesion that often plays a part in the production of eye disease, as well as of other forms of head and neck trouble. It involves the whole cervical region, often causing a lateral swerve of the cervical spine. The cervical tissues are contractured or hypertrophied upon one side more prominently than upon the other. The condition is often evident upon simple inspection from immediately behind. The fullness upon one side of the neck, and generally a corresponding depression in the tissues on the opposite side, are readily seen. In some cases the condition is better appreciated upon palpation. The fingers are readily pressed more deeply into the tissues upon one side of the posterior cervical aspect than upon the other. Contracture of the muscles may be felt here on both sides. If the vertebrae are traced down the mid-line of the back of the neck, a lateral swerve is often evident. In other cases the bony lesions are more evident by examination of each verteba with the patient lying upon his back.

Dr. A. T. Still calls attention to the fact that contracture of the cervical muscles opposite the 4th vertebra are common in eye-diseases, and that pressure here causes pain in the eye. A case is reported in which pressure between the 2nd and 3rd dorsal vertebrae upon the right side revealed tenderness at that point and also caused pain in the eye.

Without question cervical bony lesion is the most important one with which the Osteopath deals in eye-diseases.

Upper dorsal lesion may be muscular, but is usually bony. It involves chiefly the upper four or five vertebrae, but may extend as low as the 6th or seventh. The lesions of the 1st, 2nd and 3rd dorsal vertebrae are the most important here. A common abnormality of the anatomical parts here is a "hump" or prominent cushion of flesh covering the spinous processes of the upper two or three dorsal vertebrae. There is often conjoined with this condition a marked prominence of the first dorsal spine from above, as if the cervical spine had been moved a little anteriorly upon the first dorsal. This cushion is a common condition in eye-troubles of various sorts, and is sometimes connected with heart-trouble.

Among lesions of this region may be mentioned lesion of the upper ribs on either side as low as the sixth, sometimes thought to have as bearing upon nutritional disturbances of the eyes.

We are perhaps not in a position or yet to point out that special kinds or locations of lesion result in specific diseases of the eye. Cases involving deficiency somewhere in the optic tract seem to favor lesion in the upper cervical region. In the above reports, 19 cases in which probably the intrinsic apparatus of the special sense of sight, was involved such as weakness, impaired vision, blindness, etc., show lesion chiefly in the upper cervical region. All but two cases show cervical lesion, 13 of them being entirely in the cervical region; 11 at the atlas; 8 at the axis, third, or both; also the 4th, 5th and 7th were involved. The most important lesions occured about atlas, axis, and third.

Cases in which there is nutritional disturbance, as in conjunctivitis, keratitis, glaucoma, cataract, and closure of the tear-duct, also cases in which there is structural change, such as astigmatism, pterygium, etc., probably due to lack of nutrition, present atlas, general cervical, inferious maxillary, and upper dorsal lesion. Compilations of data, by which proof of these matters might be made, are lacking. Yet it seems that nutritional disturbances, involving in some way chiefly the fifth nerve, would be found tending more toward the upper dorsal region, for the anatomical reason that this nerve has important connections with the upper dorsal nerves and cord.

Motor disturbances, such as diplopia, strabismus, eye strain, etc., show less of high cervical lesion and more from about the third cervical down to the upper dorsal. In this connection it is recalled that diplopia has been caused by pressure at the 7th cervical, and strabismus by pressure at the 2nd dorsal.

This phase of the subject, inquiry how far specific lesion results in a certain form of eye disease, presents a good field for research. It is evident that at present we cannot more than indicate probabilities.

ANATOMICAL RELATIONS: There are good anatomical reasons why lesion in the upper dorsal and cervical regions causes eye disease. These portions of the spine are particularly rich in nerve-connections with the eye. These lesions act by disturbing blood nerve, or lympathic-supply of the eye. The blood-supply suffers sometimes by direct impingement, as of vertebrae upon the vertebral arteries, or by derangement of the vaso-motor control by lesion to the nerves. The lymphatics suffer by direct impingement, as by clavicular lesion damming back the lymphatic drainage from the head. The lesion affecting the eye does so chiefly, however, by distbrbance of the numerous important nerve-connections met in the upper dorsal and cervical regions.

Experience has taught the Osteopath that bony lesion in those regions causes most eye-diseases and that its removal cures them.

The superior cervical ganglion, well known to suffer by lesion of atlas, axis, or 3d cervical, sends its ascending branch to join the carotid and cavernous plexuses, thence to help form a secondary plexus about the opthalmic arteries and to contribute branches to the minute plexus of the sympathetic within the eyeball itself. Thus is established a direct path of communication between the upper cervical lesion and the eye.

The ciliary ganglion lies at the back of the orbit, between the trunk of the optic nerve and the external rectus muscle. In this situation it is readily impinged by that treatment that presses the eyeball back into the orbit. With this ganglion are connected the 3d, 5th and sympathetic nerves, it thus becoming, through the functions of these nerves, a sensory motor, and sympathetic center for the eye-ball. Neck lesion, as will be shown, may effect either or all of these nerve-connections, in this way deranging the function of the ganglion with regard to the eye.

The third cranial nerve innervates all the voluntary muscles of the eye except the external rectus and the superior oblique. It is further the nerve which contracts the pupil by supplying the sphincter function of the iris. This function is shown by the American Text-Book of Physiology to have its center in the superior cervical ganglion, where it could be affected in lesion of the upper cervical region, causing disturbance of accommodation in the eye. Neck lesions are known to cause strabismus and diplopia (cases 23 and 25), showing disturbance by such lesion of the function of the 3d nerve. (Also of the 4th and 6th) The anatomical relations in strabismus caused by lesion at the 2d dorsal, and diplopia by lesion at the 7th cervical is not well understood. The local treatment of the ciliary ganglion is important in these motor disturbances.

Fibers antagonistic to the ciliary function of the third nerve, being dilators of the pupil, are found rising in the third ventricle, whence they pass through the medulla and cervical cord to the anterior roots of upper dorsal nerves and to the first thoracic ganglion of the sympathetic. From these points they reach the eye via the cervical sympathetic cord, ophthalmic division of the fifth, and its nasal and long ciliary branches.

These facts indicate the importance of upper cervical, general cervical, and upper dorsal lesion in the causation of lack of accommodation, eye-strain, and similar troubles.

The latter sympathetic connection indicates the so-called cilio-spinal center at the 4th cervical to 4th dorsal. Quain states that these pupillo-dilator fibers pass from the 1st, 2d, and 3d dorsal nerves, sometimes also from the 7th and 8th cervical.

In addition to the above, motor fibers to the involuntary muscles of the orbit and eye-lids pass from the upper four or five dorsal nerves. Also retinal fibers leave the sympathetic at the superior cervical ganglion, pass to the Gasserian ganglion of the fifth, thence through its branches to the eye. It is shown that, acting through these fibers, stimulation of the cervical sympathetic causes constriction of the retinal arteries, while stimulation of the thoracic sympathetic causes dilatation of them. These facts indicate the importance of cervical and upper dorsal lesion in vaso-motor disturbances in the retina, as in retinitis.

The fact that many of these sympathetics, as pointed out, pass to the eye *via* the fifth nerve shows the intimate relation between the superior cervical ganglion, the cervical and upper dorsal sympathetic, and the fifth nerve, consequently the potency of cervical and upper dorsal lesion to affect the fifth nerve. This nerve sends its sensory ophthalmic division to join with the sympathetic from the cavernous plexus. It has trophic and vaso-motor fibers to the eyeball and its appendages. Green states that section of the fifth nerve is followed by keratitis and ulceration. It has charge of the nutrition of the eye-ball, supplying also the lachrymal glands, conjunctiva, skin of the lids and adjacent parts of the face. *Nutritive disturbances of the eyes, such as keratitis, conjunctivitis, retinitis, cataract, glaucoma, pteryguim, etc., must be referred to lesion affecting the fifth nerve. Likewise optic-nerve-atrophy, and other effects due to insufficient nutrition would result from lesion affecting the fifth.

Slips of the inferior maxillary articulation are thought to impinge fibers of the fifth nerve, (articular branches from the auriculo-temporal nerve) and to cause certain eye troubles   (case 33.)

A review of these various connections shows that cervical and upper dorsal lesion may affect:

1. The superior cervical ganglion and its sympathetic connection with the local sympathetic plexus of the eye-ball.

2. The various cervical nerves and through them the ganglion and the other cervical sympathetics.

3. The pupillo constrictor center in the inferior cervical ganglion.

4. The pupillo-dilator center in the same ganglion and at the lower cervical and upper three dorsal nerves.

5. The motor fibers from the upper four or five dorsal nerves to the involuntary muscles of orbit and eyelids.

*For important functions of the fifth nerve see "Principles of Osteopathy."

6. The fifth nerve by its connections with the superior cervical ganglion and cervical sympathetic.

7. Constrictors of the retinal arteries in the cervical sympathetic.

8. Dilators of the same in the thoracic sympathetic, and

Both of these at the superior cervical ganglion

It is noticable that all of these eight connections, except perhaps No.
5, may be reached at the superior cervical ganglion. This explains the
special importance of lesion to atlas, axis and 3rd cervical, before pointed
out as most frequent in eye-diseases. These upper cervical lesions affect
this ganglion. From the variety of functions represented in these various
fibres congregated in the superior cervical ganglion we must conclude that
lesion of the atlas, axis, or third, etc , affecting this ganglion, would cause
a variety of diseases of the eye.

Lesions causing stomach, kidney, and pelvic diseases may secondarily
become the cause of disturbances in the eye. The relation here is probably
entirely reflex Perhaps also in these conditions alteration of blood-pressure is a disturbing factor.

It seems that cervical lesion causing obstruction of the tear-duct,as well
as manipulation upon the nose along its course to open it, affect the mucous
membrane lining it through the distribution of the fifth nerve.

Clavicular and first rib lesion, obstructing the lymphatic drainage of
the eye by obstructing the flow from the deep cervical lymphatics into the
thoracic or right lymphatic duct, may affect the metabolism of the eye.   It
has been thought that lesion affecting the female breast may react upon the
eye reflexly.

The PROGNOSIS in eye-diseases is, generally speaking, good. Marked
results, even to cure of blindness of many years' standing, have been acquired. Very often surprisingly quick results have been attained. An examination of the case reports at the opening of this chapter will show that in
twenty-four of the thirty-three various cases reported a cure was affected.
Quick results, either as cure or benefit, were attained in seventeen cases
The cases met by the Osteopath are frequently of long standing and in bad
condition. In many cases these results were gotten after specialists had
failed. All cases cannot be cured. Many are subjects for the specialist.

The TREATMENT of eye-diseases is necessarily almost entirely upon the
neck, as it has been shown that the lesions in these cases occur here. The
removal of these various lesions is already understood from discussions in
the previous pages. The treatment looks, in general, to the establishment
of perfect circulation, and the regulation of the nerve-mechanism. The
general neck treatment, as applied is cases of insomnia, headache. apoplexy,
etc., q v., given with a specific object in view, would be the method employed (see also Chap. III and IV).

In many cases the simple removal of lesion is the only treatment required
Often this treatment, and the general neck treatment may be supplemented by

local treatment upon the eye, and about it, reaching its nerve-mechanism and blood circulation directly. (See Chap. V. A and B.) This work includes treatment to the fifth nerve as the one being in charge of the nutrition and circulation of the eye. This nerve is particularly regarded in all nutritive diseases, such as keratitis, and in all inflammatory, hyperemic or anemic conditions, such as conjunctivitis, etc.

In conjunctivitis the local irritant, if one be present, must be removed. Treatment should not be made upon the eye in these cases, but about it. The chief treatment is in the neck, especially upon the superior cervical ganglion.

In granular conjunctivities the same treatment is made. The granulations must be broken down. (Chap. V.) After this the correction of the circulation by by the cervical treatment prevents their further growth.

In keratitis treatment proceeds as in conjunctivitis. In both conditions the fifth nerve must be especially treated.

The removal of lesion and the correction of blood-flow are the essential points in these and all similar cases.

In pterygium especial treatment is made to cut off the "feeders." (V. Chap. V.) After this operation they are absorbed by the corrected circulation by means of the neck work. In some cases removal of neck lesion is followed by absorption of the growth, as in case 15. Sometimes light manipulation over the closed lid aids the absorption.

The same remarks apply to pannus.

In diplopia, ptosis, strabismus and other motor troubles, lesion must be sought as the cause of the muscular palsy, tension, etc. Treatment is applied to the lesion and to the affected nerve. These troubles sometimes yield to the correction of cervical lesion alone. The muscles may be treated direcly as in VI. Chap. V.

In cataract the treatment looks to the absorption of the cataract through increased circulation. Cervical treatment, removal of lesion, and local treatment about the eye and upon the fifth nerve, all as before described, have successfully accomplished a cure in these cases.

In the various optic nerve troubles, also, the treatments are used to affect the nerve through its blood-supply. Numerous cases of blindness from optic-nerve-atrophy have been cured in this way. The optic nerve may be stimulated by tapping or pressure upon the eyeball. (II, III, Chap. V.) Retinitis likewise yields to this treatment.

In conjugate deviation, both eyes turning strongly to ons or other side, the lesion, usually cervical, affects the the third and sixth nerves, supplying respectively the internal ructus and the external ructus of the eyeballs. The treatment is local and cervical.

DISEASES OF THE EAR.

CASES: (1) Deafness of two years' duration in a lady of forty-two, caused by displacement of atlas to the right, tightening muscles and ligaments around the ear and lower jaw. Tenderness was extreme in the cervicial region. Dry catarrh was present. There was lesion of the 2nd cervical vertebra. The patient had been injured in a railroad wreck, being confined to the bed. She could not hear a clock strike in the room, nor the playing of a piano. After three treatments the patient could hear the clock strike. After five weeks' treatment the hearing was completely restored.

(2) A case of deafness, pronounced by specialists incurable, was treated four weeks osteopathically and again examined by a specialist, who pronounced the case cured.

(3) Deafness in a young boy, due to lesion of the atlas. The deafness was complete in one ear, and almost so in the other. After one month's treatment he could hear conversation spoken in an ordinary tone.

(4) Total deafness of several years' standing much benefitted by three weeks' treatment, the patient being able to hear the street cars pass the house.

(5) In a boy of fourteen, a continuous discharge from the right ear, of ten years' standing. Lesion of the atlas and axis, luxated to the right, and contraction of the tissues. The case was cured in nine treatments.

(6) In a boy of eleven, partial deafness in, and continual discharge from one ear. The lesion was a slip of the atlas. The case was cured in one month's treatment.

(7) In a young lady, an abscess in one ear had been discharging for several months. After one treatment there was no further discharge, and after four treatments the trouble had disappeared.

The LESION in ear diseases, as illustrated by the above cases, are almost as a rule in the atlas and axis. The 3rd cervical and other cervicals may be affected, but in the vast majority of cases the atlas and axis, one or both, are affected. It is more often at the atlas than elsewhere. A luxation of the temporo-maxillary articulation, impinging probably the articular fibres of the auriculo-temporal branch of the inferior-maxillary division of the fifth nerve, and contractured tissues about the upper cervical region and the angle of the jaw may act as lesions in these diseases.

The fifth nerve supplies the external auditory canal by its auriculo-temporal branches, the upper one of which sends a branch to the tympanum. Also the vidian of the fifth sends nasal branches to the membrane of the end of the Eustachian tube. The internal throat treatment given to affect this tube, does so by stimulating these fibres, thus freeing the secretions in this portion of the Eustachian tube. Reasoning by analogy, doubtless the

secretory, trophic, and vaso-motor functions of the fifth nerve with relation
to the eye and other parts of the head and face are extended to the ear,
secretion of cerumen and circulation about the ear being to some extent
under control of the fifth.   Experience connects lesions of this nerve with
ear-diseases.   It has been shown above that the nerve suffers from lesion
of the upper cervical region, such as occur in ear troubles (see Diseases of
the Eye).   The treatment of this nerve, so important in nasal catarrh and
other inflammatory affections of the eye, nose, and parts of the head, is important likewise in these catarrhal, inflammatory, and other circulatiory
troubles, so commonly complicated with the diseases of the ear.

Vaso-constrictor fibres for the ear are contained in the cervical sympathetic.   They constitute another pathway for the effect of cervical lesion to
reach the ear.   Likewise the atlas and axis lesion may affect the blood-
supply of the ear through the medulla, which suffers from these lesions.   It
is possible that vaso-motors for the head exist in the upper dorsal nerves,
though upper dorsal lesion is rare in ear trouble.   It is likely that much of
the effect of cervical lesion upon the ears is gotten through the vaso-motors
and other sympathetics.

The claim is made that the auditory nerve may be inhibited by deep
pressure opposite and behind the third cervical vertebra.

The pneumogastric nerve has an auricular branch, and is in close connection with the fifth in relation to the ear, as well as with the cervical
sympathetic.   The petrosal ganglion of the glosso-pharyngeal is related to
upper cervical lesion by sending a branch to the superior cervical ganglion.
Its tympanic branch passes from this ganglion and contributes fibres to the
mucous lining of the middle ear, and to the mastoid cells. It sends branches
to unite with the sympathetic and form a plexus on the carotid artery in
the carotid canal-   Thus is this nerve connected both with neck lesions and
with the blood-supply to the ear.   The facial nerve, well known to be influenced by lesions of the atlas and axis, as seen in facial paralysis, has
direct communication with the auditory nerve and with the auricular branch
of the pneumogastric.

The various simple methods described in the texts on this subject will aid
one to determine the location of the trouble in the external, middle or internal ear.   The disease may be seated in the auditory nerve or in the brain,
in such case being as directly connected with cervical lesion, before shown
to affect the brain and cranial nerves.

TREATMENT: An ear syringe may be used in the ordinary ways to
cleans the ear of secretions, discharges, foreign objects, etc.

The removal of bony lesion and the cervical treatment as before described are the main osteopathic treatments applied in ear diseases. The presence of the original cause of these diseases in the form of neck lesion ne-
ccssitates practically the whole treatments being cervical. There is no iocal

ear treatment, except as in the common methods in vogue in use of syringe, etc.

Outside of removal of lesion, an almost specific treatment for eye and ear is that of opening the mouth against resistance (Chap. IV, Div. I, II, VII), and the neck treatment, with the object of increasing circulation through the carotid arteries. Due attention is given to the cervical sympathetics and vaso-motors in this connection.

The internal throat treatment (p. 24) may be used, the finger being directed about the opening of the Eustachian tube to stimulate the local points of the fifth nerve, the mucous membranes, and thus the secretions. This aids in freeing the tube, an object that is well accomplished by the aid of the external throat treatment upon the carotids, etc.

GOITRE

CASES: (1) In a lady of twenty-five, a bilateral, vascular goitre of about three months' standing, growing rapidly, causing considerable dyspnea and discomfort. The treatment consisted merely of stretching the muscles and ligaments attached to the sternal end of the clavicle, raising it, and depressing the first rib. Marked improvement followed the treatment at once. Two months later the enlargement and other symptoms had disappeared.

(2) Exophthalmic goitre and nervous prostration of one months' standing. The trouble followed nervous strain and over-work. The goitre was as large as a hen's-egg, and the usual symptoms of exophthalmic goitre were present. The case yielded rapidly to treatment and at the end of two weeks the goitre had disappeared and the eyes were normal. In one month she had recovered from the goitre and nervous prostration, and had gained twenty pounds in weight.

(3) In a boy of fourteen, a goitre of two years' standing. Lesion existed as a lowering of the right clavicle and muscular contracture in the lower cervical and upper dorsal region. One treatment a week for twelve weeks cured the case.

(4) A case of goitre treated by raising the clavicles, relaxing the tissues surrounding the gland, and opening circulation to and from the gland. After one month there was no perceptible change; after two months the growth had begun to get smaller, and after three months the condition was cured.

(5) In a lady of thirty-four, a large exophthalmic goitre with all the usual symptoms marked. The general system was in bad condition. Lesion was luxation of the fourth cervical vertebra; the spine was irregular. The case was cured in six months.

(6) Exophthalmic goitre and eczema of the face and neck in a young lady of twenty-six cured in six weeks' treatment.

(7) In a lady, a goitre of one year's standing. No bony lesions were found. After one month's treatment the diameter of the neck had been decreased one and one-half inches.

DEFINITION:—Goitre is defined as "a chronic hypertrophy or hyperplasia of a portion or the whole of the thyroid gland. It is of obscure origin, involving one or more of the structural tissues, and is subject to various degenerative changes."

This so called simple goitre is met in various forms; simple hypertrophic, follicular, fibrous, vascular, cystic, degenerative, etc. They are most frequently met and treated osteopathically.

Exophthalmic goitre (Grave's or Basedow's disease) is quite a different condition. It is defined as, "a chronic neurasthenic neurosis characterized by rapid heart-beat, enlarged thyroid, protrusion of the eye balls, and various neurasthenic or vaso-motor symptoms."

Osteopathy simply regards goitre as an enlargement of the thyroid gland due to a specific, usually bony, lesion which interferes with the proper blood and lymph circulation of that body. This leads to congestion, engorgement, and hypertrophy. In some cases, especially in exophthalmic goitre, the lesion may act chiefly upon the innervation of the gland, producing the various phenomena marking the disease.

The LESIONS bear, in conformity with the above view, a close anatomical relation to the disease. They are generally bony lesions of the cervical and upper thoracic regions, consisting in displacements of middle and lower cervical vertebrae, of the clavicle, or of the first rib. Yet various muscular, and other tissue, contractures are often found as the lesions in the case. These commonly occur together with bony lesion, but may be independent of such. They occur mostly in the anterior region of the neck, involving the infra-hyoid muscles and the soft tissues down to the root of the neck. The scaleni muscles are often involved. The posterior cervical and upper dorsal muscles are sometimes found contractured and acting as lesion.

The chief bony lesions in simple goitre are of the clavicle and first rib, while in exophthalmic goitre lesions of the cervical vertebrae are more frequent. Yet either form of lesion may occur in either case. The clavicle and rib lesion, and the contracturing of the anterior cervical tissues act specifically by obstructing arterial, venous, and lymphatic currents to and from the gland. The inferior thyroid artery arises from the thyroid axis, which, lying behind the clavicle and scalenus anticus muscle may suffer pressure from them when abnormal in position. The superior thyroid artery is related to the infra-hyoid muscles, and may suffer from their contracture. But the interferences of these lesions with the lymphatic and venous drainage of the gland are doubtless most potent in causing goitre. The lymphatics of the gland are large and numerous, emptying upon the right into the lymphatic duct, upon the left into the thoracic duct, both avenues of lymphatic drainage, therefore, lying where derangement of clavicle or of first rib may obstruct them.

Just as clavicular and first rib lesion has been known to obstruct lymphatic drainage of the breast and result in so-called cancer, the same kind of lesion may prevent lymphatic drainage and cause goitrous enlargement of the thyroid.

In a like manner the venous return becomes abridged. The superior and middle thyroid veins are in relation to the inferior hyoid muscles, and suffer pressure from their contracture. They both empty into the internal jugular vein which may be obstructed by clavicular lesion. The chief venous flow is through the three or four large inferior thyroid veins, and it may be impinged by clavicular and anterior cervical lesion. This view of

lesion is well supported by the fact that simple goitres often rapidly disap
pear after treatment, restoring clavicle and first rib to position, relaxing anterior cervical tissues, and reestablishing perfect circulation of all fluids to
and from the thyroid. This has been observed in some cases, probably of
vascular goitre, by Dr. Still, in which the facts strikingly illustrate the correctness of the osteopathic etiology. In these cases he saw, in a few hours,
a great reduction in the volume of the gland follow removal of such obstructions to the vessels. The gland seemed to have been rapidly emptied
and the goitre drained away by the the renewed drainage.

The nerve-supply of the thyroid gland is from the middle and inferior
cervical ganglia of the sympathetic. Consequently various vertebral lesions
are found, especially in exophthalmic goitre. Such lesions have been found
from the 2nd to the 7th cervical vertebra. In discussing diseases of the eye
and of the heart the connections of the cervical sympathetic mechanism
with both of these organs has been pointed out. The lesions occuring thus
to the innervation of the thyroid, cervical lesions, are likewise closely related anatomically to the innervation of eye and heart, accounting in part
for the related disturbance of these organs in exophthalmic goitre.

This disease has been regarded by medical writers as due to disturbed
innervation of the gland, or to an affection of the sympathetic nerves. It
has been sometimes thought that the seat of the disease is in the medulla,
and that the disturbance of the thyroid function causes the gland to throw
into the blood substances that irritate the nerves and cause the various
neurasthemic symptoms accompying the condition. It is readily seen that
cervical lesion may disturb the innervation of the organ, set up the smypa-
thetic disturbance, and derange the function of the thyroid. This disturbance of the sympathetic innervation is further evident in the vascular condition of the gland, its arteries being dilated, and in the paralysis of the
orbital vessels, which become distended with blood and cause the exoph-
thalmos. Dana explains all symptoms upon the theory of vaso-motor and
cardio-motor paresis, a result that may readily be due to the operation of
cervical lesion upon the sympathetic.

The PROGNOSIS is good in all cases. It is to be noted that according
to Anders the prognosis in goitre (simple) is but guardedly favorable as to
life, but unfavorable as to cure, while but few cases of exophthalmic goitre are
expected to be cured. Yet under osteopathic treatment very numerous
cases of both kinds have been cured. A cure is often effected, even in long
standing cases which have tried all the known remedies.

The prognosis is most favorable in younger and shorter cases, and in
those in which the gland is soft. Under treatment, signs of softening in a
part of the gland are indications of progress. In the vascular and parenchymatous forms the progress is good. The former promise the most for
quick results. In the hard, fibrous forms, and in those in which degeneration of the tissues, or calcareous infiltration has taken place, the prognosis
is not favorable.

Some cases of goitre yield quickly; some are very slow. From one to three months' treatment is usually necessary.

The TREATMENT looks at once to the removal of lesion, and to the free opening of lympathtic and venous drainage. All the cervical muscles must be relaxed. This direction applies especially to the deep anterior cervical and the hyoid muscles, as well as to the tissues about the gland.

Pressure is made downwards over the goitre, out about its edges, and along the course of the veins draining it. All the tissues about the root of the neck anteriorly, and about clavicles and first ribs, must be relaxed. The ribs and clavicles should be separated, elevating the latter and depressing the former.

Close attention should be given to all the cervical vertebral articulations, seeing that they are perfectly adjusted.

In exophthalmic goitre one must look particularly to the cervical sympathetics, toning them to overcome the vaso-motor paresis. Inhibitory cardiac and local eye treatment may be applied as before directed. A moderate pressure of the eye-ball back into its orbit aids in emptying the blood from the distended vessels. For a similar reason pressure upon the gland, in exophthalmic and in vascular forms of goitre, is a good measure. In the former kind one should look well to the constitutional condition and to that of the general nervous system.

NEURALGIA.

CASES: (1) Severe facial neuralgia of two weeks' standing, with inflammatory eruption upon the affected side, the right, and inflammation of the right eye. The usual treatments had been tried for two weeks without avail. The lesion was a marked displacement of the atlas to the left. It was corrected and the case cured in one treatment.

(2) Facial neuralgia affecting the right side of the face and head, especially the forehead over the right eye. The lesion was luxation of the atlas to the left. The case was cured in one treatment.

(3) Facial neuralgia of two years' standing was greatly relieved by one treatment and was cured in six weeks, the patient gaining twenty-two pounds during that time.

(4) Facial neuralgia and pains between the shoulders. The lesions were contraction of cervical muscles and lateral luxation of the fourth and fifth dorsal vertebrae. Four treatments cured the case.

(5) Brachial neuralgia, involving the left arm and the left side as low as the fifth rib. The pain was intense, and the case was of more than one years' standing. The arm was wasted and the pain continuous. Lesions were a lateral luxation of the second dorsal vertebra, and contraction of the muscles of the whole upper spinal region as low as the sixth dorsal vertebra,

drawing together the upper five ribs on the left side and causing intercostal neuralgia in this region. In two weeks the pain was overcome and the arm began to develope. The case was cured.

(6) Brachial neuralgia of more than one year's standing. The pain affected the right arm and rendered it almost useless. The lesion was of the right first rib, pressing upon the brachial plexus. At the third treatment the rib was set and the pain ceased.

(7) Cervico-brachial neuralgia in the right arm, shoulder, and chest, due to lateral luxation of the 5th cervical and third dorsal vertebrae and muscular contractures of the cervical and left intercostal muscles. The case was practically cured in four months.

(8) Intercostal neuralgia of several years' standing, cured in less than one month.

(9) Intercostal neuralgia due to heavy lifting, so severe that the patient was unable to sit erect without great pain. Lesion was depression of 3rd and 4th ribs on both sides. Immediaie relief followed treatment, and the case was cured in four weeks.

(10) Intercostal neuralgia of ten years' standing, causing an intense pain in the left side, extending to the abdomen. Lesion was a luxation of the 8th left rib, and the case was cured by replacing it.

(11) Spinal neuralgia of a number of years' standing, due to lesion of the 4th dorsal vertebra. The case was cured in two months.

(12) Neuralgia in the head, of eight years' standing, lasting continually thirty-six hours during each menstrual period. Lesion was at the atlas, with muscular contractions in the lower dorsal and lumbar region. The case was cured in one month.

(13) Neuralgia of the stomach of three years' standing, the attacks coming on after each meal. At the time of examination so serious had the condition become that the patient had not taken solid food for more than two weeks. Lesion was a lateral twist of the spine between the sixth and seventh dorsal vertebrae Improvement followed one treatment, and the case was cured in about one year.

(14) Ulnar neuralgia, accompanied by swelling of the arm and of the ulnar side of forearm, hand, and third and fourth fingers. The trouble was of two years' duration, spinal lesion was found at the origin of the brachial plexus, and a contraction of the muscles in the upper dorsal region. After four treatments there was no further pain, and the case was dismissed cured in one month.

(15) Neuralgia in the third finger of the right hand, of several years' standing. Lesion was at the third cervical vertebra, which was corrected in a few treatments, removing the condition.

(16) Tic Douloureux of twelve years' standing. The pain would occur spasmodically in the infra-orbital terminals of the fifth nerve, at intervals of from three to ten minutes. Lesion was found in a displaced atlas, which was corected in six weeks, curing the case.

DEFINITION: "Neuralgia is a pain in the course of a nerve, unaccompanied by structural charges. It is due to irritation, direct or indirect, of the nerve." Often this irritation is from pressure of a displaced bony part or of contractured tissues.

The LESIONS found causing this condition are usually bony, and these act by pressing directly upon a nerve, or by affecting centers or sympathetic connections. In case 6 above, the brachial neuralgia was due to direct pressure of the first rib upon the brachial plexus, of nerves. In case 1 or 2 it is evident that lesion of the atlas was too low to affect the nerve involved, the fifth cranial, by direct pressure. Here the effect may have been upon the medulla, thus affecting the center in which certain roots of origin of the fifth arise, but more probably the effect was upon the nerve through its numerous sympathetic connections in the upper part of the cervical region, as pointed out in the discussion of the fifth nerve in diseases of the eye, q. v.

In intercostal neuralgia the pressure is usually directly upon the nerve by a displaced rib, but may be due to vertebral lesion.

The commonest bony lesion in neuralgia is a luxated vertebra, such a cause having been known to produce neuralgia in any part of the body. (See cases 1, 5, 7, 11, 13.) It is probable that in such cases the vertebra brings direct pressure upon the nerve as it emerges from the spinal canal.

Any bony part in the body in relation to nerves may become displaced and impinge upon the adjacent nerve, causing neuralgia. Frequently the cause of irritation is pressure of contractured tissues upon the nerve. This occurs at the foramina of exit of the various branches of the fifth nerve upon the face. The tissues at and about the foramen become congested or contractured, pressing upon the nerve. These contractures may occur along the spine, as in case 4. Contracture of the intercostal muscles may draw the ribs together, irritate the nerves and cause the neuralgia. Contractures are often the direct irritating cause in cases of neuralgia due to exposure, tranmatism, etc.

The lesion may be one causing a primary disease, as rheumatism, gout, or specific infectious disease, allowing of the generation of poisons in the system, which affect the nerves by circulating in the blood.

In TIC DOULOUREUX the lesion is usually at the atlas, but often is found among the other upper cervical vertebrae. Contracture of the cervical muscles and of the tissues about the foramina are often the causes.

In CERVICO-OCCIPITAL neuralgia the lesions are usually among the upper four cervical vertebrae.

In INTERCOSTAL neuralgia occur lesions of vertebrae at the origin of the nerves affected, of the ribs, and of the spinal and intercostal muscles.

MASTODYNIA, or neuralgia of the breast, occuring generally in women, is due to similar lesions as intercostal neuralgia. Commonly one finds rib lesion in the region affected.

LUMBO-ABDOMINAL neuralgia, marked by pain in the lumbar region, hyphogastrium, buttocks, or genitals, is caused by lesion in the lower dorsal and lumbar spine.

CERVICO-BRACHIAL neuralgia is due to lesion of the lower cervical vertebrae, of the first rib, clavicle, and of the upper dorsal vertebrae. It may be caused by vertebral lesion anywhere from the atlas th the sixth dorsal.

Neuralgia in the LOWER LIMBS is due to lumbar, sacral, or innominate lesions. VISCERAL NEURALIGA, as of stomach or intestines, is caused by vertebral lesion of the corresponding spinal region. COCCYGODYNIA is caused by displacement of the coccyx.

The PROGNOSES is good in all kinds of neuralgia. Cases of long standing often yield at once. A few treatments, or a single treatment, commonly, at once relieve the poin. Permanent cure is usually accomplished.

The TREATMENT is simple. Often the removal of lesion is at once sufficient to entirely cure the condition. The lesion should always be removed as soon as possible. Likewise any causes of irritation must be removed, as an ulcerated tooth, a cicatrix, a growth in the nose, etc. Constitutional conditions giving rise to neuralgic states must be met according to the case.

Relaxation of all contractured tissues must be accomplished. The manipulatiou is carried over the course of the affected nerve, relaxing the tissues about it. The pain of the disease does not prevent this local treatment. Inhibition of the pain is accomplished, not by pressure, but by light manipulation. The main treatment is usually upon a lesion at the origin of the affected nerve, or in its path.

The above method of treatment is applied to any special variety of the disease. Tic Douloureux often yields at once to light manipulation over the course of the affected branches upon the face. (Chap. V. B.)

RHEUMATISM.

CASES. (1) Inflammatory rheumatism, off and on, for sixteen years. The effect was general, but the body below the waist was worse, hip and lower limbs being very bad. Lesion occured at the 4th lumbar vertebra. The inflammation began to subside with the first treatment. The patient, confined to the bed, was able to sit up in one week, and was cured in five weeks.

(2) Inflammatory rheumatism of three years' standing, cured in two months.

(3) Inflammatory rheumatism of one month's standing, the patient being confined to the bed. The hands, feet, elbows, and knees were affected and very painful. Under the first treatment the pain and swelling were much relieved; the second day the patient was out of bed, and in a short time he was cured.

(4)   Rheumatic fever of twelve weeks' standing cured in three weeks.

(5)   Muscular rheumatism of three years' standing in a man of seventy. The left lower limb was affected. The case was cured in three weeks.

(6)   Muscular rheumatism and swelling of the lower limbs in a woman of seventy-four. The case was cured in five treatments.

(7)   Muscular rheumatism, in the form of torticollis, following malarial fever. The condition was of one month's standing. It improved from the first treatment, and was cured in three weeks.

(8)   Muscular rheumatism in the shoulder, the patient having been unable to raise her hand to her head for seven months. The first rib was found party dislocated at its head. The arm could be raised to the head after one treatment, and the case was cured in one month.

(9)   Acute articular rheumatism in a lady of eighty-three, of three months' standing. Lesions occured in the upper dorsal and lumbar regions of the spine. The hips and knees were affected. One month's treatment had greatly improved the case.

(10)   Acute articular rheumatism in a lady of eighty-two, who had suffered with attacks of this disease most of her life. Both knees were much swollen, and the patient had been in bed for two weeks. Improvement followed the first treatment, and in ten days she could get about very well. The case was cured in several weeks.

(11)   Articular rheumatism affecting the foot, of six years' standing, and due to an upward dislocation of the tarsal end of the first metatarsal bone. The case was cured by reducing the d'slocation.

(12)   Chronic rheumatism of three years' standing, occuring in the spring and fall. The whole body was affected. Three months' treatment had greatly benefited the case.

(13)   Chronic rheumatism of eight months' standing. The patient was unable to raise his hand to his head or to dress himself. After one treatment he could do both, and the case was pratically cured by four treatments. Lesions were found at the third cervical vertebra, 1st to 4th dorsal, and 4th lumbar.

(14)   Lumbago, in occasional attacks, one of which had been brought on by bicycling. Lesion was found in a lateral luxation of the 4th lumbar vertebra. The case was relieved by one treatment, and was cured in three treatments.

(15)   Lumbago, brought on by a muscular strain, showed lesions at the lumbo-sacral and sacro-iliac articulations. The case was cured in a few treatments.

LESIONS: In the three forms; Acute Articular Rheumatism, or Rheumatic Fever, or Inflammatory Rheumatism, Chronic, or Chronic Articular Rheumatism, and Muscular Rheumatism, various bony and muscular lesions are found.

In Rheumatic Fever special bony lesions may be lacking. Often spinal lesions affecting liver and kidneys are found, and muscular contractures may be present at lesion. Bony lesions are apt to occur at the origin of the nerves supplying the affected points. Contractured tissues due to climatic effects are common.

In Muscular and Chronic Rheumatism specific lesion is much more definite than in Rheumatic Fever. Local bony lesions play an important part in the production of muscular rheumatism, as do also muscular contractures. Both may be due to physical strains. Contractures may likewise be due to exposure to inclement weather, etc.

It is common in muscular rheumatism of shoulders and arms to find luxation of the lower cervical and upper dorsal vertebrae, one or several, together with contractures in the fibres of the trapezius muscles in these regions. So in rheumatism of special muscle groups bony lesion is quite generally found at the origin of the nerves supplying them. This is equally true for chronic articular rheumatism. For example, in these very numerous cases in which the joints of the lower limbs are affected, it is almost the rule to find lumbar or innominate lesions obstructing the nerve-supply to the limbs.

In rheumatic affections of special localities as, for example, the wrist, ankle, etc., it is common to find a local bony part out of place, as carpal, tarsal, or metatarsal bone. In lumbago there is almost invariably luxation of lumbar vertebrae, irritating the nerve-fibres supplying the muscle-bundles of the erectors spine.

The contracturing of tissues as the result of chronic rheumatism is often sufficient to draw a joint out of place, as in case of the hip-joint.

Lesions in rheumatism act by deranging blood and nerve supply, locally or generally. In inflammatory rheumatism the effect is a constitutional one, acting upon the system through lesions which derange the functions of liver and kidneys, also of the central nervous system. Yet this condition is often a good deal like "catching cold," and presents, therefore, no constant lesion.

In the other forms of rheumatism, local derangement of nerve and blood-supply is the result of the lesion. This lesion may be present at the exact locality of the effect, or in the course or at the origin of the nerves supplying the part. In the case of muscular rheumatism particularly, the fact that the pathology is indefinite, that no structural changes occur in the muscles, and that many authors regard it as nuralgia, well supports the osteopathic theory that it is due to bony or muscular lesions irritating the nerve-supply of the muscles affected. This effect is especially well shown in that form of muscular rheumatism known as Lumbago, in which vertebral lesion, irritating the local nerve-fibres, is regarded as the cause, osteopathically. As a matter of fact one meets numerous cases diagnosed as either rheumatism or neuralgia, or to which these terms are applied interchangably. From an osteopathic point of view it makes but little difference which view of the case is taken. The essential fact is lesion irritating nerve-supply, its removal being the necessary therapeutic measure.

The PROGNOSIS, in all forms of rheumatism, is good. Even the so-called incurable chronic rheumatism is often cured. The prognosis is especially good in inflammatory and muscular rheumatism. In such cases one expects to give relief at one treatment. Quick cures are often made in them. In chronic cases the progress is slow because of the deformity, the deposit in the joint, and the thickening of the local tissues. Many of these cases are incurable but may be benefitted. Up to a certain point the deposits may be absorbed, the deformity overcome, and the joint be put in good condition. It is the rule, however, that the enlargement or deformity of the joint cannot be much relieved, though the progress of the disease may be stayed.

The TREATMENT of these cases must be persistent, but not severe. In inflammatory rheumatism the extreme pain, which cannot tolerate the slightest jarring of the floor, or movement of the bed-clothes, must be considered. Yet it does not prevent treatment of the case. Delicacy of manipulation enables one to soon overcome the patient's fear and to manipulate the joints at will. The beneficial effect of this treatment becomes at once apparent in reduction of the pain and inflammation. Cases should not be treated too often or too long at a time.

In these cases, especially in rheumatic fever, special attention must be given to stimulating the activities of kidneys, liver, digestive system, and skin, to remove poisons from the system and to improve the condition of the blood. Often the treatment is at first confined to these parts, so important is it to gain control of their functions.

A general spinal treatment is necessary in rheumatic fever, for constitutional effects. A close watch must be kept upon the general health, and lungs and heart must be kept well stimulated. Careful stimulation of the heart will prevent the disease reaching that part. It is particularly necessary to provide against the heart being affected.

The circulation to the joint, muscle, or part affected, must be kept free. This is accomplished by work along its vessels, by removal of bony lesion and muscular contracture, but especially by springing the bones of the joint so as to separate them and allow of free circulation of the blood to the membranes. It is in this way that the deposits are removed and the membranes restored to normal condition.

In acute inflammation of a joint, also, its blood-supply must be kept free and itself be lightly manipulated, to take down the inflammation.

In muscular rheumatism the muscles should be stretched and manipulated gently to stimulate the metabolism of the local tissues, aiding them to throw off the poisonous substances supposed to collect in them.

In any case the nerve-supply of the part must be treated from its origin, and the lesion be removed.

In Lumbago the affected muscles must be relaxed, and the lesion be reduced. It is readily affected. The patient may sit upon a stool,while the practitioner stands in front and passes his arms about the body, clasping either side of the spine well down toward the sacrum. He now raises and slightly rotates the trunk, first to one side, then to the other, relaxing the muscles, separating the vertebræ, and relaxing rhe nerve-fibres from impingement.

In inflammatory rheumatism one should look after the hygiene of the sick chamber. Cold baths and sponging with tepid water are allowable for the fever, but are not usually necessary under the osteopathic treatment. The patient should be between blankets, which absorb the perspiration and prevent chill. The joint should be well protected by being wrapped in some soft, warm material, such as cotton. The diet should be light and nutritious. Chronic cases should be protected from toil, exposure, etc.

Diseases of Women from page 220.
(13) Prolapsus of the uterus with retroversion in a woman of 40 of several yrs. standing. Lesion was a slight displacement of the innominate. The case was cured by local and spinal treatment. Lesion was corrected.
(14) Leucorrhea in a married woman of 30. Lesion: slight deviation of lower D & L vertebrae to the left. Upon correction of spinal lesion in less than one month, the case was cured.
(15) Leucorrhea, congestion of the ovaries are. painful menstruation of three yrs. standing. Left innominate luxated, and lesion at 10th & 11th D. Case cured in 4 mos.

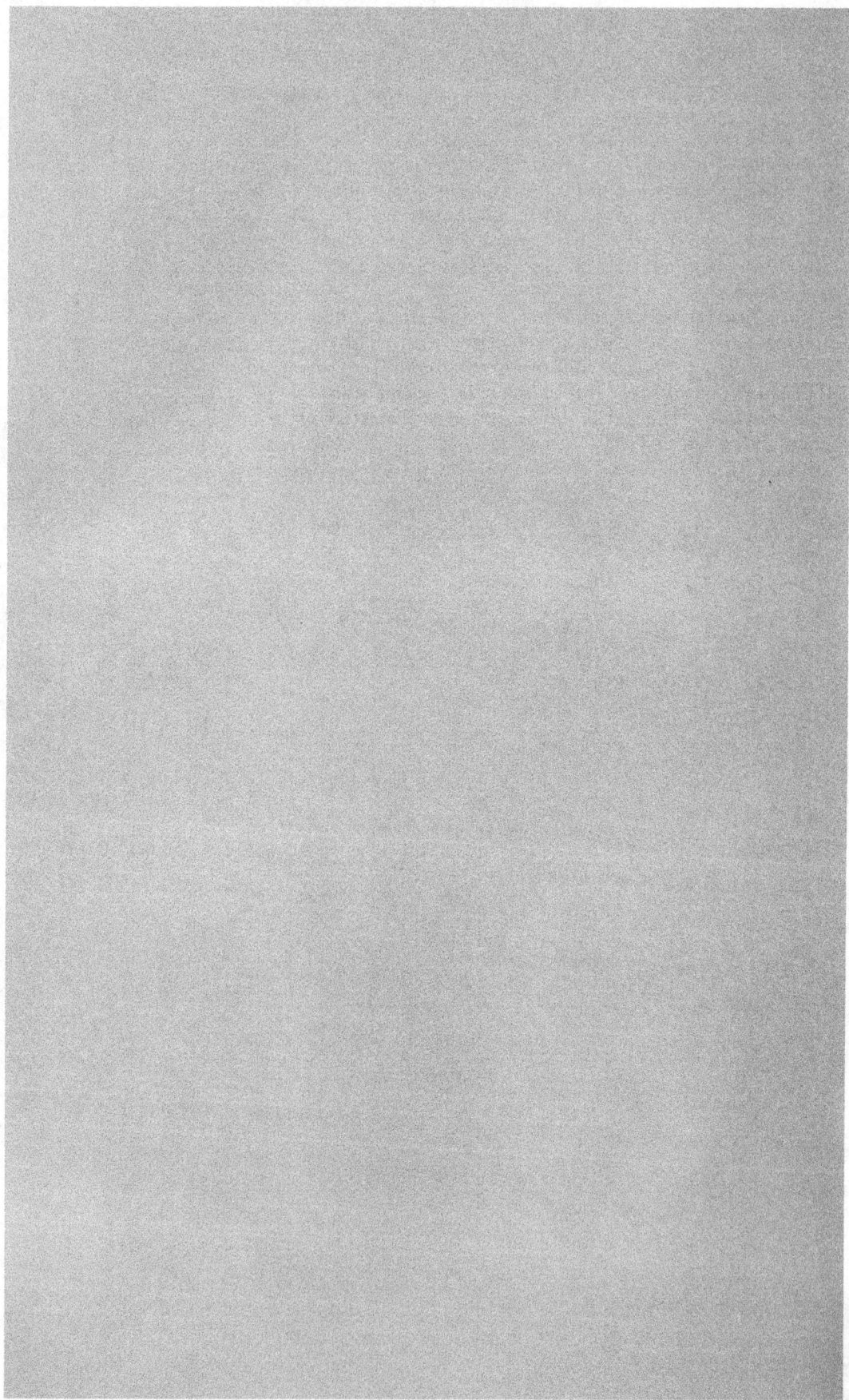

DIABETES MELLITUS AND DIABETES INSIPIDUS.

CASES: (1) Diabetes Mellitus in a man of thirty four. The disease was well established by urinalysis and the characterictic symptoms. The patient was a great sufferer from pain in the lower dorsal and lumbar regions, and showed bony lesions at the 12th dorsal, second and fifth lumbar vertebrae. He was discharged cured after eight months' treatment, and has since passed the medical examination for life insurance, being pronounced a good risk.

(2) Diabetes Mellitus in a young man of nineteen, who had been given up to die. He was passing nine pints per day of urine of a sp. gr. of 1054. In one week it was reduced to 1043, and four pints per day. He gained strength daily, and was practically cured at the time of report.

(3) Diabetes Mellitus in a lady of fifty-six. The patient had lost eighty pounds in six months, and her symptoms were very marked. The case was expected to die. Lesions were found in the upper cervical vertebra. also of the 2nd and 3rd dorsal, and lower dorsal and upper lumbar vertebrae. The sp. gr. of the urine was 1043, sugar 4 per cent, and quantity from 10 to 18 pints *per diem*. Improvement was continuous from the first, and in five months the case was cured.

(4) A case of Diabetes Mellitus showed, under treatment, continual diminution of the quantity of urine, and a complete disappearance of the sugar in a few weeks. Some months later the patient was still in good health.

(5) Diabetes Mellitus in a lady of fifty-six. She passed about 200 ounces of urine each day, containing a large percentage of sugar. A depression of the right ribs over the region of the liver. The case showed marked improvement under the treatment. In four months the general symptoms were much improved, and the quantity of sugar was less than half as much as at first.

(6) Diabetes Mellitus, in which lesions were found in the lower dorsal and lumbar region. Also in the cervical region and at the atlas. Marked improvement took place under treatment, but the treatment was discontinued before a cure was affected.

(7) Diabetes Mellitus showing lesion in the lower dorsal and lumbar regions. The treatment was continued for four months, and the case was completely cured, the patient passing a medical examination for life insurance.

(8) Diabetes Mellitus in a girl of sixteen. The case was in an advanced stage, showing a large percentage of sugar. The case was cured in five months.

(9) Diabetes Mellitus in a man fifty-one years of age. Lesion was a posterior condition of the spine from the sixth dorsal to the second lumbar

vertebra. At the time of report, one month's treatment had been taken, and improvement was made.

(10) Diabetes Mellitus showing lesion in the cervical and lower dorsal regions. The urine contained two percent of sugar. Complete cure was made.

LESIONS causing diabetes are usually bony lesions along the spine from the middle dorsal to the lower lumbar region. McConnell notes the fact that in a number of cases there was a posterior swerve of the spine form the middle dorsal to the upper lumbar region.

Sacral lesion has been noted in these cases, some showing a slip of the ilium, some lesion of the fifth lumbar. Cervical lesion, chiefly in the upper cervical region is sometimes found in diabetes mellitus. Sometimes a rib lesion, as in case 5, occurs in the region of the liver or of the splanchnics.

Lesions of the dorsal and upper lumbar region involve the innervation of these organs, derangement of which is thought to be most closely associated with diabetes. Through their effects upon the splanchnics and solar-plexus, they derange the functions of the liver, pancreas, and intestines, all thought to be implicated in this condition. It is well established that pancreatic disease is usually closely associated with diabetes, that a glycolytic ferment secreted by this gland is necessary to normal metabolism. This being disturbed results in sugar in the urine. Such a result is doubtless affected by such lesions as above, interfering with the innervation of the organ by way of the solar and splenic plexuses.

It has already been shown how closely are such lesion associated with derangement of the liver innervation, the glycogenic function of the organ being disturbed in diabetes.

It may be that these lesions likewise aid the condition by deranging the activities of the intestinal villi. According to Pavy's view of diabetes a disturbance in the functions of the cells of the intestinal villi is the essential feature in the causation of diabetes. Lesion to the vaso-motor innervation of the portal vessels, arising from the 5th to 9th dorsal may have something to do with such a disturbance. Lesion to the upper region may aid this effect.

The influence of the general nervous system in diabetes is well known, but not well understood. It is shown that lesions to the medulla, cord and sympathetic system cause diabetes. The various spinal and cervical bony lesions dobutless could do the mischief resulting in diabetes, as it has been shown frequently that these lesions may injure cord, medulla, or sympathetic system, as in paralysis, etc. In this connection one sees the importance of upper cervical lesions, which may affect the medulla. Here, in the floor of the fourth ventricle, lies the so-called diabetic center. It is a point, puncture at which results in diabetes. The effect is doubtless gotten through the vagi nerves, whose origin is from this point. With regard to this fact, also to the well known participation of the vagi in liver functions, it seems that cervical and spinal lesion, affecting the vagi through their sympathetic cervical connections, or through their connections with the solar plexus, may in this way produce a part of the effect of lesion in diabetes.

PROGNOSIS. Although diabetes mellitus is a grave, and, by ordinary methods, an incurable disease, the outcome under osteopathic treatment is usually more encouraging. A fair percentage of cures has been shown, there being no room for doubting the facts in such cases. In accounts of twenty-six cases gathered by Dr. C. W. Proctor, thirteen improved continually under the treatment; seven were entirely cured; others were yet under treatment.

It may be well said that in such cases our prognosis for recovery is fair, and for benefit is good.

The TREATMENT is mainly, as far as the specific treatment is concerned, upon that portion of the spine most affected with lesion, namely along the splanchnic and lumbar regions. It is of course necessary to remove the lesion as soon as possible. Treatment at the above mentioned regions is particularly for restoring to normal the functions of pancreas, liver and small intestine.

As the heart, kidneys, lungs and spleen undergo pathological changes, it is necessary to give special attention to their condition, according to methods before given. The skin and general excretory system must be stimulated to aid in excreting the sugar from the blood. The bowels must be treated for the constipation which is usually present.

A thorough general systemic treatment is given for the purpose of affecting the various organs involved in the disease, stimulating and increasing the general nutrition of the body, which is much affected, and of upbuilding the general nervous system.

It is necessary to give close attention to the diet and regimen of the patient. Carbobydrates must be excluded from the diet as thoroughly as passible, no sugars nor starches being allowed in any form. Meats, fish, poultry, eggs and green vegetables which do not contain starch(string-beans, lettuce, water-cress, spinach, young onions, tomatoes, olives, celery,) are allowed. So, likewise, are milk, cream, butter and cheese. The patient should drink plenty of water, especially such alkaline mineral waters as Vichy, Carlsbad, etc.

He should take light exercise, but should avoid fatigue, particularly inimical to his weakened condition. For the same reason, while warm and steam baths are recommended, they should not be prolonged for fear of a weakening effect.

In DIABETES INSIPIDUS the lesions are usually found in the lower splanchnic area, affecting the kidneys. Some cases show lesion of the superior cervical vertebrae. In the latter case the effect may be upon the medulla, or upon the sympathetic system. There is a point in the floor of the fourth ventricle, puncture at which causes diabetes insipidus.

These various bony lesions may cause it by affecting the cord, since is is known that injuries to the cerebro-spinal axis result in the disease. Anders regards the condition as a vaso-motor neurosis, usually of central. sometimes of reflex origin. It is also thought to be due to a vaso-motor relaxation of the kidneys. It is readily seen that spinal lesion to the renal splanchnic could result in this vaso-motor neurosis and give rise to the disease.

The PROGNOSIS is good under osteopathic treatment, although the condition is regarded as incurable. A fair number of cases are cured.

The TREATMENT is mainly local for the kidneys, by removal of lesion at the splanchnic areas and by the various special ways of affecting the kidneys as pointed out in considering diseases of the kidneys.

Some general treatment for the nervous system may be necessary.

* * *

DIPHTHERIA.

Numerous cases have been treated successfully by osteopathy.

The LESIONS usually found in such cases are muscular and bony lesions in the neck. Dr. Still regards the important cause a contraction of the tissues of the throat and neck, including the scaleni muscles, drawing the first rib backward under the clavicle and thus disturbing its articulation with the first dorsal vertebra. These contractures about the throat interfere with the venous circulation through the pharyngeal and internal jugular veins, favoring a congested or a catarrhal condition of the mucous membranes of the throat, and leading to diphtheria. It is well known that catarrhal conditions preispose to the disease.

Bony lesions and muscular contractures in the cervical region interfere with the innervation of the muscles and mucous membrane of the throat. The sympathetic innervation is from the superior cervical ganglion. This distribution unites with fibres from the pneumogastric, glosso-pharyngeal, and external laryngeal nerves, forming the pharyngeal plexus. Hence upper cervical lesion may, by affecting the superior cervical ganglion, derange the sympathetic vaso-motor supply of the pharyngeal mucous membranes and lead to the disease.

The PROGNOSIS is good. The case is usually readily cured.

In the TREATMENT the main idea is to keep open the circulation about the throat and to thus prevent the formation of the membrane, or to prevent its further growth. A thorough relaxation of the muscles and anterior tissues of the neck must be maintained. The tissues at the root of the neck, and about the clavicle and first rib must abso be kept free and loose. The clavicle should be raised. The first rib should be pressed downward and forward, working at its central articulation to correct the position of its head. By the process of these treatments the venous and lymphatic drainage from about the throat is kept open. This regulates the vaso-motor disturbance of the membranes, tends to loosen the membrane already formed, and, by preventing further exudation, stops the further growth of the membrane.

The splanchnics, liver, kidneys and bowels should be treated twice daily, to keep free the excretion of poisons from the system, and to aid nutrition, to keep up the strength of the system.

Cervical bony lesion should be removed, and treatment should be given to the vagi, superior cervical ganglion, and cervical sympathetics to correct circulation and aid in gaining vaso-motor control.

The internal throat treatment should be given to aid in gaining the same end. Proper precautions should be taken to protect the finger so that the child may not wound it with his teeth. The finger is inserted and swept down over soft and hard palate, fauces and tonsils, to relieve the local inflammation by starting the circulation.

In laryngeal diphtheria an external treatment about the larynx and down along the trachea is good. (Chap. III, A. V.)

A general systemic treatment should be carefully given to build up the strength. The heart and lungs should be kept carefully stimulated to avoid complications in them. The case should be carefully looked after for some time, to strengthen the heart and to overcome the weakness of the throat.

The general treatment aids in preventing paralysis, particularly apt to occur about the throat, sometimes in other parts of the body.

The patient should be isolated and the usual antiseptic pecautions should be practiced. The patient should be kept upon a liquid diet. Milk ice cream, broths, and the like are used.

CROUP.

(Spasmodic Croup, Catarrhal Croup, or Laryngismus Stridulus.)

DEFINITION: This is a disease peculiar to children and held to be chiefly of nervous origin, but it is often associated with acute catarrhal laryngitis. It is associated with paroxysmal coughing, difficulty of breathing, and attacks of threatened suffocation.

Numerous cases have been successfully treated by Osteopathy.

The LESIONS of greatest importance in croup involve contracturing of the muscles and tissues of the throat, irritating the pneumogastric nerves, and their recurrent and superior laryngeal branches. These contractures likewise prevent proper circulation to and from the larynx, and favor the catarrhal condition in this way. The irritation of the pneumogastrics and their branches is accountable for the spasmodic condition of the larynx during the paroxysms.

Dr. Still ragards as important sacral and lower spinal bony lesions in croup. He also finds a contracture of the omohyoid muscle, drawing the hyoid bone down and back upon the superior laryngeal nerve, irritating it, and causing the spasm In croup, as in other throat diseases, he finds that the contracture of the cervical tissues and scaleni muscles draws the first rib back under the clavicle, draws it upward, and deranges its articulation with the first dorsal vertebra. This condition is important in shutting off venous and lymphatic drainage from the larynx, and favors the inflammation of the mucous membrane.

Various contractures of the posterior cervical muscles, as well as those bony lesions common in laryngitis, as of atlas, axis, and 3rd cervical vertebra, are sometimes present, acting to disturb sympathetic innervation, vagi, and circulition.

One must, however, chiefly regard those contractures and bony lesions about the throat and neck anteriorly. Arising from exposure, cold, etc., they become the chief cause of croup

The PROGNOSIS is good. Immediate relief is given by the treatment. The spasm, stridulous breathing, and threatened suffocation are overcome at once by the treatment during the attack.

The chief TREATMENT is to at once relax all the anterior cervical tissues, to free the circulation and to relieve the irritation to the superior and recurrent laryngeal nerves. The treatment should begin well up beneath the inferior maxillary bone, being made especially about the hyoid bone and muscles, and should be carried down along the throat and trachea.

The hyoid bone should be grasped and manipulated laterally, forward, and upward, relaxing the omo-hyoid and other muscles. (Chap III, A. III. Chap. IV, III.)

The process of freeing the circulation is materially aided by working along the course of the carotid arteries and internal jugular veins, raising the clavicle, and relaxing the surrounding tissues.

Treatment may be made close along the larynx and trachea. (Chap. III, A. V). This is helpful during the spasm.

Inhibition may be made upon the superior laryngeal nerve by pressure immediately below and behind the greater cornua of the hyoid bone, and upon the recurrent laryngeal at the inner side of the sterno-mastoid muscle at the level of the cricoid cartilage. This is likewise useful during the spasm.

Anders notes the fact that sometimes the epiglottis becomes wedged into the rima glottidis, and must be helped out by the use of the index finger.

The spasm may be lessened by manipulation about the region of the diaphragm, relaxing it, and by treatment of the phrenic nerves in the neck. (Chap. III, A. VIII.)

Due attention must be given to the tissues and bony lesions of the posterior cervical region.

All sources of reflex irritation, as intestinal parasites, dentition, indigestion, etc., must be looked after. The child should not be allowed to over-eat or drink.

In spasmodic croup the attack is sometimes relieved by easing an overloaded stomach. Tickling the fauces with the finger will cause the vomiting. Cold applications may be used over the throat and chest. A warm bath is a convenient means to employ to break up a spasm.

WHOOPING-COUGH.

(PERTUSSIS).

DEFINITION: An acute, highly contagious disease, occuring chiefly in children, and characterized by a catarrhal inflammation of the mucous membrane of the respiratory tract, and by a peculiar spasmodic cough ending in a whooping inspiration.

Its true, nature is not known, but that theory that regards it as a lesion of the phrenic, pneumogastric, sympathetic, or recurrent laryngeal nerve, or perhaps of the medulla, best accords with the osteopathic view of the etiology.

The PROGNOSIS is good. The course may be aborted if taken early, but if the disease is well started but little more than alleviation can be accomplished. The case is safely carried through, and the danger of complications is minimized.

The LESIONS In whooping-cough, as in croup, the contraction of the omo hyoid muscle drawing the hyoid bone against the pneumogastric nerve is important, as is also the contracturing of the cervical tissues drawing the first rib back, and disturbing its central articulation.

Cervical bony lesions are found at the upper, middle, and lower cervical vertebrae, and bony lesions are also found about the first and second dorsal vertebrae, the first rib and clavicle.

The upper cervical lesion affects sympathetics and vagi in ways before pointed out. The middle cervical lesion affects phrenics and diaphragm, sometimes important in this condition. The contractures of throat tissues, lesion of clavicle and first rib retard venous and lymphatic drainage, and lead to catarrhal conditions, well known to be of much importance in producing the condition. The mucous membranes are thus weakened and laid liable to the action of the specific infection.

Lesions of the upper dorsal vertebrae and of the upper two or three ribs may derange the sympathetic connections of the laryngeal innervation.

The TREATMENT is much the same as in croup. The prime point is to free the circulation about the larynx and whole respiratory tract, as there is a catarrhal condition of the whole tract. This object involves the relaxation of all the anterior cervical tissues, treatment of the hyoid bone and relaxation of the omo-hyoid, raising the clavicle, etc. All bony lesions of the cervical, upper dorsal, and upper thoracic region must be overcome, together with existing contractures, in order to remove all sources of irritation to the laryngeal innervation. The ways in which these lesions act, and the method of their removal has before been sufficiently explained.

For the cough, treatment should be made down along larynx and trachea, and about the angle of the jaw.

Dr. Still mentions, also, treatment to the phrenic nerves and diaphragm to relieve the condition.

The lungs may be stimulated, and all the upper ribs be raised, to ease respiration. The lungs, heart, kidneys, and general system must be carefully looked after and thoroughly treated to avoid the complications and sequelae that may arise in the form of broncho-pneumonia, pleurisy, pericarditis, acute nephritis, etc.

INFLUENZA.

(LA GRIPPE—EPIDEMIC CATARRHAL FEVER.)

CASES : (1)   Four cases in one family restored to usual health within a week.

(2)   Four cases cured in four or five treatments, no bad results following the disease.

(3)   La Grippe, attacking the throat and complicated with a severe tonsilitis, was cured by several treatments.

(4)   A severe attack of la grippe cured in four days by treatment directed to bowels, kidneys, and splanchnic nerves.

(5)   A list of thirty-five cases, one of which had been cured by one treatment, and the remaining cases cured by several treatments, none requiring over four.

(6)   A report of a number of cases of la grippe, all with mared symptoms. In every case the patient was able to be up in from one to three days No complications nor sequelae arose.

(7)   A lady of seventy-one had been confined to her bed for two weeks with la grippe and rheumatism. After seven treatments she was about, the la grippe being cured and the rheumatism much improved.

(8)   A case of la grippe cured in four treatments.

LESIONS : While no specific bony lesion has yet been mentioned as occurring in Influenza, there is yet a specific condition of lesion doubtless closely associated with the invasion of the disease into the system. This condition is a general contracturing of the spinal muscles, most marked in the upper dorsal and cervical regions, but affecting the whole spinal system. This may be regarded as the specific lesion in Influenza. Dr. Stil.

regards it as shutting down upon the whole vascular and nerve systems of the body, through the constricting affect of these contractures upon the spinal nervous system through its posterior distribution. The result is a sluggish condition of all the vital fluids, lymphatic, blood, and nerve.

While it is doubtless true that the bacillus of Pfeifer is the infecting agent, it yet remains to account for the sudden invasion of the system by this germ, since it is known that the germs of disease cannot attack healthy tissues and that a body in perfect health is immune.

In this connection it is significant that debilitated persons fall the easiest victims to the malady. In a majority of such individuals it is doubtless true that various osteopathic lesions already exist and so weaken the system in one way or another.as to lay it liable to the invasion of the the germ.

Just so, the general muscular contracture found as the characteristic lesion in la grippe, acts upon the vital forces of the system to debilitate them and lay the body liable to invasion. Tnis theory would appear entirely reasonable in the light of the fact that Pepper thinks it likely that the germs exists everywhere, but depends upon certain extraordinary atmospheric or telluric conditions for occasion to break out into virulence. It is quite reasonable to hold that some special set of circumstances, it may even be these same extraordinary atmospheric conditions, results in these spinal contractures which, occurring coincidentally with the periods of virulence of the germ, allow of the invasion of the system.

La grippe is most frequent in bad weather, and it may be that then exposure to cold may set up these contractures. While it is true that the authorities hold the disease to be entirely independent of climate and season, it is yet true that a person may "catch cold" at any time and place, these contractures being well known to result.

It is probable that the presence of various lesions, bony and otherwise, in the body. determines the disease to a special part of the system, resulting in the peculiar manifestation of the disease which disguishes it as the abdominal type, the cerebral type, the thoracic type, etc.

Probably, too, such lesions are responsible for the various complications and sequelae which constitute so marked a feature of the attack, as affections of lungs, heart and nervous system.

The PROGNOSIS under osteopathic treatment is particularly good. One, or a few treatments being usually all that are necessary in uncomplicated cases. When the case is taken in time complications do not ensue. If present they are usually readily overcome by the treatment. It is a well known fact that the mortality is influenza is due chiefly to its complications, consequently not the least satisfactory result of osteopathic treatment is in overcoming danger of these. The distressing sequelae, especially affecting lungs, nervous system, and eyes and ears, do not occur.

The TREATMENT indicated is a thorough general one, as for a bad cold, including particularly the complete relaxation of all the spinal tissues, thus restoring the equilibrium of the vascular and nervous systems. This object accomplished, a long step toward recovery has been taken.

During this process occasion is taken to strongly stimulate heart and lungs, regulating circulation, sweeping out congestions, inducing perspiration and lessening fever, and sustaining these organs themselves against the effects the disease is likely to produce in them. This treatment embodies raising the clavicle and ribs, work over the chest anteriorly, stimulation of the vaso-motor and accelerator innervation in the upper dorsal region, etc., all described in considering the diseases of heart and lungs.

The liver, kidneys, bowels and fascia are likewise kept well stimulated.

It is well, especially in the rheumatoid type, to carry the relaxing treatment over all parts of the body, flexing and rotating the thighs, working about shoulders, upper limbs, neck, etc. This overcomes the distressing general aching and soreness in the muscles.

Careful abdominal treatment is called for, particularly if the disease shows a tendency to settle in that region. Work upon the liver, bowels, solar and hypogastric plexuses, and splanchnics in the usual way will meet these requirements.

The general spinal and cervical treatment both aids the general affect and provides against affection of the central nervous system, brain, and organs of special sense.

The general health must be carefully guarded, the patient must be kept from exposure, be prevented from going out too soon, and be kept upon a light, nutritious diet. This should be largely fluid in case the patient confined any length of time to his bed.

The fever, headache, pains in the eye-balls, and other manifestations of the disease are treated specially in the usual ways.

SCIATICA.

Sciatica is a disease in which Osteopathy has secured particularly brilliant results. Great numbers of cases have been cured, many of them having tried previously every known means of treatment.

The PROGNOSIS is good. Usually immediate relief is given upon the first treatment. Often the case is soon cured, though many cases call for a patient continuance of the treatment.

The LESIONS are almost always of such a nature as to bring irritation upon the nerve, either by direct pressure upon the nerve, or upon certain fibres contributing to it. Derangement of its blood-supply may play a part in producing the condition.

The common lesions are bony ones along the lumbar and sacral regions. Lesions of the 4th and 5th lumbar vertebrae, lesions of the first and second sacral nerves by contracture of the tissues about them, innominate displacement, slipping of the sacro-ilac joint and derangement of its ligaments, displacement of the sacrum, and derangement of the coccyx, are all important forms of lesion producing sciatica. These lesions impinge the fibres contributing to or connecting with the sacral plexus. Some may directly press upon the nerve.

A frequent cause of sciatica is contracture of the pyriformis muscle upon the trunk of the sciatic nerve. The tissues about the sciatic notch may be contractured and irritate it. It is said that lesion along the cord, anywhere from the 2nd dorsal down, may cause sciatica. McConnell states that downward displacement of the 11th or 12th rib may cause it.

The TREATMENT is simple. It calls for the immediath removal of the source of pressure or irritation by correction of lesion, A general relaxation of tissues about the nerve and about its connections is done, due attention being given to relaxation of ligaments, as at the sacro-iliac articulation.

This relaxation of the tissues should be carried along the femoral vessels, often thus relieving the condition in an important manner. The tissues along the course of the nerve, at the sciatic notch, at the back of the thigh, and behind the knee should be relaxed also. Strong internal circumduction is used to relax the pyriformis muscle.

The sciatic nerve should be well stretched by one of the methods described. (VI, p. 49.)

MALARIA.

Malaria is a disease which, although due to the activities of a specific germ, the Hematozooan of Leveran, yet presents marked bony lesions, which account for the manifestations of the germ within the system.

The LESIONS are mostly in the splanchnic area, disturbing the sympathetic and vaso-motor innervation of liver, spleen and kidneys. McConnell notes lesion as a marked lateral deviation at the 9th and 10th dorsal vertebrae, and a resulting downward luxation of the 10th rib, also lesion of the 9th to 11th dorsal vertebrae or in the corresponding ribs.

Dr. Still points out lesion at the first lumbar, at the sacrum, at the splanchnics, and in the cervical region.

These various bony lesions must produce a marked affect upon the sympathetic system resulting in vaso-motor disturbance.

The PROGNOSIS is good. Dr. Still says that he never needs to give a patient a second treatment. Usually a few treatments overcome the difficulty, and quick results are often shown. Yet it often happens that but slow progress is made. Complications, however, are prohibited by the treatment. Marked relief is at once given during the paroxysm.

The TREATMENT is directed particularly to the splanchnic area, and to opening of the abdominal blood-supply. By the splanchnic and abdominal treatment liver, kidneys, spleen, and bowels are kept in an active state. This is the chief object of the treatment.

Treatment is given at any time, during or between the paroxysms.

The specific treatment employed by Dr. Still in cases of malaria is as follows: With the patient sitting facing him, he passes his arms beneath the axillae and grasps the spine with both hands, one on either side of the spinous process, at the fourth dorsal vertebra. He now draws the patient's body toward him, though not moving the patient from his position on the chair, thus stretching the spine and bringing pressure upon the 4th vertebra. He closes this manoeuvret by twisting or rotating the trunk slightly, first to one side and then to the other, all the time continuing the pressure at the vertebra. This simple process is repeated at the 12th dorsal for the renal splanchnic. In this way the splanchnics and renal splanchnics are stimulated.

He concludes the treatment by momentarily bringing pressure with his thumbs down upon the femeral arteries. The time of this pressure is merely long enough to allow one heart-beat to elapse. His idea is that this momentary damming back of the femeral currents upon the heart causes it to give a sudden strong beat to overcome the resistance, rousing it to activity and stimulating the system.

A general spinal, cervical, and stimulative treatment to heart and lungs may be given for the chill. This overcomes the intense vaso-motor constriction of the surface of the body, collateral with an inward congestion, and equalizes the circulation. The abdominal treatment aids this process.

This general treatment likewise aids in taking down the fever. The more specific treatment may be given as indicated, in the cervical region, upon the chief vaso-motors, and vaso-motor center of the medulla, via the superior cervical ganglion.

No specific treatment is called for to allay the sweating, as this is itself a relief to the patient's condition. The general method of treatment described may be properly applied during this stage or during the intermission.

TYPHOID FEVER.

CASES: (1) A case taken in the usual way, and presenting the usual symptoms. The fever was 103° at 4 p. m. when the Osteopath was called. The next morning the fever was below 102°, rising that evening to 103.5°. On the succeeding evening it was again 103.5°, but this was the highest point reached. Thereafter, instead of the temperature remaining about 104° for two weeks, as is typical, the gradual decent began immedeately, and in two weeks the patient was well. As early as five days after treatment began most of the symptoms had disappeared. Fourteen days after treatment began the evening temperature was normal. Five days later the patient was out upon the street.

(2) This case, when first seen, had a pulse of 102, a temperature of 105°, and all the usual symptoms marked, even deleruim being present, and the stools and urine passing involuntarily. He had been ill with the fever for two weeks. Gradual descent of the temperature began immediately upon treatment. It became normal seventeen days after treatment began. The symptoms began to abate with the fever, all but the weakness having disappeared in twelve days.

(3) A case seen on the day after it had taken to bed, with a temperature of 101°. In two days the symptoms began to abate. On the fourth day the fever had risen to 104°, falling, then rising on the seventh day to 104° again. After this there was a gradual descent, until on the evening of the twenty-fifth day the temperature was normal. The usual period of high temperature had thus been prevented.

(4) A case of typho-malarial fever which had been ill fonrteen days when the Osteopath was called. The temperature was 103°. After six treatments the case was discharged cured.

(5) Typhoid Fever and Pueumonia, showing a temperature of 105°, having been ill thirteen days when the Osteopath was called. But one treatment was given in this case. It recovered entirely.

(6) In a girl of nine, who had suffered from typhoid fever, the lingering effects of the disease, suffered from five years before, were very marked. The difficulty took the form of acute attacks commencing with pain in the eyes, followed by intense headache and delerium, and a rash upon the skin. As this rash disappeared, swelling and pain in the joints would follow. These attacks would recur about every two weeks. The child was emaciated and suffered from involuutary micturition. She had been under

skilled medical care, and the case had attracted such attention that it was discussed before a convention of physicians in Denver.

Being treated osteopathically during an attack, she recovered this time without the usual swelling and rheumatic symptoms. After two months' treatment the case was discharged cured.

The only bony lesion was a lateral luxation of the third cervical vertebra, but all of the spinal muscles were intensely contractured.

These few cases are quite typical of the many treated.

LESIONS: Dr. Still describes, as the characteristic "typhoid spine," a posterior prominence of the lower lumbar region, caused by backward displacement of the 3rd, 4th and 5th lumbar verthbrae. He holds that the results produced by these lesions is a paralysis of the lymphatic supply of the bowels, by pressure upon the spinal nerves at their exit from the intervertebral foramina. Thus is produced the essential typhoid condition of the small intestine characteristic of the disease.

He notes also lesions along the upper dorsal region, at which point he makes treatment upon the lungs, correcting the activities of the lymphatic system, thus, as he says, making water to put out the fire of the fever.

In general, the lesions found in typhoid fever are rib, vertebral, and muscular lesions affecting the splanchnic and lumbar regions of the spine, irritating spinal nerves, and through them disturbing the sympathetic, vaso-motor, and lymphatic supply of the small intestines.

As before pointed out in detail (see diseases of stomach and intestines), these portions of the spine suffering from lesion give origin to the visceral nerves of the intestines. The vaso-motor supply of the abdominal vessels, according to Quain, is from the splanchnic and lumbar portion of the cord. These include the vaso-motors of the jejunum and ileum, the seat of ulceration in the disease.

Pathologically, the process in the first two stages of typhoid, infiltration and necrosis of the patches, is regarded as a vaso-motor disturbance. The first stage is an intense inflammation, involving to a greater or less degree the whole mucosa. The second stage is the result of an obstructed circulation to the parts of the intestine involved In view of these facts it is evident that successful therapeutic measures must gain vaso-motor control. It is an indication to the Osteopath that he must do spinal work upon the vaso-motor area supplying the bowels, removing the lesion that is obstructing the natural play of forces necessary to health.

The PROGNOSIS is good, yet one must not forget to be upon his guard, constantly, against the complications and intercurrent maladies that so often carry off the typhoid patient. Under osteopathic treatment, however, complications and sequelae are quite prevented. Indeed, much fine osteopathic work has been done upon paralytic and various other forms of the sequelae following a former attack of typhoid fever.

If taken within a week or ten days the course can be usually aborted to a marked degree. Often cases gotten early have had their course terminated within a few days. Bad cases, taken under the treatment after so late as the fourteenth day, commonly at once show marked improvement.

The characteristic course of the temperature is entirely changed. It is usual to notice, no matter in what stage the case may be when it comes under the treatment, that the temperature begins at once to gradually decline. When the case is taken before the second week, the usual period of high temperature is prevented.

TREATMENT: The main object of the treatment, as pointed out, is to gain vaso-motor control of the intestinal blood-supply, and to restore the intestinal lymphaties to normal activity. Consequently the main treatment in these cases is spinal. It must be devoted particularly to the correction of the malpositions of the 3d, 4th and 5th lumbar as described above, and to the removal of any spinal, muscular, rib, or vertebral lesion present.

Most of the treatment in these cases must be done upon the spine, leaving the abdomen almost entirely free from manipulation.

All the spinal muscles should be relaxed, this, with a careful cervical treatment, quieting the nervous system, and relieving the jerking of the *subsultus tendinum.* This treatment is carefully made while the patient is lying upon one side. The patient must not be moved into various positions anymore than can be avoided. It is important to avoid fatiguing him.

Lungs and heart should be kept gently stimulated by work in the usual place in the upper dorsal. This aids in keeping up the patient's strength and in preventing complicating diseases of these organs. Treatment at the renal splanchnics should be given to keep the kidueys active.

The main treatment being along the splanchnic and lumbar regions, these portions of the spine are treated by careful relaxation of all contractures, by gently springing the spine for the relaxation of ligaments and for the freedom of the nerves, and in removing the bony lesions mentioned.

The correction of the lesion to 3d, 4th, and 5th lumbar controls the diarrhoea. It may be treated in the usual way.

The spleen and liver are reached by spinal work at their innervation.

The abdominal treatment is almost nil. Any manipulation made here should be with extreme gentleness. It is best to confine this treatment to the iliac regions, raising the intestines slightly, with the idea of straightening them in the iliac fossae. (IV. Chap. VIII.)

The fever is treated by work at the superior cervical ganglion in the usual way, thus regulating the systemic circulation by affecting the general vaso-motor center in the medulla. The treatment to the heart and lungs aids this process by equalizing the circulation, as does also the general spinal work and the treatment given along the spine for intestinal circulation specifically. The heart beat should be slowed by inhibition at the 2d to 5th dorsal, on the left.

In case of rapid beating of the heart, persisting sometimes for a long period, Dr. Hildreth finds that correction of the left 5th rib gives relief.

The hiccough is treated in the usual way.

In case of hemorrhage the patient should be kept perfectly quiet, have no solid food, and an ice-bag should be applied over the caecum. The foot of the bed should be elevated. Inhibition of peristalsis should be done by work from the 9th dorsal down along the lumbar region.

In case of perforation, hot applications, or the ice-bag, are applied to the abdomen to relieve the patient.

The usual precautions should be taken for the hygiene of the sick room, the disinfection of the linen, the sterilizing of the stools, and urine and general cleanliness.

The patient's body, a part at a time, should be sponged with tepid water daily. The Brand system of baths is much used at the present day.

In regard to diet the usual observance of a strictly liquid diet is followed. Some are using light, easily digested food the first week or ten days, until danger of perforation has arrived. The claim is made that the patient's strength is in this way much better preserved. It would be safe for an Osteopath to carry a case through on such a diet providing he got it early enough to prevent the danger of perforation.

After first taken the patient should not be allowed to get up from his bed. A bed-pan and urinal should be used.

During convalescence the patient's condition should be carefully watched. The return to a hearty diet should be gradual in spite of his great appetite. After a liquid diet the semi-solid food should not be allowed until the temperature has been normal a week.

ERYSIPEAS.

(ST. ANTHONY'S FIRE. "THE ROSE.")

Erysipelas is a disease frequently treated and cured osteopathically. The PROGNOSIS is good.

The LESIONS are various forms of obstruction to the circulation of the part affected. The lesion may be bony, or a contracture of muscles or other tissues. It may directly press upon veins and lymphatic vessels, preventing the proper drainage of the part, or it may derange the vaso-motor innervation and the sympathetic innervation of the lymphatics. For example a case of erysipelas in a lower limb was cured by turning the head of the femur well in the socket, and in raising tne abdominal viscera up from the region of the crural arch, where they were pressing upon the blood vessels and preventing drainage from the limb through the femoral vein and lymphatics. By thus relaxing the tissues and removing direct impingement from the vessels, the blood-flow was restored and the case was cured.

Another case in which the eruption appeared upon the face, was cured by springing the temporol-maxillary articulation with the assistance of corks placed between the molar teeth, as one would set a dislocated jaw. In this way various tissues about the jaw may have been relaxed, or impingement of the fibers of the fifth nerve removed, restoring circulation.

The most usual lesions in erysipelas are found preventing the circulation from the head, as the face is the part most frequently attacked. Lesions of cervical vertebrae and muscles affect the vaso-motors and sympathetics regulating the blood and lymphatic circulation of the face, and lead to inflammation by obstructing these fluids, the specific germ being present and attacking the part thus rendered liable to its action. Clavicle and first rib lesion may directly obstruct the jugular veins and the cervical lymphatics, leading to same result.

McConnell notes lesion of the 2d, 3d, 4th and 5th dorsal vertebrae, and of corresponding ribs and surrounding muscles, causing erysipelas in the face, by disturbing sympathetic innervation.

The TREATMENT is simple, calling for removal of lesion and re-establishment of venous and lymphatic drainage of the affected part. This involves relaxation of muscles and other tissues, restoration of bony parts to position, freeing of nerve connections, etc., as already pointed out, according to the part affected.

It is not necessary to manipulate the inflamed part.

As erysipelas is a dermatitis the need of gaining vaso-motor control is apparent. The special treatment of the neck to affect free circulation to and from the head and face has been sufficiently discussed in the treatment of diphtheria and of the eruptive fevers.

A general spinal treatment must be given to strengthen the general nervous system against the various nervous complications and sequelae that may arise, such as delerium, coma, subsultus tendinum, etc. Bowels must be kept free, and liver and kidneys kept active to get rid of the poison of the disease which is deranging the constitutional condition. The kidneys must be especially supported against albuminuria and uremia.

Among the hygienic measures and domestic remedies recommended, are isolation of the patient, drinking of plenty of cold water, cold spongings of the part, or applications of iced cloths, and the application of collodion over the eruption. Carbolized vaseline may be used to anoint the affected part.

The diet is important. The patient should be liberally fed on a light, nutritious diet. Anders states that liberal feeding of the patient is of greater service to the patient than any of the recognized forms of medicinal treatment, and that lack of attention to the diet during the primary attack tends to increase the frequency of relapse

MEASLES.

(MORBILLI, RUBEOLA.)

Very numerous cases have been successfully treated.

The Prognosis is good. The danger of complications and sequelae is minimized, as these cases recover quickly and thoroughly under the treatment.

While it is held that measles, once started, must run its course, yet the period of convalescence is shortened and the child is about earlier without danger of complications.

Lesions: Dr. Still describes in this disease a general congestion of the lymphatics and of the superficial fascia, insufficient lymphatic drainage of the skin becoming evident as a cutaneous rash. This general congestion is due to spinal muscular contractures all along the spine, irritating the spinal distribution of nerves, and through them deranging sympathetic vaso-motor and lymphatic nerve-supply.

This general congestion of the spinal muscles appears as lesion in measles. The clavicle may be found with its sternal end displaced backward against the vagus nerve, causing the cough, and aiding to cause the catarrhal condition of the bronchi. Upper rib lesions may be found, their correction relieving the cough. Weakened children, especially those presenting upper spinal and thoracic rib lesions, are apt to become victims of pulmonary tuberculosis after measles. The clavicle and first rib lesion, as well as various cervical bony lesions and muscular contractures, probably account for complications and sequelae in eye, ear, nose and throat. These effects come largely through obstructed lymphatic drainage from the neck, a fact well illustrated by the marked enlargement of the cervical lymph glands as a complication or sequel of the disease.

In the Treatment the first step, especially if the rash has not developed, is a thorough stimulation of the cutaneous system, including a general spinal treatmennt, with particular attention to atlas and axis, for effect upon the vaso-motor center in the medulla; upon the second dorsal and fifth lumbar, cutaneous centers. In tardy cases one such treatment suffices to bring out the rash abundantly, a desirable result, since upon its appearance the headache and fever disappear, and the patient feels better.

This treatment would include a general relaxation of the spinal muscles, correcting the lymphatic obstruction.

An important effect of the general spinal and cervical treatment, together with some special treatment to heart and lungs, is to correct the general circulation, calling away from all the viscera the abnormal amount of blood retained in them as a congestion, in this disease. For this purpose these should be added treatment of the splanchnics, solar plexus, liver, kidneys, and abdominal circulation generally.

The usual treatment of the throat, internal and external; of the neck; of clavicle and first rib; of the upper anterior chest, raising the ribs, and working in the anterior intercostal spaces against the costal cartilages; and of the face and nose, should be given to overcome the catarrhal condition of the respiratory tract, just as a cold and a bronchitis are treated.

The lungs should be kept well supported by the treatment, to avoid the danger of bronchitis and pneumonia. Likewise kidneys, eye, ear, nose, and throat should be guarded against effects in them.

The cough is relieved by relaxing the throat tissues, treatment along the larynx and trachea, correction of first rib and clavicle, and raising of the upper ribs.

The patient should remain in bed until desquamation is well along, should be in a darkened room for the sake of the eyes, and should be kept upon a light diet of milk, bread, light soups, etc.

The general spinal treatment, and treatment of the cutaneous system and centers, will aid in allaying the itching of the skin. For this purpose, also, a daily warm bath may be given.

RUBELLA.
(FRENCH OR GERMAN MEASLES.)

VARICELLA.
(CHICKENPOX.)

To these conditions we may apply the same general remarks concerning lesions and treatment, osteopathically, as made in considering measles.

The very mild symptoms accompanying these conditions call for but little treatment aside from the general constitutional one, pointed out in detail in measles. These points of treatment may be applied as necessary.

Due attention must be given to avoid exposure, the dangers of complication, etc. In rubella the enlargement of the cervical lymphatics calls for attention in the manner pointed out. The slight fever and catarrhal symptoms are readily overcome. In both conditions due attention must be given to the cervical and general spinal treatment, and to the maintenance of the activities of the various viscera. Usually the spinal muscles are contractured, and must be relaxed. These contractures doubtless effect the general lymphatic system by way of the spinal nerves. For example, in varicella the superficial lymph glands are sometimes visibly enlarged.

In varicella the usual precaution of preventing the child's scratching off the scabs by putting mittens or bandages upon the hand and wrists, and of painting the scab over with collodion may be observed.

SCARLET FEVER.
(SCARLATINA.)

Numerous cases have been successfully treated osteopathically. The PROGNOSIS is good, but must be guarded in cases complicated with diphtheria. The experience is to bring these cases safely through the attack, free from complications and sequelae.

The LESIONS are, in general, the same as described for the various acute, specific fevers. Contractured spinal and cervical muscles are noted. One must expect various bony lesions, accounting for the weakness of the special parts attacked by complications or sequelae, as for the kidneys, throat, and general nervous system by the usual bony lesions found present in diseases of these parts.

The TREATMENT proceeds along the lines already laid down. In this case there is especial need of thorough constitutional treatment on account of the multiplicity of symptoms and the variety of organs sometimes affected.

The general spinal treatment is given, relaxing muscles, stimulating the splanchnics, etc. Particular attention must be given to lesions affecting the kidneys, and to the thorough treatment of the innervation of them, throughout the course of the disease, for the purpose of avoiding the post-scarlatinal nephritis, so common a complication.

For a like reason one must give especial attention to the treatment of the throat to avoid diphtheria.

The cervical treatment must be carefully carried out. The marked enlargement of the lymphatic glands that sometimes occurs may be avoided or controlled by the usual treatment. Relaxation of all the anterior and posterior muscles and tissues, treatment along larynx and trachea, raising the clavicles, etc., must be done. This treatment frees the lymphatic and blood-circulation through the neck, and keeps eye, ear, and throat in good condition.

The heart must be kept well supported The fever is treated in the usual way. When the patient's system is kept well supplied with moisture by allowing him a plentiful supply of cold water, daily treatment of the sub-maxillary salivary glands will aid in keeping the mouth and lips moist.

The irritation of the skin may be relieved by the treatment indicated for that purpose in measles. Daily tepid sponging and warm bathing, as well as anointing of the skin with an animal fat or with cocoa butter, are useful for this purpose.

The patient should be isolated, the scales shed in desquamation should be carefully collected and burned, and the room should be disinfected after convalescence. The diet should be light. Plenty of milk and alkaline water may be used.

TUMORS.

CASES: (1) Ovarian tumor, upon which operation was advised, cured by two months' treatment.

(2) Uterine fibroid tumor, the patient having for sixteen years suffered intensely at period. Surgeons were about to operate upon the case,

when it was decided to try Osteopathy. After four treatments the period was passed without any discomfort. After three months' treatment the tumor had disappeared.

(3) Intestinal fibroid tumor. There was a history of constipation, and colicky pains for a number of weeks, constantly increasing in severity and and frequency, and leading finally to spasms.

The abdomen was much distendad with feces and gas; the 10th, 11th, and 12th left ribs were displaced downward. The tumor could be deeply palpated in the left side of the abdomen, at the level of the crest of the ilium.

The colon was cleared with repeated enemas of water and oil. As the tumor still remained an operation was decided upon. But, before the day set, the tumor loosened under osteopathic treatment, and was passed from the rectum. It was in size 1¾ by 1¼ inches. It was examined by leading physicians who pronounced it fibroid tumor.

(4) A tumor upon the back of the neck, due to a much enlarged sebaceous gland, had been growing for ten years. Treatment was directed to softening the contents of the gland until able to pass through the duct, the passage being facilitated by removal of the hair into the follicle of which the gland emptied. Under the treatment the tumor had been much reduced at the time of report.

(5) A case in which an abdominal tumor in the region of the stomach, and an epithelial cancer upon the nose were nearly removed by the treatment.

(6) A tumor of the brain, so called, was a condition found to be due to a displacement of the atlas and a great contraction of the cervical muscles. The head was drawn backward, and giddiness, insomnia, and ocular disturbance were present. The condition seemed likely to lead to insanity, and leading physicians diagnosed it as tumor upon the brain. Correction of the lesions cured the case, and the diagnosis of cerebral tumor was shown to be wrong.

(7) An abdominal tumor in a lady, the waist measuring 46½ inches, and increasing at the rate of 1 in. per week. Lesion was found at the 5th dorsal, also at the 11th, and the left ribs were luxated. The tumor appeared to be as large as a cocoanut. At the end of one months' treatment the growth had been stopped and the waist measurement was reduced 1 in.; at the end of 2 months, 13½ in., and had reached nearly her normal size. The treatment was continued for three months longer, and the case was discharged cured.

(8) A tumor of the breast, about the size of a walnut, very hard and involving the center and deep portion of the gland. Sharp pains radiated in all directions from the tumor, but mostly toward the axillaryregion.

The condition was found to be an engorgement due to obstructed lymph vessels, with which the gland is richly supplied. The lesion was a twist of the clavicle, narrowing the space between the clavicle and first rib, and caused by using a crutch for a lame leg upon the same side as the lesion. Thus was caused an obstruction to the lymphatic drainage of the breast, and the growth resulted. As a preliminary measure the limb was cured and the use of the crutch was dispensed with. The clavicle was righted and the growth began to be absorbed. The case was cured in seven weeks.

(9) A case thought by the physicians a cancerous nodole in the breast, and for which operation was advised, was cured by the treatment.

(10) A tumor just external to the vaginal orifice, of four month's standing. There was a fluid contained in the tumor, and it varied in size, becoming smaller after the patient had remained in a recumbent position for a few days. There was prolapsus of the uterus and lesion among the lumbar vertebrae. The case was cured in two mouths.

(11) An ovarian tumor in a patient, from whom, two years previously, the left ovary and a tumor weighing twenty-five pounds had been removed. A few months later a tumor appeared upon the right ovary, and operation was advised. After a month and a half of treatment the tumor had disappeared.

(12) Fibroid tumors of the uterus in a patient who had, four years previously, been injured in the left side by a viscious cow. The patient was suffering from heart and bowel troubles, and female diseases. Various spinal lesions were found. By four treatments the tumors were loosened and passed, there being several of them, varying in size from that of a hen's-egg to that of a walnut,

The PROGNOSIS, generally speaking, to benefit or cure various tumors by osteopathic treatment is good. Numerous cases have been saved by this means from the surgeon's knife. While many tumors cannot be cured, the treatment merits a trial in every case before operation be submitted to.

The LESIONS are various bony, muscular, and other obstructions to blood and lymph flow, or to nerve-supply. Some lesions cause tumorous growths by direct irritation of the tissues. A frequent cause of tumors is found in lesion to the lymphatic drainage of a part, through direct pressure upon its lymphatic vessels or by constrictor effect upon them by lesion to the vaso-motor and sympathetic nerve supply. Tumors of the breast are very often due to such a cause. (cases 8 and 9).

The common lesions in tumor of the breast are found at the clavicle, first rib, among the upper five or six ribs, or among the corresponding vertebrae. Abdominal tumors are commonly caused by lower rib and lower vertebral lesions, uterine tumors by sacral or lumbar lesions, etc.

The simple TREATMENT is to remove lesion, correct lymphatic and blood drainage, or remove any source of direct irritation upon the tissues. Correcting anatomical relations is the main point, and commonly no manipulation directly upon the tumor is required, yet such a measure is sometimes employed to soften a fatty tumor and aid in its absorption, or to loosen a fibroid growth, several such having thus been loosened and discharged *per rectum* or *per vaginam*. One instance is recorded in which external treatment upon the nose loosened and caused the discharge of a cancer in the upper nasal passage.

It is a point worthy of note that in many instances fibroids, according to all evidences, have been absorbed by the renewed blood-currents. It indicates that new fibrous tissues, once formed, may be absorbed under the treatment.

INDEX.